Atlas of
Urogynecological
Endoscopy

Atlas of Urogynecological Endoscopy

Edited by

Peter L Dwyer MBBS FRANZCOG FRCOG
Director of Urogynecology
Mercy Hospital for Women
Associate Professor
University of Melbourne
Melbourne
Australia

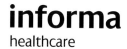
informa
healthcare

© 2007 Informa UK Ltd

First published in the United Kingdom in 2007 by Informa Healthcare, Telephone House, 69–77 Paul Street, London EC2A 4 LQ. Informa Healthcare is a trading division of Informa UK Ltd. Registered Office: 37/41 Mortimer Street, London W1T 3JH. Registered in England and Wales number 1072954.

Tel: +44 (0)20 7017 6000
Fax: +44 (0)20 7017 6699
Website: www.informahealthcare.com

Although every effort has been made to ensure that all owners of copyright material have been acknowledged in this publication, we would be glad to acknowledge in subsequent reprints or editions any omissions brought to our attention.

Although every effort has been made to ensure that drug doses and other information are presented accurately in this publication, the ultimate responsibility rests with the prescribing physician. Neither the publishers nor the authors can be held responsible for errors or for any consequences arising from the use of information contained herein. For detailed prescribing information or instructions on the use of any product or procedure discussed herein, please consult the prescribing information or instructional material issued by the manufacturer.

A CIP record for this book is available from the British Library.

Library of Congress Cataloging-in-Publication Data

Data available on application

ISBN 10 1 84184 540 X
ISBN 13 9781 84184 540 1

Distributed in North and South America by
Taylor & Francis
6000 Broken Sound Parkway, NW, (Suite 300)
Boca Raton, FL 33487, USA
Within Continental USA
Tel: 1 (800) 272 7737; Fax: 1 (800) 374 3401
Outside Continental USA
Tel: (561) 994 0555; Fax: (561) 361 6018
Email: orders@crcpress.com

Distributed in the rest of the world by
Thomson Publishing Services
Cheriton House
North Way
Andover, Hampshire SP10 5BE, UK
Tel: +44 (0)1264 332424
Email: tps.tandfsalesorder@thomson.com

Composition by C&M Digitals (P) Ltd, Chennai, India
Printed and bound in India by Replika Press Pvt Ltd.

Contents

Contributors

Anita Clarke MB BS FRACS
Consultant Urologist
St Uincent Hospital and Mercy
Hospital for Woman
Melbourne
Australia

Alison De Sousa
Department of Urogynecology
Mercy Hospital for Women
Heidelberg
Victoria
Australia

Peter L Dwyer MBBS FRANZCOG FRCOG
Director of Urogynecology
Mercy Hospital for Women
Associate Professor
University of Melbourne
Melbourne
Australia

Brigitte Fatton MD
Urogynecology Unit
Department of Obstetrics and Gynecology
University Hospital of Clermont-Ferrand
France

Christopher F Maher
Urogynecology Unit
Royal Women's and Mater Hospitals
Brisbone
Australia

Peter J Maher
Director, Endoscopy Gynecology
Department of Endoscopic Gynecology
Mercy Hospital Women
Melbourne
Australia

Jack R Robertson MD
Professor Emeritus
Departments of Obstetrics and Gynecology and
    Urogynecology
University of Nevada Medical School
Reno, NV
USA

Anna Rosamilia MBBS FRANZCOG FRACOG CU PHD
Urogynecologist
Department of Obstetrics and Gynaecology
Monash Medical Center
Clayton
Victoria
Australia

Lore Schierlitz MBBS FRANZCOG
Department of Urogynecology
Mercy Hospital for Women
Heidelberg
Victoria
Australia

Tan Poh Kok
Consultant Obstetrician and Gynecologist
Department of Obstetrics and Gynecology
Consultant Urogynecologist
Female Urinary Incontinence and Pelvic Floor
    Reconstructive Surgery Unit
Singapore General Hospital
Singapore

Foreword

Two important procedures underpin urogynecology – cystoscopy and laparoscopy; both are diagnostic and also *therapeutic*. As correct diagnosis should always precede treatment, it is important that the skills for these two procedures should be learnt by all gynecologists and *urologists* interested in urogynecological conditions, and their trainees.

The *Atlas of Urogynecological Endoscopy* has many attributes: first, it is edited and authored by Peter Dwyer, the doyen of urogynecologists in Australia, with a national and international reputation. He is recognized by his peers for his teaching, clinical skills, and experience, together with impressive research and publications, which he condenses here for this Atlas. Secondly, the Atlas is unique in that it fills a void in the library of practical manuals in gynecology and urogynecology. Thirdly, Peter Dwyer has drawn together a host of international experts to co-author with him, a tribute to his standing in urogynecological circles.

It is as a teaching manual that this Atlas succeeds. As well as full coverage of urogynecological conditions, for which cystoscopy and laparoscopy are relevant, the book emphasizes the correct equipment and the training requirements for endoscopy. Although these skills are best learnt in the operating room, this Atlas is vital for understanding the indications, techniques, and complications of cystoscopy and laparoscopy and the care of these instruments.

The Atlas is well written and beautifully illustrated (most of the pictures having been taken by the author) and should find a place in every urogynecological library. I commend this book and wish it every success.

Stuart L Stanton
Professor of Urogynaecology (London)

Preface

The lower urinary tract has for a long time been of special importance to both gynecologists and urologists in the treatment of urogynecological conditions. Howard Kelly, Professor of Obstetrics and Gynecology at Johns Hopkins Hospital in Baltimore, pioneered the use of cystoscopy and ureteric catheterization, particularly in the United States, and described operations for stress incontinence and vaginal prolapse. His successor at Johns Hopkins, Guy Hunner, continued his interest and was the first to clearly describe the condition of interstitial cystitis. However, these skills and interest were lost to most gynecologists until Jack Robertson pioneered the air cystourethroscope and its use in the evaluation of urinary incontinence and urethral pathology. Jack has been appropriately described as the father of American urogynecology and I am honored to have him as co-author for the first chapter of this book: 'History of endoscopy of the female urinary tract'. My mentors, Stuart Stanton and Robert Zacharin, were international leaders in the discipline of urogynecology and pelvic floor disorders. Both men believe that endoscopy of the lower urinary tract is integral to the management of female urinary incontinence and pelvic floor disorders. However, they are the exceptions, and expertise in endoscopy of the lower urinary tract has been lost to most gynecologists and neglected in the curriculum of gynecological training programs. The introduction of stress incontinence procedures, including the minimally invasive sling procedures (such as TVT) and long needle urethral suspension operations (Pereira or Stamey), has increased the numbers of gynecologists performing cystourethroscopy in their surgical practices. Cystourethroscopy is integral to the safe performance of these procedures and is also being increasingly used to recognize urinary tract complications intraoperatively and lessen the risk of medicolegal consequences. However, because gynecologists have little exposure to cystourethroscopy or lower urinary tract disorders during gynecological training, this has caused new problems. Gynecologists are frequently faced with cystoscopic findings with which they are unfamiliar. These might be benign conditions such as squamous metaplasia or cystitis cystica, where they have had to call a urologist or unnecessarily refer the patient for a second cystoscopy; more importantly, serious conditions such as malignancy may be misdiagnosed or missed through ignorance or incomplete examination.

The purpose of this book is primarily to educate gynecologists and urologists in the instrumentation of the lower urinary tract and pelvic endoscopy, and how it is used in the diagnosis and treatment of lower urinary tract and pelvic floor disorders. Endoscopy is very much a visual endeavor with 'a picture worth a thousand words.' This book is liberally illustrated with case reports and cystoscopic photographs to enhance learning and condition recognition. The majority of photographs used in this book I have collected over the last 15 years since the introduction of modern imaging technology and three-chip cameras. Photographs with case reports are used liberally to encourage learning. I would also like to thank James Scurry for his histopathological photographs and Richard Millard for his photographs of bladder cancer.

Finally, I would like to thank all my co-authors, especially Jack Robertson and Stuart Stanton, who are the present-day equivalents of Kelly and have, in their own ways, pioneered modern urogynecology. The other co-authors have all worked with me at the Mercy Hospital for Women, Melbourne and have made excellent contributions. Peter Glenning, another one of my mentors in urogynecology and life, proofread all chapters, and made helpful suggestions. My thanks also go to the publishers, Informa Healthcare, and especially Commissioning Editor Oliver Walter, for valuable advice and keeping me on track, and Kathryn Dunn, Senior Production Editor. Finally, special thanks go to Geraldine Rhoderick, my hardworking and patient secretary; my wife Pam for the many interruptions to family life, and to my son Patrick, my IT expert, who always answered my many calls for help with good nature.

Peter L Dwyer

1

History of endoscopy of the female urinary tract

Jack R Robertson and Peter L Dwyer

When one tries to imagine the thrill the first endoscopists felt, the realization that they could actually see for the first time inside the living body, this exhilaration could not be described better than Marion Sims, when he said about 1845:

> Before I could get the bent spoon handle into her vagina, the air rushed in with a puffing noise, dilating the vagina to the fullest extent. Introducing the bent handle of the spoon, I saw everything as no man has ever seen before. The fistula was as plain as the nose on a man's face. The edges were clear and well defined and distinct, and the opening could be measured as accurately as if it had been cut out of a piece of plain paper.[1]

Of the pioneers who led the way, Bozzini, a German physician, documented in 1804 the need to examine deeply seated organs, including the bladder and urethra. He advocated the inspection of all 'interior cavities' by looking through natural openings or at least small wounds. He designed a number of long thin funnels, which he called a 'lichtleiter' (light conductor), with illumination provided by a light reflected from a box containing a wax candle. He presented his instrument to the Faculty of Medicine of Vienna, but they were reportedly alarmed at such a contraption. They severely ridiculed Bozzini's lichtleiter, which effectively halted endoscopic development for many decades. There is no evidence that it was used in a human.[2]

However, his ideas predicted the development of diagnostic and operative endoscopy of the urinary tract (cystourethroscopy) and abdominal cavity (laparoscopy) both of which play such as important part in the management of female pelvic floor disorders. He wrote:

> Surgery will not only develop new and previously impossible procedures, but all uncertain operations which rely on luck and approximation will become safe under the influence of direct vision, since the surgeon's hands will now be guided by his eyes.

In 1826 Pierre Segalas had some success with a simplified version of Bozzini's instrument. It was a funnel with a polished interior to reflect light. It was used to illuminate the bladder and ureteral orifices. Illumination was from candles. A concave mirror focused the light. This was one of the 'keyhole' instruments which afforded not more than 3 mm of aperture.[3]

In 1853 Antonin Jean Desormeaux, a French surgeon used a modified lichtleiter to examine his patients with urinary problems. A system of mirrors and lenses improved visualization. For illumination, he used a much brighter lamp flame burning a mixture of alcohol and turpentine instead of a wax candle. Although this caused a number of burns, it was considered reasonably successful.

Max Nitze, a German physician is generally credited as the 'father of the modern cystoscope.' He, with Josef Leiter in 1869, devised a combination of lenses which enlarged the field of vision, and illuminated the inside of the bladder as never before. Light was from the glow of a platinum wire. He filled the bladder with ice water to prevent thermal injury.[4]

Thomas Edison's incandescent lamp was a giant step in cystoscopy. The heat of the bulb still required a water medium.[5]

It is important to discuss the contribution of Marion Sims at about this time. It was not endoscopy, but the positioning of the patient to get a better view. Sims wondered about the possibility of placing patients with vesicovaginal fistulae in the knee-chest position. This convinced him that cure was possible. In 1852 he announced the cure of 252 fistulae out of 320 attempts.[6]

Josef Grünfeld (Figure 1.1) born in Gyorke, Hungary, was the first to successfully catheterize the ureters under vision, using malleable catheters introduced into the bladder alongside his glass-ended endoscope in 1876. He was also the first surgeon to remove a bladder tumor by cystoscope in 1881 after developing an endoscopic loop threader, scissors, forceps and knives.

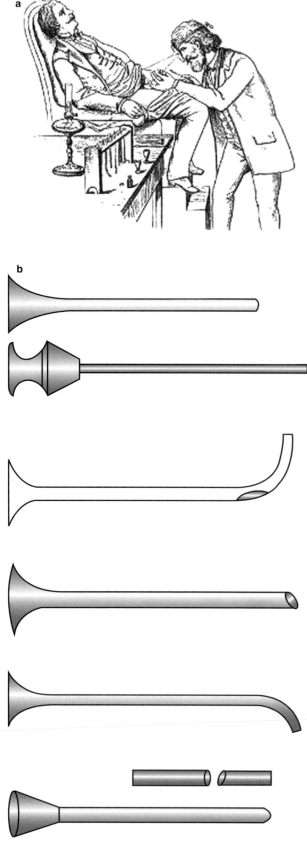

Figure 1.1
Josef Grünfeld with a male patient (a) and his endoscopes (b).

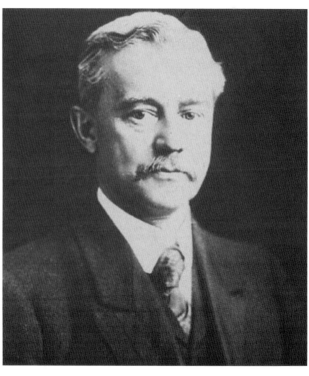

Figure 1.2
Howard A Kelly, 1911.

In 1893 Howard A Kelly (Figure 1.2) invented a cysto-scope which was simply a handled, hollow tube with a glass partition, which accidentally broke. Kelly wondered, like Sims, if the bladder could be distended with air. He inserted the broken cystoscope. With the removal of the obturator, the bladder ballooned with air. He was then able to insert a ureteral catheter under direct vision, and was said by some to be the first, a gynecologist, to do so.[7] However Hunner, a protégé of Kelly, later concluded that 'Grünfeld of Vienna' was the first to pass a metal catheter into the ureter under direct vision.

The American Surgical Society, later the American College of Surgeons, met in Baltimore in 1900. A contest was held between Howard Kelly and Hugh Hampton Young, who is often considered the father of modern urology. Using his air cystoscope, Kelly inserted ureteral catheters in a female patient in just 3 minutes. Young equaled this time in a male patient, using the catheterizing cystoscope developed by Leopold Casper of Berlin.[8] So began the friendly compet-itive rivalry between gynecologists and urologists in the area of female urology and urogynecology.

Guy Hunner (Figure 1.3) was the first of Howard Kelly's resident gynecologists to graduate from the Johns Hopkins Medical School in Baltimore and later also became profes-sor of gynecology at Johns Hopkins. He followed Kelly in his interest in endoscopy of the female urinary tract and female urology. In 1914 Guy Hunner described the condi-tion of interstital cystitis (IC) in a manuscript titled: 'A rare

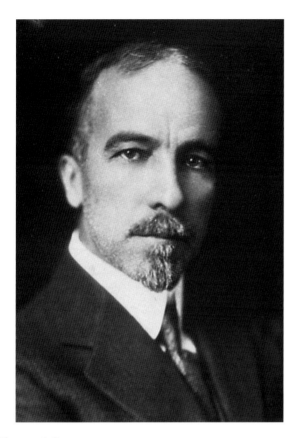

Figure 1.3
Guy L Hunner, 1916.

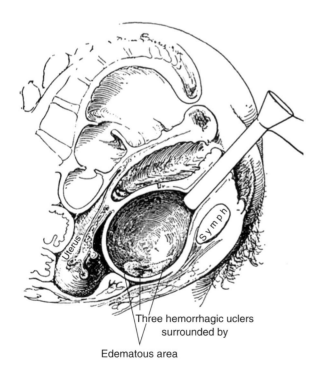

Three hemorrhagic uclers surrounded by

Edematous area

Figure 1.4
The Kelly cystoscope used by Hunner to diagnose interstitial cystitis with the patient in the knee-chest position.

type of bladder ulcer in women; report of cases' in the *Boston Medical and Surgical Journal*.[9] He used the Kelly method of air cystoscopy with the patient in the knee-chest position, as described by Sims, to visualize the bladder (Figure 1.4). In this and his subsequent publications in 1918 (Figure 1.5), he eloquently describes the appearance of the bladder in women with IC, as seen through the Kelly air cystoscope, the presenting symptoms, etiology, differential diagnosis, pathology, and treatment. Hunner described 'the congestion oozing blood' and the classical fissuring and bladder ulceration of IC, which today still bears his name – 'Hunner's ulcer'. His descriptions have stood the test of time and can be even more clearly seen today using the modern cystoscope. (see Chapter 3).[10,11]

At the beginning of the 20th century, endoscopy was rare, mostly because the instrumentation was imperfect, and the skills needed to thread large tubes through various orifices often resulted in injuries. The invention of the rod lens system and flexible fiberoptic endoscopes opened a new world of diagnosis and treatment.

Air cystoscopy is a simple, inexpensive method of examining the female bladder, but it has three disadvantages: external illumination, lack of a lens system, and it is necessary to position the patient in the knee-chest position. In 1951 Ridley tried indirect air cystoscopy with a female in the knee-chest position, but found the urethrovesical junction and urethra were difficult to visualize because of heat from the light bulb and not having a straightforward lens.[12]

Urinary incontinence is one of life's miseries, and its cure remains a challenge. The specialization of medicine created an artificial division in the female pelvis. Embryologically, anatomically, and functionally, the lower urinary tract and the female genital tract are united. The female urethra was not considered the source of pathology because it could not be adequately examined. Anomalies of the genital tract frequently accompany those of the urinary tract due to their close embryological structures.

Jack Robertson (Figure 1.6) had realized women were being treated as second-class citizens. They were being examined with male instruments by urologists, who were largely untrained in urogynecology. There were no instruments designed for the female urinary tract.

In 1968 the first joint meeting of the American College of Surgeons and the German Surgical Society was held in Munich. At that meeting Robertson met the German instrument maker Karl Storz, of Tuttlingen. Robertson had designed a female urethroscope, 8 inches long with a straightforward view. He convinced Karl Storz, who had just acquired the breakthrough fiberoptic technology, invented by Professor Harold H. Hopkins, to make that first female urethroscope, the Robertson CO_2 endoscopy telescope (Figure 1.7). The scope fits into an airtight handle, through which the CO_2 is insufflated from the CO_2 endoscopy monitor, which allows urethral and bladder pressure studies to be accomplished during endoscopy with a variable flow rate from 30 to 120 cc/min. The

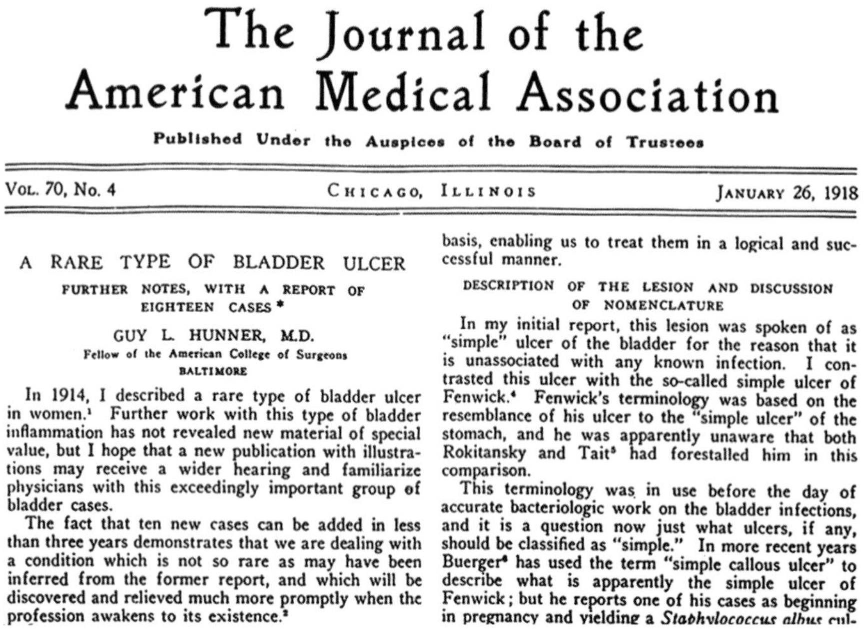

The Journal of the American Medical Association

Published Under the Auspices of the Board of Trustees

VOL. 70, No. 4	CHICAGO, ILLINOIS	JANUARY 26, 1918

A RARE TYPE OF BLADDER ULCER

FURTHER NOTES, WITH A REPORT OF EIGHTEEN CASES *

GUY L. HUNNER, M.D.
Fellow of the American College of Surgeons
BALTIMORE

In 1914, I described a rare type of bladder ulcer in women.[1] Further work with this type of bladder inflammation has not revealed new material of special value, but I hope that a new publication with illustrations may receive a wider hearing and familiarize physicians with this exceedingly important group of bladder cases.

The fact that ten new cases can be added in less than three years demonstrates that we are dealing with a condition which is not so rare as may have been inferred from the former report, and which will be discovered and relieved much more promptly when the profession awakens to its existence.[2]

basis, enabling us to treat them in a logical and successful manner.

DESCRIPTION OF THE LESION AND DISCUSSION OF NOMENCLATURE

In my initial report, this lesion was spoken of as "simple" ulcer of the bladder for the reason that it is unassociated with any known infection. I contrasted this ulcer with the so-called simple ulcer of Fenwick.[4] Fenwick's terminology was based on the resemblance of his ulcer to the "simple ulcer" of the stomach, and he was apparently unaware that both Rokitansky and Tait[5] had forestalled him in this comparison.

This terminology was in use before the day of accurate bacteriologic work on the bladder infections, and it is a question now just what ulcers, if any, should be classified as "simple." In more recent years Buerger[6] has used the term "simple callous ulcer" to describe what is apparently the simple ulcer of Fenwick; but he reports one of his cases as beginning in pregnancy and yielding a *Staphylococcus albus* cul-

Figure 1.5
Guy Hunner's classical description of interstitial cystitis in the *Journal of the American Medical Association*.

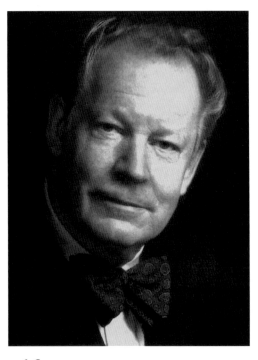

Figure 1.6
Jack Robertson.

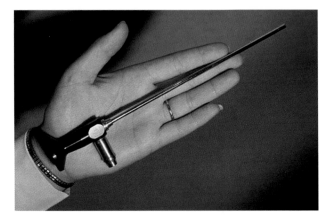

Figure 1.7
The Robertson CO_2 female air urethroscope.

endoscopy monitor uses an X-Y recorder to chart the pressure (in cmH_2O) and the volume of gas (in cubic centimeters) with the sensations experienced during bladder filling.[13]

Although a variety of tubes had been used to look in the bladder, the female urethra had just been the place on which to rest them. For the first time, a physician could view the working of the internal urethral sphincter and could actually see a urethral diverticulum, which previously had been rarely diagnosed.

The female urethroscope became the prototype for the first arthroscope. The scopes proliferated to access every orifice and, like the laparoscope, are able to be introduced through minute punctures. Now with magnetic resonance imaging (MRI) and computed tomography (CT) scans, anatomy can be visualized without a scope. The newest ultrasounds are proving even more sensitive and diagnostically revealing.

Women are no longer second-class citizens in medicine.

Endoscopy of the urinary tract is a developing science, with new endoscopes to visualize the upper urinary tracts, and new instruments to perform procedures that previously required open surgery, such as the removal of calculi or foreign bodies. The flexible cystoscope is an example of a recent development that utilizes the fiberoptic lens system to provide a scope that is smaller and pliable, increasing patient comfort and the range of vision. This has been particularly valuable in the male, allowing flexible cystoscopy using only lidocaine gel as outpatient cystoscopy with local anesthetic for a procedure previously only comfortably performed in women, with their shorter urethra.

References

1. Sims JM. The Story of My Life. New York: Appleton, 1894.
2. Herman JR. Urology. A View through the Rectrospectroscope. New York: Harper and Row, 1973.
3. Pousson A, Besnos E (eds.). Encyclopedie Francaise d'Urologie. Paris: Doin et Fils, 1914–1923.
4. Macalpine JB. Cystoscopy and Urography, 2nd edn. Baltimore: William Wood, 1936.
5. Encyclopedia Britannica, Thomas Edison.
6. Sims JM. On the treatment of vesico-vaginal fistula. Am J Med Sci 1852; 23: 59–82.
7. Kelly HA. Medical Gynecology. New York: Appleton, 1908.
8. Young HH. A Surgeon's Autobiography. New York: Harcourt, 1940.
9. Hunner GL. A rare type of bladder ulcer in women; report of cases. Boston Med Surg J 1915; 172; 660.
10. Hunner GL. Elusive ulcer of the bladder. Further notes on a rare type of bladder ulcer, with a report of twenty-five cases. Am J Obstet Gynecol 1918; 78: 374.
11. Hunner GL. A rare type of bladder ulcer. Further notes with a report of eighteen cases. JAMA 1918; 70: 4.
12. Ridley JH. Indirect air cystoscopy. South Med J 1951; 44: 214.
13. Robertson JR. The Robertson method. In: Genitourinary Problems in Women. Springfield, Illinois: Charles C Thomas, 1978: 42–64.

2

Functional anatomy of the lower urinary tract

Alison De Souza and Peter L Dwyer

Introduction

The aim of this chapter is to provide a clear understanding of the anatomy and function of the female lower urinary tract and the pelvic floor for the pelvic surgeon and uroendoscopist.

The functional anatomy of the urinary organs encompasses:

- the urethra, which conducts urine from the bladder to the exterior
- the bladder, which temporarily stores and expels urine
- the ureters, which convey urine from the kidneys.

The endopelvic fascia, ligaments, and the pelvic muscles support the pelvic organs and play an important role in the maintenance of continence and the prevention of prolapse. An understanding of the normal anatomy and function of these structures is integral in the diagnosis and management of disorders of the urinary tract and pelvic floor. These structures will be discussed in the order they are encountered via the cystoscope.

Urethra

The female urethra is a fibromuscular tube that is approximately 4 cm long and 6 mm in diameter, with its axis parallel to the vagina (Figure 2.1). The vagina supports the urethra posteriorly and is fused with it at the distal third.[1,2]

The external urethral orifice is an anteroposterior slit that is located in the vestibule of the vagina and approximately 2 cm below the glans clitoris. The internal urethral orifice is found at the junction of the urethra and the bladder and lies approximately opposite the middle of the symphysis pubis.[2]

The pubourethral ligaments extend from the inferoposterior aspect of the symphysis pubis to the junction of the middle and upper third of the urethra and firmly support it anteriorly.[3] These ligaments contain fibers of the bladder detrusor muscle and assist in maintaining the urethra's stability during micturition when the detrusor contracts.[1] The most medial fibers of the pubococcygeus muscle support the urethra laterally. These muscle fibers do not attach to the urethra but insert into the lateral walls of the vagina and are known as the sphincter vaginae. These fibers increase urethral resistance, thereby contributing to continence.[2]

The wall of the urethra consists of an inner mucous membrane and an outer muscle layer. The epithelium at the external urethral meatus is keratinized stratified squamous epithelium (Figure 2.2) and is continuous with the skin of the vestibule. Passage through the urethra reveals the longitudinal folds of mucous membrane lining, which are

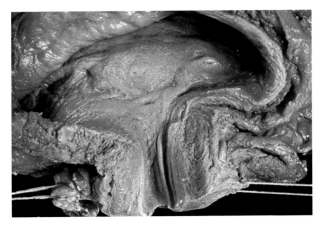

Figure 2.1
Female urethra and bladder opened anteriorly to demonstrate the posterior urethra and urethral crest, and the trigone. (Reproduced with permission from Gosling et al.[1])

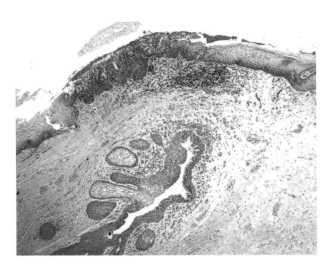

Figure 2.2
Keratinized stratified squamous epithelium changing to
non-keratinized stratified squamous epithelium with urethral
glands in distal urethra.

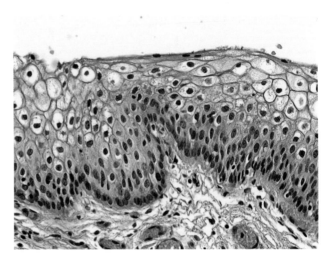

Figure 2.4
Histology of normal squamous mucosa frequently
found in bladder trigone, urethra, vestibule, vagina,
and cervix.

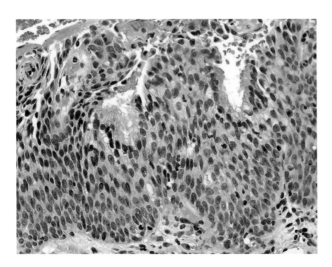

Figure 2.3
Pseudostratified mucosa seen overlying urethral glands in the
distal urethra.

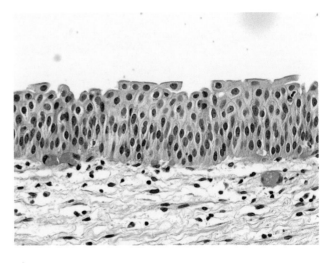

Figure 2.5
Normal transitional mucosa (present in renal pelvis, ureter,
bladder, and urethra), with lamina propria containing
numerous thin-walled veins.

non- keratinized stratified squamous epithelium and its
supporting lamina propria (Figure 2.3). As one moves
proximally, the urothelium changes from stratified squamous (Figure 2.4) to transitional in the urethra (Figure 2.5),
although the stratified squamous epithelium may extend
onto the trigone of the bladder (Figure 2.6). Stratified squamous epithelium is a normal variation seen in pre- and
postmenopausal women and is sometimes referred to as
squamous metaplasia. The cystoscopic appearance may
vary from flat and opaque to a raised sugar-coated appearance (Figure 2.7). This histological variation is not associated with pathological urinary symptoms.[3]

The lamina propria of the urethral wall contains a
prominent vascular plexus of longtitudinally orientated
blood vessels (arterioles and thin-walled venules) in a
stroma of collagen and elastin fibers. These vascular
cushions contribute to passive urethral closure pressure
and provide a watertight urethral seal (Figure 2.8). Along
the posterior urethral lumen is a midline ridge known as
the urethral crest, which projects anteriorly and gives the
lumen a crescentic slit appearance in transverse section[2]
(see Figure 2.1). Many small mucous urethral glands and
lacunae open into the urethra (see Figure 2.2). Near the
lateral margins of the external urethral orifice, a group of

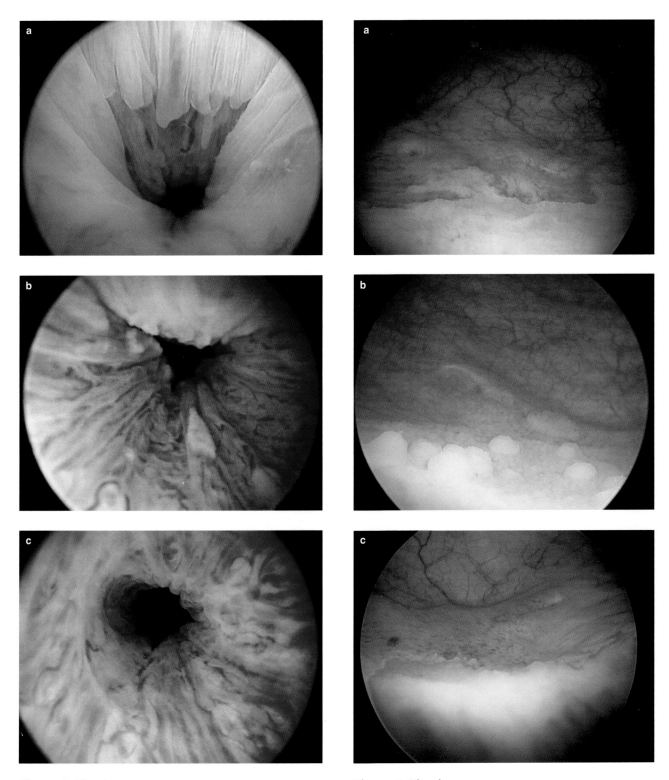

Figure 2.6(a–c)
Variations in urethroscopic appearance of stratified squamous and transitional mucosa within the urethra.

Figure 2.7(a–c)
Variations in cystoscopic appearance of stratified squamous epithelium (squamous metaplasia) on the trigone from flat opaque to raised sugar-coating appearance.

glands open together into the paraurethral duct (Skene's gland). If these become blocked or infected, a cyst or abscess can develop (figure 2.9).

The muscular wall of the urethra is made up of an outer striated muscle, which forms the urogenital sphincter muscle, and an inner smooth muscle layer. The striated

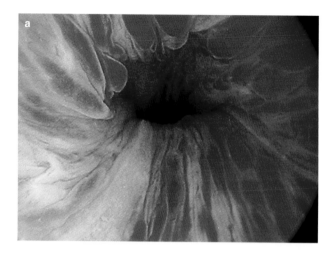

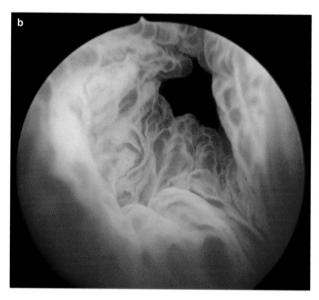

Figure 2.8(a,b)
Urethroscopic view of prominent vascular plexus of longitudinally orientated blood vessels providing vascular cushions which contribute to passive urethral closure pressure and a watertight urethral seal.

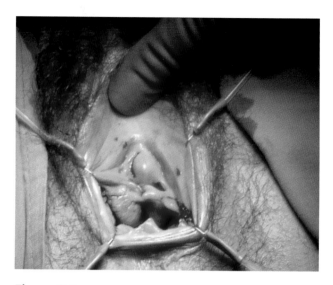

Figure 2.9
Paraurethral Skene's abscess.

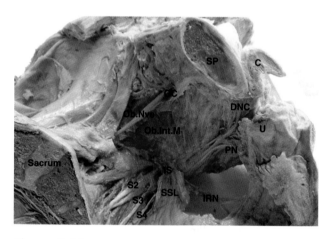

Figure 2.10
Left hemipelvis. The arcus tendineus levator ani and levator ani muscles have been removed. The Alcock's canal was opened and the ischiorectal fossa was dissected to demonstrate the branches of the pudendal nerve: the inferior rectal nerve (IRC), the perineal nerve (PN), and the dorsal nerve of clitoris (DNC). C=clitoris; IS=ischial spine; OC=obturator canal; Ob.Int.M=obturator internus muscle; Ob.Nve=obturator nerve; SP=symphysis pubis; SSL=sacrospinous ligament; U=urethra. (Reproduced from Achtari et al,[8] with permission.)

urethral sphincter muscle has two components: namely, a circular proximal layer, which is sometimes deficient posteriorly (urethral sphincter), and a distal portion of two over-arching circular striated muscles which lies next to the perineal membrane and is called the compressor urethra and the urethrovaginal sphincter.[5] The external sphincter muscle fibers are all slow twitch, and can exert tone over prolonged periods. The muscular fibers of the urogenital sphincter muscles are anatomically separate from the adjacent pubococcygeus muscle which assists with urethral support.[2]

The smooth muscle layer extends the entire length of the urethra. Proximally at the bladder neck, it is continuous with the non-striated detrusor muscle. Distally, the smooth muscle ends in the fatty tissue surrounding the external urethral meatus. The urethral smooth muscle has an extensive parasympathetic cholinergic nerve supply which is the same as the detrusor muscle. This muscle is active during micturition and shortens and widens the urethral lumen.[1]

Nerve supply of the urethra and the pelvic floor

The urethra obtains its nerve supply from both the autonomic and somatic nervous systems. The parasympathetic system is dominant during urine storage and the sympathetic system during urine evacuation.

The external urethral sphincter (outer striated muscle) has motor cell bodies which lie in the intermediolateral columns of S2, S3 and S4 of the spinal cord. Parasympathetic fibres travelling from these motor cell bodies via the pelvic splanchnic nerves stimulate sphincter contraction resulting in urethral occlusion. Additional somatic motor fibres from the perineal branch of the pudendal nerve (S4) provide supply to the sphincter urethrae.[6]

The nerve supply to the smooth muscle of the urethra is divided into proximal and distal. The smaller proximal region is supplied by the sacral sympathetic trunks via the superior and inferior hypogastric plexuses. This motor nerve supply is continuous with the smooth muscle of the bladder neck and fibres of the superficial trigonal muscle. The remaining majority of the smooth muscle of the urethra is innervated by the parasympathetic nerves which also supply the detrusor muscle.[1,2,6]

The lamina propria of the urethral adventitia contains sensory nerves originating from the perineal branch of the pudendal nerve which also supplies the vaginal mucosa.[1,6]

The pudendal nerve originates from S2–S4 and has three main branches (Figure 2.10). The inferior rectal nerve (S2,3) arises at the beginning of the pudendal canal and enters the ischiorectal fossa where it gives motor branches to supply the external anal sphincter and sensory branches to the anal canal and perianal skin.

The perineal nerve (S4) arises from the middle of the pudendal canal and is motor to the perineal muscles: ischiocavernosus, bulbospongiosis, superficial and deep transverse perinel and the sphincter urethrae (pubourethralis) This nerve therefore provides some voluntary motor control to the mechanism of continence.

The dorsal nerve of the clitoris is the terminal branch of the pudendal nerve which crosses the infrapubic canal and supplies the sensory innervation to the clitoral area.[6,7]

Bladder

External anatomy

The bladder is a reservoir for urine and therefore varies in size, shape, and location according to its capacity and that of the nearby structures. When empty, the bladder is located in the lesser pelvis lying posterosuperiorly to the pubic bones and separated from them by the retropubic space. The bladder is mobile in the extraperitoneal subcutaneous fatty tissue, except the bladder neck, which is held in place by the pubovesical ligaments.

The pubovesical ligaments are the superior portions of the pubourethral ligaments and, along with the levator ani and the vagina, are the main supports of the bladder.[1,2]

As distention with urine occurs, the bladder extends anterosuperiorly into the greater pelvis and abdominal cavity. The bladder is tetrahedral in shape (like an anterior boat hull), with an apex, base, and neck, and has a superior and two inferolateral surfaces.

The apex of the bladder is the anterior end, and points towards the superior edge of the pubic symphysis. It is from the apex that the median umbilical ligament extends to the umbilicus behind the anterior abdominal wall.[2]

The base of the bladder is triangular and posteroinferior and is closely related to the anterior vaginal wall. It extends between the ureteric orifices posterosuperiorly and the bladder neck inferiorly (Figure 2.11a) and expands only slightly in size as the bladder fills.[1] The trigone is located on the internal aspect of the bladder base. The ureteric orifices will be seen to undergo peristalsis periodicaly and eject urine (Figure 2.11b), sometimes with particulate matter (Figure 2.11c,d).

The neck of the bladder is where the base and the inferolateral surfaces meet. It is the lowest point and the most fixed. The triangular superior surface of the bladder's body extends from the apex to the ureteric orifices and is completed by the posterior border joining them. This superior surface varies the most in shape during filling as it expands anterosuperiorly into the abdominal cavity. During cystoscopy, this surface is often referred to as the fundus or dome and an air bubble is visible, which assists the operator with orientation[2,8,9] (Figure 2.12a).

Internal anatomy

The interior of the bladder is visualized after passing through the internal urethral orifice. There is a smooth transition on entry to the bladder, as there is no internal sphincter at the bladder neck (in contrast with the male). The muscle fibers of the bladder are longitudinal and continuous with the wall of the urethra.[1,2]

Entry into the bladder reveals a smooth triangular area of mucosa called the trigone (see Figure 2.11a). The internal urethral sphincter forms the anteroinferior angle of the trigone (the apex) and the ureteric orifices form the boundaries posterolaterally. The ureteric orifices are usually shaped as an oblique slit and are joined by a slightly raised area called the interureteric ridge. The smoothness of the trigonal mucosa is due to its adherence to the underlying smooth muscle layers. The remainder of the bladder is lined by the vesical mucosa, which is folded into rugae (Figure 2.12b) when the bladder is empty and smooths out as the bladder fills[1,2] (Figure 2.12a).

A ridge exists superiorly along the trigone running between the ureteric orifices (Figure 2.11a). This is created by the continuation of the longitudinal smooth muscle of the ureters 'musculus interuretericus' and is known as the

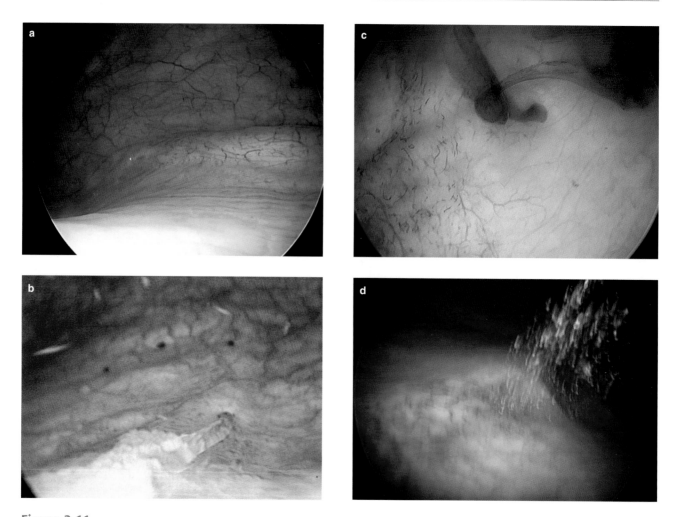

Figure 2.11
(a) Cystoscopic view of trigone, right ureteric orifice, and interureteric ridge; (b) left ureteric orifice with peristaltic jet of urine, (c,d) ureteric jets with particulate matter.

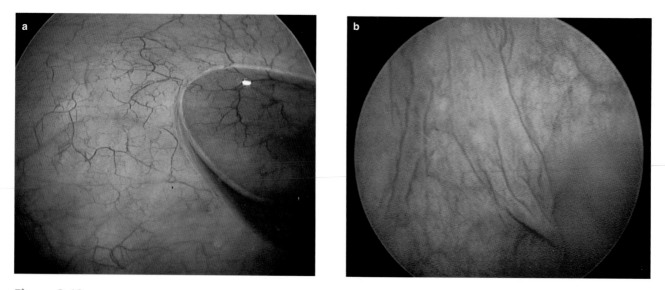

Figure 2.12
(a) Smooth mucosa of bladder dome with air bubble following cystodistention; (b) flaccid bladder wall folded into rugae with the bladder near empty.

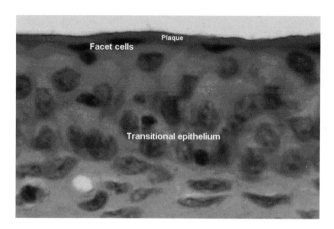

Figure 2.13
Histology of the urothelium showing stratified transitional epithelium with superficial facet or 'umbrella' cells with large nuclei covered by a mucoprotein plaque.

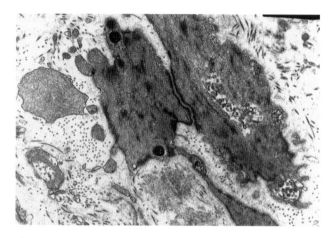

Figure 2.14
Electron micrograph of two detrusor muscle cells with cell borders tightly abutted to one another (an adherens junction). These junctions facilitate mechanical coupling and provide rapid communications between cells for the propagation of action potentials to ensure a coordinated single detrusor contraction.

interureteric crest or ridge. This ridge extends laterally beyond the ureteric openings and forms the ureteric folds. This is created by the end of the ureters running obliquely through the bladder wall.

Histology

Histologically, the bladder consists of three layers: an inner mucous membrane, the detrusor muscle, and the outer adventitia. The bladder is also covered with a serosal layer of peritoneum when distended.[1,2]

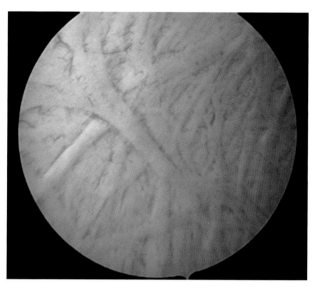

Figure 2.15
Cystoscopic view of mildly trabeculated bladder dome showing the hypertrophic interlacing smooth muscle fibers.

The mucous membrane consists of urothelium supported by lamina propria. The thickness of the urothelium varies according to the distention of the bladder, with the exception of the flat trigone which is only ever two to three cell layers' thick. The urothelium is a stratified epithelium consisting of superficial capping or 'umbrella' cells with large nuclei which are joined to each other by tight junctions. This, together with a mucoprotein covering, provides an impermeable barrier to urine and bacterial colonization (Figure 2.13). If colonization of these superficial cells occurs with urinary tract infection, they are extruded into the urine, giving it a cloudy appearance.

Disruption of this mucoglycan layer has also been suggested as a possible cause for painful bladder disorders, including interstitial cystitis.

There are several normal morphological variations in the bladder mucosa. The most commonly seen variation at cystoscopy in adult females is non-keratinizing squamous metaplasia, which is visualized over the trigone. Proliferation of urothelial cells into the underlying lamina is known as Brunn's nests. Mucus-secreting glands may also be present and are near the ureteric and internal urethral orifices.[1]

Smooth muscle cells are long spindle-shaped cells with a single nucleus and are connected to each other by adherens junctions (Figure 2.14). These facilitate mechanical coupling and provide rapid communications between cells for the propagation of action potentials. These cells are arranged in muscle bundles or fascicles that are grouped together by larger bundles separated by connective tissue. The bundles are not clearly arranged in distinct layers, but run in all directions in the detrusor muscle (Figure 2.15). This structure enables the bladder to contract in all dimensions to expel urine efficiently. Autonomic nerve fibers form a dense plexus amongst these smooth muscle cells and are largely cholinergic in type. There are only few sympathetic noradrenergic nerves, which extend to the detrusor muscle via the bladder's vascular supply.[1]

The trigonal smooth muscle is continuous with the detrusor muscle but has a different histology and embryology. The trigone is derived from the caudal ends of the mesonephric ducts, while the rest of the bladder is derived from a segment of the urogenital sinus (see Chapter 3). The trigone is made up of two distinct layers. The deep layer is consistent with the main detrusor muscle and can be thought of as the 'trigonal detrusor muscle'. The superficial trigonal layer is morphologically distinct and consists of smaller smooth muscle cells. This layer is continuous proximally with the intramural ureters and inferiorly with the proximal smooth muscle of the urethra. The superficial trigonal muscle forms only a small portion of the muscle mass of the bladder neck and proximal urethra.[1,2]

At the uretovesical junction, 1–2 cm of the distal ureter is surrounded by detrusor muscle. This forms a sleeve, known as the sheath of Waldeyer, and assists in the prevention of urinary reflux when the bladder muscle contracts.[1] The ureteric muscle, which has no parasympathetic innervation, becomes continuous with the superficial trigonal muscle at the ureteric orifices.[2]

The bladder neck muscle is also histologically distinct from the remaining detrusor muscle. Smaller tightly packed smooth muscle cells interspersed with connective tissue extend into the urethral smooth muscle. There is a rich cholinergic nerve supply in this area which shortens and widens the bladder neck during micturition.[1,2]

Nerve supply of the bladder

The nerves supplying the bladder form the vesical plexus and consist of both parasympathetic and sympathetic afferent and efferent fibers. Efferent parasympathetic fibers supplying the bladder are derived from the pelvic splanchnic nerves, S2–S4, of the spinal cord. The efferent sympathetic fibers travel from T11 through to L2 segments of the spinal cord.[6]

The vesical plexus consists of pre- and post-autonomic ganglionic fibers and cholinergic nerve cell bodies. The fibers from this plexus pass lateral to the rectum, genital tract, and bladder before they ramify in the detrusor muscle wall. In addition to the vesical plexus branches, there are many small groups of autonomic neurons throughout all regions of the bladder wall which are mainly excitatory cholinergic (parasympathetic) in type.[1] The parasympathetic supply is motor to the detrusor muscle and inhibitory to the sphincter.[10] The peripheral location in the bladder wall of the postganglionic cell bodies of the motor neurons means that surgical nerve damage results in

decentralization rather than denervation of the bladder muscle. Pelvic surgery such as a radical hysterectomy or colectomy injures the preganglionic motor neurons, resulting in a poorly compliant acontractile bladder rather than bladder atony,[9] similar to other upper motor neuron disorders such as spina bifida.

The detrusor muscle has a very sparse sympathetic supply of noradrenergic nerves. These nerves generally accompany the vascular supply to the bladder but rarely extend among the smooth muscle cells of the detrusor. However, they are found in the superficial trigonal muscle and support the theory that this muscle is not vesical in origin. The superficial trigonal muscle may contract during micturition, closing the vesical orifices of the ureters and assisting in the prevention of vesicoureteric reflux.[2]

A number of other neurotransmitters have been detected in the bladder wall, including somatostatin, which provides a further non-cholinergic, non-adrenergic nerve-mediated autonomic effect on the bladder.[1] The vesical afferent fibers relay information regarding bladder distention and pain. When these fibers are stimulated by stretching, the bladder contracts reflexively, the sphincter relaxes, and urine flows. With toilet training, we learn to suppress this reflex when we do not wish to void. The reflex afferents follow the course of the parasympathetic fibers from the inferior surface of the bladder, as do those transmitting pain sensations such as that from overdistention.[10] Pain fibers from the superior bladder surface follow the sympathetic fibers retrogradely to the spinal ganglia of T11 to L2.[2]

Pelvic ureter

Lying in extraperitoneal tissue, the ureter enters the pelvis by crossing anterior to the common or external iliac arteries. On the pelvic side wall, it is anterior to the internal iliac artery and immediately posterior to the ovary in the peritoneum, forming the posterior boundary of the ovarian fossa. The fascia of obturator internus is situated laterally and it crosses and is medial to the umbilical artery, the obturator nerve, artery and vein, the inferior vesical and middle rectal arteries.[2,6]

The ureter continues anteromedially and is related to the uterine artery, cervix, and vaginal fornices (Figure 2.16). The uterine artery initially lies laterally to the ureter and runs a short parallel course along the pelvic side wall. The ureter then travels inferomedially in the broad ligament of the uterus where the uterine artery is anterosuperior for approximately 2.5 cm. The uterine artery then crosses the ureter to its medial side to ascend alongside the uterus. As the ureter descends into the pelvis, it courses anteriorly and superiorly to the uterosacral/lateral cervical ligament complex (see Figure 2.16). The ureter turns anteriorly approximately 2 cm above the vaginal fornix and lateral to the uterine cervix. It then moves medially to reach the

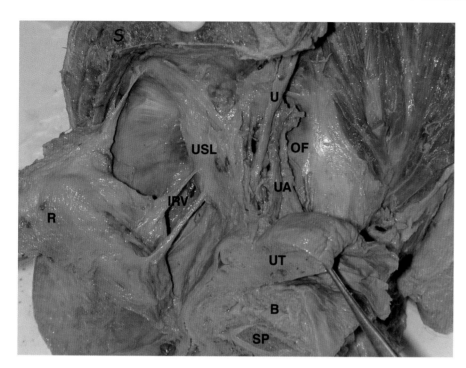

Figure 2.16
Left hemipelvis displaying the course of the left ureter (U) and its relationship to the uterine artery (UA) and uterosacral/lateral cervical ligament complex (USL) and uterus (UT). Other structures are sacrum (S), rectum (R), inferior rectal vessels (IRV), obturator fascia (OF), bladder (B), and pubic symphysis (SP).

bladder, approaching its opposite counterpart before entering the bladder posteriorly. The ureter courses medially for 1.5 cm in the intramural and submucosal segments of the bladder wall before entering the bladder at the ureteric orifices of the upper trigone. The uterus and vagina are commonly deviated to one side of the midline; therefore, one ureter may be more closely related to the cervix and vagina than the other.[2,6,8]

Histologically, the wall of the ureter, like the urethra and bladder, is composed of three layers: the external adventitia, the smooth muscle layer, and the inner mucous membrane. The adventitia is loose connective tissue which merges with the retroperitoneal fatty tissue. The smooth muscle of the ureter is a complex mesh of muscle fibers with distinct layers indistinguishable. At the ureterovesical junction, the fibers become longitudinal and develop into the muscular component of the interureteric ridge, eventually merging with the superficial trigonal muscle. The mucosa consists of extensively folded urothelium, giving a stellate outline supported by lamina propria.[1,2]

The ureterovesical junction and the pelvic brim are points of constriction of the ureter and are potential sites for obstruction by stones. The ureter may also be obstructed at the pelvic brim by the gravid uterus.[2]

Nerve supply of the pelvic ureter

The pelvic ureter receives autonomic supply from sympathetic, parasympathetic, and peptidergic nerves of the adjacent autonomic superior and inferior hypogastric plexuses. The functional significance of these different types of autonomic nerves in relation to smooth muscle activity is not fully understood, as nerves are not essential for the initiation and propogation of ureteric contraction waves. This occurs via the intercellular 'gap' junctions between muscle cell to muscle cell.[1,2] The nerves, however, may exert a modulating effect on the contractility of ureteric smooth muscle. Nerves present in the lamina propria of the ureter are thought to be sensory in function and follow sympathetic fibers retrogradely to reach the spinal ganglia and spinal cord segments T11 through to L1 or L2.[1,2,6]

Functional considerations of the lower urinary tract

The function of the lower urinary tract is to maintain continence with the bladder, acting as a reservoir of urine, and to allow micturition to occur at an appropriate time and place.

Continence

For urinary continence to be maintained, intraurethral closure pressure must be greater than bladder pressure. There are both active and passive forces which maintain this urethral pressure. The lamina propria of the urethra contains a significant amount of elastic and collagen fibers, which together with vascular plexus turgor, provide passive urethral resistance. The external urethral sphincter corresponds anatomically to the region where maximal urethral closure pressures are recorded in the midurethra. The striated muscle of this sphincter maintains tone over long periods without fatigue and thus has a main active role in urethral occlusion. During episodes of increased intra-abdominal pressure such as coughing and sneezing, additional motor fibers are likely to be recruited to increase the occlusive force of the urethra and maintain its closure.[1,2]

The smooth muscle of the proximal urethra is continuous with that of the bladder neck. The longitudinal orientation of the fibers suggests that they are active in allowing micturition rather than promoting continence.[1,2]

The periurethral fibers of the pubococcygeus muscle (levator ani) are innervated by the pudendal nerve. They contain fast- and slow-twitch fibers and are under voluntary muscle control. These fibers form an important active occlusive force on the urethra especially during episodes of increased intra-abdominal pressure. This force is strongest just distal to the maximal urethral closure pressure of the external urethral sphincter.[2]

Micturition

Micturition, whether voluntary or involuntary, occurs as a result of the coordinated synchronous act of urethral relaxation and detrusor muscle contraction. The fall in urethral resistance is partially due to the action of the 'musculus dilator urethrae', the longitudinal smooth muscle system in the bladder neck and proximal urethra[9] and the relaxation of the external urethral sphincter. The pressure rise is due to the contraction of the detrusor muscle. The smooth muscle's complex meshwork acts synchronously to reduce all dimensions of the bladder and effectively empty it. It is

this pressure that overcomes the passive resistance of the elastic fibers of the urethra and contributes to its tone during continence.[1]

References

1. Gosling JA, Dixon J, Humpherson JA. Functional Anatomy of the Urinary Tract. An Integrated Text and Colour Atlas. London: Gower Medical, 1983.
2. Dyson M. Urinary system. In: Williams PL, ed. Gray's Anatomy, 38th edn. London: Churchill Livingstone, 1995: 1837–45.
3. Zacharin RF. The anatomic supports of the female urethra. Obstet Gynecol 1968; 32(6): 754–9.
4. Maizels M. Normal development of the urinary tract. In: Walsh PC, Gittes RF, Perlmutter AD, Stamey TA, eds. Campbell's Urology, 5th edn. Philadelphia, PA: WB Saunders, 1986: 1545–95.
5. Oelrich TM. The striated urogenital sphincter muscle in the female. Anat Rec 1983; 205: 223–32.
6. Sinnatanby CS. Anatomy: Regional and Applied, 11th edn. Edinburgh, UK: Churchill Livingstone, 2006: 306–23.
7. Schraffordt SE, Tjandra JJ, Eizenberg N, Dwyer PL. Anatomy of the pudendal nerve and its terminal branches: a cadaver study. ANZ J Surg 2004; 74: 23–6.
8. Achtari C, McKenzie B, Hiscock C et al. Anatomical study of the obturator foramen and dorsal nerve of the clitoris and their relationship to minimally invasive slings. Int Urogynecol J 2006; 17: 330–4.
9. Moore KL, Dalley AF. Clinically Orientated Anatomy, 4th edn. Baltimore, MD: Lippincott Williams & Wilkins, 1999: 332–415.
10. Moore KL, Agur AM. Essential Clinical Anatomy, 2nd edn. Baltimore, MD: Lippincott Williams & Wilkins: 2002: 209–74.
11. O'Callaghan D, Dwyer PL. Clinical and urodynamic follow-up of women with established urinary dysfunction after radical hysterectomy. Aust NZ J Obstet Gynaecol 1994; 34: 557–61.

3

Cystourethroscopic instrumentation and equipment

Tan Poh Kok and Peter L Dwyer

Introduction

Since Bozzini first proposed that the inside of a human bladder could be viewed with a cystoscope over 200 years ago, there have been many technical improvements in the instrumentation of urinary tract endoscopy that have allowed the clinician to see more clearly, diagnose more accurately, and do procedures that had to be performed previously as open operations. The history of female cystourethroscopy is discussed in Chapter 1. Any surgeon operating in the pelvis today requires the skills to perform cystourethroscopy efficiently and safely: therefore, a good understanding of the cystoscopic instrumentation and how it is used is required.

Cystourethroscopy refers to the endoscopic examination of the lower urinary tract. It allows direct inspection of the bladder and urethra, confirmation of ureteral patency, and diagnosis of a wide range of lower urinary tract disorders. This chapter describes the basic instrumentation of cystourethroscopy used in the diagnosis and treatment of lower urinary tract disorders, and the newer equipment for video imaging which provide clearer pictures for viewing, analysis, teaching, and medical records. Cystourethroscopes are available as the traditional rigid instruments or the more recently developed flexible fibercystoscopes.

Rigid cystoscopes

Rigid cystoscopes are manufactured in many sizes from different manufacturers, but basically they are similar and consist of the following parts: the sheath, the obturator, the bridge, and the telescope (Figure 3.1).

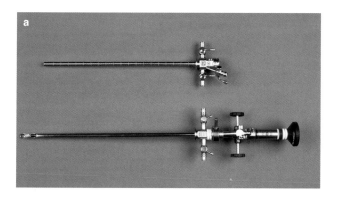
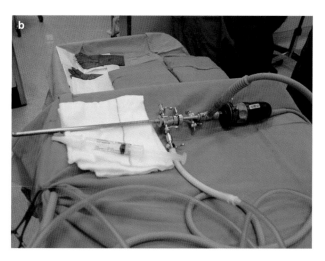

Figure 3.1
(a) Cystoscope (70°) with Albarran deflecting bridge and fenestrated shealth (below) and Sasche straight sheath (above).
(b) Cystoscope with camera and irrigation fluid attached, and lubricant lidocaine gel; ready for action.

Sheath

The sheath is the outer, most rigid part of the instrument (Figure 3.2). It serves to protect the interchangeable telescopes which are delicate and expensive, and can be damaged if bent or dropped. The sheath also provides an access for introducing distending media (irrigation) and a channel for working instruments (working or operating channel). The proximal end of the sheath has two irrigation ports, one for the introduction of the irrigation medium and the other for its egress. The distal end of the cystoscope sheath is cut away in a fenestration (Figure 3.3) to permit the use of operative instruments and angled 70° and 30° cystoscopes. Opposite the fenestration, the sheath is beveled to enhance the comfort of introduction of the cystourethroscope into the urethra.

Because irrigation fluid leaks at the urethral meatus until the fenestrated tip is completely inserted, this design makes urethroscopy difficult. Unlike cystoscope sheaths, urethroscope sheaths (Sasche sheath) are cut flush at the distal end, having a shorter beak and no fenestration. This allows distention of the distal urethra and more complete visualization of the urethral walls.[1]

Sheaths are available in various calibers, which are measured by their diameter, usually using the French (Fr) scale.[2] This is calculated by measuring the diameter of the scope in millimeters and multiplying by 3. The sizes range from the short delicate pediatric sheath (8–12 Fr), to the larger (25–28 Fr) sheath capable of accepting a telescope and two working instruments. In practice for adults, the smallest diameter sheath (17 Fr) is useful for diagnostic purposes and the larger caliber (21 Fr) provides space for the placement of instruments into the irrigation-working channel. Flexible cystoscopes are in the order of 15–18 Fr, even with working channels.

Obturator

Obturators can be introduced into the sheath to provide a smooth tip for insertion into the urethra. The *closed* obturator provides a solid intact tip for introduction of the instrument in a tactile blind fashion. A *visual* obturator accommodates a telescope and fills the space between the telescope and the sheath to provide a smooth surface against the urethra and allows the sheath to be introduced under vision.

Bridge

The bridge serves as a watertight connector between the telescope and the sheath. It may have one or two angled side-arms for introduction of instruments (e.g. biopsy or diathermy) into the irrigation-working channel. A deflecting bridge (Albarran bridge) may be inserted into the sheath to allow the use of flexible instruments (Figure 3.4).

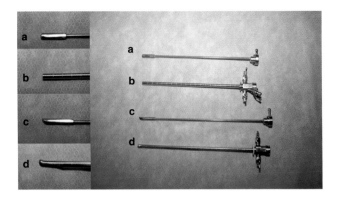

Figure 3.2
Cystoscopic obturators (a, c) and sheaths (b, d). a,b is a Sasche sheath and obturotor and c,d is a normal farestrated sheath with bereled obturator.

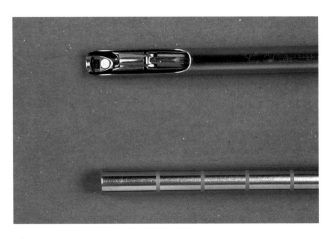

Figure 3.3
Fenestrated sheath with 70° scope (above) and Sasche sheath (below).

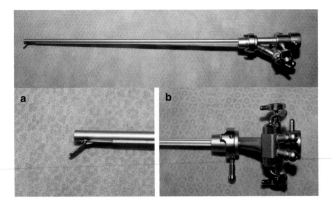

Figure 3.4
Cystoscopic sheath with (a) Albarran lever and (b) Albarran bridge.

Deflection at the instrument tip is controlled with a wheel at the proximal end of the bridge. The Albarran bridge is particularly useful for directing a ureteral catheter into a ureteral orifice, a needle for injection (e.g. Botox), or a flexible instrument (e.g. biopsy forceps) towards the dome of the bladder (Figure 3.5).

Telescope

Telescopes have evolved over many years to the accurate, well-illuminated refined visual instruments that are available for general use today. The telescope carries the fiberoptic illuminating system which extends from the tip of the instrument to the point of attachment of the light bundle just beyond the eyepiece. The light of the visual image is collected at the objective lens and transmitted through a rod–lens system to the eyepiece. The system is sealed against moisture to prevent obscured vision.

Cystoscopic telescopes are available with several viewing angles, which are determined by the lens angle relative to the instrument's long axis (Figure 3.6). Lenses focused to look directly forward are 0° telescopes. A 30° telescope provides a forward oblique view, the 70° a lateral view, and the 120° a retrograde view. The different angles facilitate the inspection of the entire bladder wall. The 30° lens provides the best view of the bladder base and the posterior wall, whereas the 70° lens is preferable for operative cystoscopy and allows inspection of the anterior-lateral walls, bladder dome, and ureteric orifices, particularly following urethral suspensions. The 0° lens is good for urethroscopic viewing of the urethra and bladder neck, but is insufficient for cystoscopy and full visualization of the bladder.

The telescope is the most delicate portion of the entire instrument system. The lenses, including the eyepiece and the objective lenses, are made of glasses which are easily damaged by dropping, bending during placement, or removal of the telescope from the sheath or by any sudden blow. They must be handled with care and treated with the respect due to a fine-precision optical instrument.

Lubricant

Lubrication of the outside of the sheath is recommended to minimize friction or trauma during the passage of the cystourethroscope into the urethra and can be either a water-soluble or oil-based lubricant. Oil-based lubricants have the advantage of lasting longer for long procedures. However, they have the disadvantages of causing local irritation, lacking solubility in urine or aqueous irrigation fluid, and obscuring vision by their tendency to coat the lens.[2]

The most commonly used lubricants in practice are the water-soluble ones containing methylcellulose, which tends to be non-irritating, dissolve readily in urine within the bladder, and wash from the urethra with urine flow. Other lubricants contain anesthetic agents such as 2% Xylocaine (lidocaine) in sodium carboxymethylcellulose or 0.75% cyclomethycaine sulfate in hydroxypropylmethylcellulose.

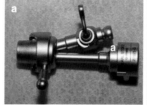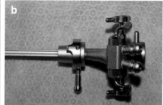

Figure 3.5
Bridges with (a) single channel and (b) dual channels.

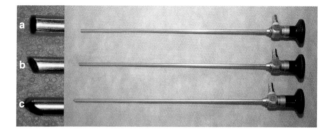

Figure 3.6
Cystoscope lenses (a) 0°, (b) 30°, (c) 70°.

Anesthetic activity is induced by absorption through the urethral mucosa after intraurethral instillation.

Flexible cystoscopy

Unlike the rigid cystoscope, the flexible cystoscope (Figure 3.7) combines the optical systems and irrigation-working channels in a single unit. The optical systems consist of flexible bundles that transmit light and images. The optical fibers are connected to a lens system that magnifies and focuses the image. A focusing knob is located just distal to the eyepiece. A deflecting mechanism allows the deflection of the distal tip of the cystoscope of up to 290° in a single plane. The flexible tip is about 15–18 Fr in diameter and 6–7 cm in length.[3] The use of the working channel with operative instruments restricts the tip deflection. Because of the delicate optical fibers (5–10 μm in diameter), the flexible cystoscope is very susceptible to damage, which will compromise the image or light transmission. Despite advances in fiberoptic technology, flexible cystoscopes still do not offer the field of visualization, the clarity, and the light-carrying capacity of the rod–lens systems in the rigid cystoscopes.

The main advantage of the flexible cystoscope is the improved patient comfort which applies largely to male patients, who often require general anesthesia for diagnostic cystoscopy with a rigid cystoscope. In the female patients, because of the lack of prostate and the short length of the urethra (3–4 cm), rigid cystoscopy is usually well tolerated and in most cases can be performed painlessly using only anesthetic lubricant.

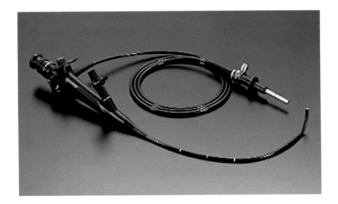

Figure 3.7
Flexible cystoscope and camera.

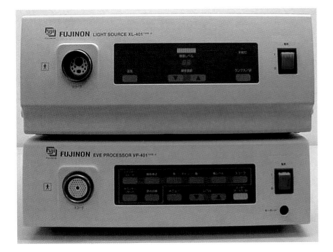

Figure 3.8
Light source and video processor.

Light source

The light source which provides illumination during cystoscopy can be provided by a halogen or xenon lamp (Figure 3.8). The simplest light source is a 150 W halogen lamp for direct viewing and is suitable for office endoscopy. Xenon bulbs generate higher light intensity (up to 300 W) and last longer than halogen lamps, but are more expensive to replace. Xenon light sources with variable illumination are recommended for video monitoring and photography during cystoscopic procedures.

Fiberoptic light cables

Light cables attach to the telescope at the eyepiece. They transmit light from the light source to the endoscope and can be either fiberoptic or fluid-filled cables. The fluid-filled cables are more durable but tend to be more expensive. The disadvantage of the fluid-filled cables is that they add a slight tint to the light. Fiberoptic cables, which are more commonly in use, contain flexible bundles of coaxial glass fibers similar to those of the flexible cystoscope and are prone to damage.

Light cables vary in length from 6 to 12 feet and in diameter from 3.5 to 4.8 mm. The light intensity carried by the light cable is inversely proportional to its length: the longer the fiberoptic light cable, the less light it delivers, with approximately 10% loss for every foot of cable over 6 feet. A 6–9 foot cable is sufficient for the purpose of video recording. Although the light intensity increases with the thickness of the cable, it is more important to choose the appropriate cable thickness for the size of the telescopic lens. For example, a cystoscope generally performs better with a 3.5 mm diameter cable than with a 4.8 mm cable, which is more suited for a 10 mm laparoscope.[4]

Only one-third of light generated by the lamp exits the distal end of the endoscope.[2] Thirty percent of lamp light is lost because core fibers constitute only 70% of the diameter of the fiberoptic cable.[5] Another 20% light loss is due to reflection at air–glass interfaces, such as fiber ends and the light cable couple. A further 20% is lost at the light cord and endoscope couple.

Broken and burned-out fibers decrease light transmission. Broken fibers are easily recognized by seeing light shining sideways along the length of the cable or unilluminated fibers when the cable is viewed on end at low light levels. A light cable should be replaced when more than one-third of the fibers are broken or burn out.

Accessory instruments for the lower urinary tract

Besides simple diagnosis of lower urinary tract disorders, cystourethroscopy also allows a variety of operative procedures to be performed on the female lower urinary tract. This includes minor procedures that are easily carried out during diagnostic cystoscopy such as biopsy of bladder mucosal lesions, removal of foreign bodies such as bladder stones and intravesical sutures. Cystourethroscopy is also used to inject bulking agents into the urethra (Figure 3.9) or Botox into the bladder wall, assess urethral coaptation during periurethral injection, or to facilitate surgical repair of urinary tract fistula and diverticulum and to evaluate damage to the bladder mucosa or ureters during bladder neck or pelvic floor reconstructive surgery. In gynecology, ureteral catheterization can be performed to assess potential ureteral obstruction[6,7] and to place ureteral catheters to act as markers prior to surgery in women with high potential for ureteral injury such as radical pelvic surgery and surgery with abnormal pelvic anatomy.[8]

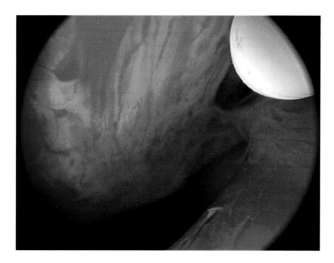

Figure 3.9
Transurethral injection of collagen into the anterior urethral wall through a long needle.

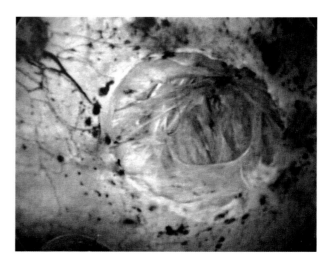

Figure 3.11
Bladder wall biopsy site exposing interlacing detrusor muscle fibers.

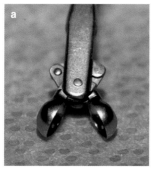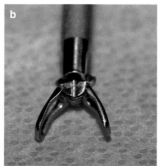

Figure 3.10
Cystoscopic forceps: (a) bladder wall biopsy forceps; (b) grasping forceps.

A wide range of instrumentation is available for use through a cystoscope. Instruments commonly used by urogynecologists include the grasping forceps with either a rat tooth or alligator jaws, biopsy forceps, and scissors, which come in different diametzers and are available in semirigid or flexible form. A flexible monopolar ball electrode (Bugby) is also available for electrocautery. Long needles can be used to inject material into the urethra and bladder.

Biopsy forceps

Bladder biopsy may be necessary to confirm or exclude a diagnosis: e.g. bladder tumor. Any bladder mucosal lesions that are suggestive of malignancy with a papillary, irregular, or erthythematous mucosa should be biopsied. However, it is important that pelvic surgeons can differentiate variations of normal (e.g. metaplasia), and benign conditions (e.g. cystitis cystica) from premalignant and malignant pathology. Biopsy forceps vary in sizes from 5 to 9 Fr.[2] They can be either flexible or rigid (Figure 3.10). The *flexible* forceps can biopsy a lesion at an angle away from the instrument and is particularly useful for lesions at the dome of the bladder. The size of the cup of a flexible forceps is small and samples are minute: e.g. the 5 Fr forceps obtains a specimen of less than 2 mm in diameter. Therefore, for satisfactory result, multiple biopsies are recommended. The risk of perforation with flexible forceps is usually small and they can be used safely in females and younger patients. Unlike the flexible forceps, which have to be withdrawn through the sheath to 'bite' the tissue, the *rigid* forceps are capable of sharply amputating the tissue without crushing it. The rigid forceps also allow biopsy of larger tissue specimen (up to 6 mm in diameters). Perforation of the bladder wall is more likely, especially if full thickness is taken (Figure 3.11); in these cases we would leave a urethral catheter in situ overnight. Despite their straight design, they can reach most regions in the bladder except the dome and the anterior wall.

Instruments to remove foreign bodies

Foreign bodies can be removed from the bladder endoscopically using *grasping* forceps, scissors, or screws (Figure 3.12). These instruments can be flexible or rigid. The grasping forceps are quite similar to the biopsy forceps except for the serrations or teeth on their jaws to provide a grasping surface. The grasping forceps are generally not suitable for taking biopsy because the tissue specimen that is not sharply amputated will pull through the teeth of the forceps.

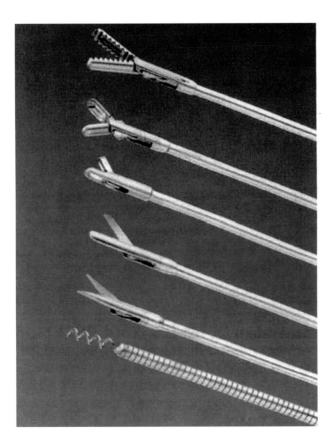

Figure 3.12
Cystoscopic grasping and biopsy forceps and screw for removal of intravesical foreign bodies.

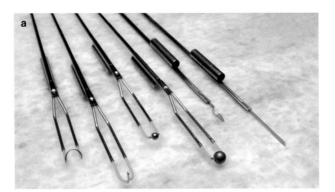

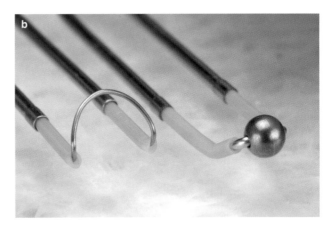

Figure 3.13
Electrocautery cystoscopic instruments for resection and diathermy.

The size of the foreign body removed by the endoscope is limited by the size of the sheath, the flexibility of the foreign body, and the ability to divide the specimen. If the foreign body is a calculus, the specimen can be fragmented into smaller pieces using forceps, vibrators, or lasers.[2]

Electrodiathermy electrodes (fulguration)

Fulguration can be used to stop minor bleeding (such as that resulting from biopsy) or destroy very small mucosal lesions such as papillomas. When the tip of the electrode is applied, satisfactory fulguration is observed when the tissue turns white or brown when coagulating current is applied to the electrode tip. Although numerous fulguration electrodes are available, the commonest designs are the 'ball' Bugbee types or coagulation electrodes (Figure 3.13).

Distending media

Irrigation with a distending medium through a cystoscope is essential to distend the bladder and the urethra for examination. Distending media can be divided into three categories: non-conductive fluids, conductive fluids, and gases. Although cystourethroscopy has been performed with carbon dioxide and popularized by Robertson in the 1970s (see Chapter 1), most practitioners today prefer to use a liquid medium (Table 3.1).

The choice of the irrigation fluid depends on the likelihood of fluid absorption, which is in turn determined by the type of procedure performed. Any of the commonly available irrigation fluids (e.g. normal saline or sterile water) can be used if there is minimal chance of fluid absorption: e.g. simple diagnostic cystoscopy. Normal saline is less irritating to bladder mucosa and may be preferable when fluid absorption is anticipated. An iso-osmotic solution such as saline or a non-hemolysing solution such as glycine or sorbitol is often used if the possibility of fluid absorption is significant (e.g. transurethral resection of the prostate). Systemic absorption of free water may alter serum electrolytes and cause intravascular hemolysis. Non-conducting solutions such as water or glycine are used with electrocautery.[9]

The irrigation liquid is usually instilled by gravity from a 1 or 3 L fluid bag through a standard intravenous infusion set connected to the cystoscope. The fluid bags should hang no more than 60 cm above the bladder to avoid

Table 3.1 Distending media for cystourethroscopy

Fluid

Non-conductive:
  Water
  Glycine (aminoacetic acid) 1.5%
  Sorbitol 3.0%
  Mannitol 5.0%
Conductive:
  Saline (sodium chloride) 0.9% or 0.45%
  Lactated Ringer's solution

Gas
  Carbon dioxide

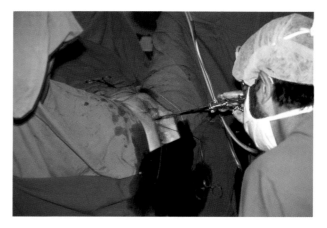

Figure 3.14
Cystoscopic examination by direct visualization is performed prior to introduction of the video camera.

vesicoureteral reflux.[1] Distending media may be warmed to 37° C, but should not be cooler than room temperature. Care should be taken to avoid air from passing with the irrigation fluid into the cystoscope, because excessive air bubbles can obstruct or distort the field of view during cystoscopic examination. However, a small amount of air is usually introduced, which gives a dome air bubble that acts as a useful marker for orientation within the bladder.

Equipment for cystourethroscopic imaging

The continuous advances in imaging technology offer clinicians a wide range of options to view and record normal anatomy, pathology, and cystoscopic procedures. Recordings either in stills or videos are valuable in capturing information for the purposes of patient education, clinical teaching of residents or physicians, and contributions to scientific literature. Although cystoscopic procedures can be performed with direct visualization using the eyepiece (Figure 3.14), the modern video system has eliminated the awkward positioning of the patient for direct visualization and allowed simultaneous viewing by the physicians, health personnel, and the patients. Visualization is also possible during bladder emptying. This is especially important in the diagnosis of interstitial cystitis to detect petechial hemorrhages which are only seen during emptying of the bladder. The video monitoring system consists of a video camera, a video monitor, a light source, light cables, and recording devices.

Video camera

The video camera consists of a camera head, a camera head cable, and a camera processor (Figure 3.15 and 3.16).

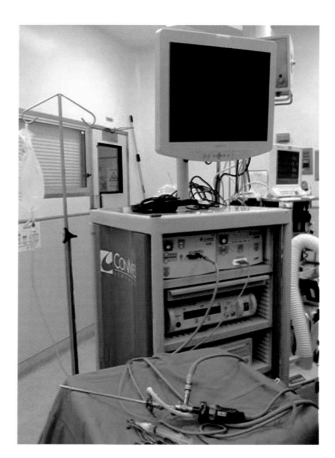

Figure 3.15
Full cystoscopic set-up with monitor, camera, and scopes.

The camera head contains a lens and light-sensitive imaging chips called charged couple devices (CCDs). The camera lens focuses the image on the CCDs. The video cameras can have one or three CCDs, which determine the quality of the color and resolution of the image the

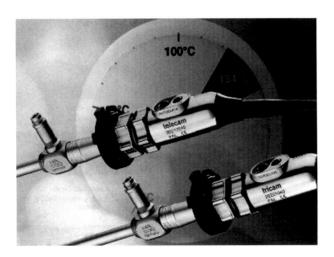

Figure 3.16
Autoclavable scopes and cameras.

cameras produce. Single-chip cameras have one CCD to reproduce color and recreate an image. They are more compact and less expensive than the three-chip cameras (with three CCDs), which contain a prism to refract light into three primary colors (red, green, and blue). Each chip picks up one color, providing an image of better color quality. The three-chip cameras also provide better resolution (up to 750 horizontal lines per inch compared with 300–450 lines in a single-chip camera), resulting in a sharper image.[4]

An adapter (endocoupler) connects the camera head to the eyepiece of the cystoscope and it contains optical lenses and the focusing mechanism, which is available in different focal lengths (25, 30, 38, and 50 mm). A longer focal length produces a larger picture but requires a greater light intensity to produce a good video image on the monitor. The camera head cable connects the camera head to the camera processor.

The camera processor or camera control unit (CCU) contains the camera's operating controls, including the power switch, white-balance, and a light boost or 'gain' to compensate for low light conditions.

Video monitor

The video monitor provides the images during cystoscopic examination (see Figure 3.15). The resolution of the monitor should match that of the video camera. For example, a three-chip camera should ideally have a monitor with 750 horizontal lines of resolution. In surgery, a monitor with a wider screen (e.g. 19 inch vs 14 inch) allows better visualization because of the larger images, although they may be brighter on a smaller screen.

Recording devices

Several choices for capturing or storing images during cystourethroscopy are available. This is a valuable adjunct for teaching undergraduate and postgraduate students. Also, it is an important part of the patient records and medicolegal documentation. Video images can be captured either as still pictures or recorded in moving images. A video printer stores a still image from a video camera and then produces a high-quality print. A premium printer allows printing of high-resolution pictures at high speed with multiple frames (e.g. 8 or 16 frames) of memory. Still pictures can also be stored in a digital still recorder where they can be displayed on a screen and selected and archived for documentation. The main advantage of the digital recorder is the capability it provides to select the desired images and erase the others. Moving images during cystoscopic procedures can be recorded digitally on storage media such as magneto-optical disks, CD recordable disks, or DVD disks.

Sterilization of urogenital instrumentation

Effective infection control should prevent transmission of infection from patient to patient or between healthcare workers and patients and is important in the management of urogenital instrumentation. There are different levels of microorganism eradication available in processing of instruments and equipment. Sterilization means the complete destruction and eradication of microorganisms, including bacterial spores, and should be used where there is penetration of skin, mucous membranes, or other tissues. Sterilization can be achieved by autoclaving (steam under pressure). For heat-sensitive equipment which cannot be autoclaved, other alternatives are ethylene oxide, peracetic acid (Steris system), and hydrogen peroxide plasma (Sterrad system) sterilization. High-level disinfection is inactivation of vegetative bacteria, viruses, and fungi but not necessarily of bacterial spores. Methods used for high-level disinfection include thermal disinfection, a minimum of 5 minutes uninterrupted boiling, or chemical disinfection (20 minutes immersion in 2% activated glutaraldehyde and rinsing in water before patient use, as glutaraldehyde is highly irritant). Glutaraldehyde is a cold disinfectant and is bactericidal, fungicidal, and slowly sporicidal. Cleaning of the instruments prior to sterilization removes soil and reduces the number of microorganisms present; it is an essential step prior to sterilization or disinfection.

Endoscopy of the urinary and genital tract involves contact with intact mucous membranes which may occasionally be breached so the level of risk warrants a high-level disinfection and preferably sterilization of instruments should be performed.[10]

Rigid cystoscopes are readily autoclavable, which is the preferred sterilization method. Certain types of camera heads and cables are now also autoclavable or disposable sterile sleeves and covers can be used. Flexible fibercystoscopes that cannot be autoclaved can be sterilized in the peracetic acid system (Steris system), which is a relatively low-temperature sterilization system: the active ingredient, peracetic acid, is a liquid chemical sterilant which is an effective biocide with no toxic residue and is suitable for heat-sensitive endoscopic equipment. Glutaraldehyde has traditionally been used for high-level disinfection of endoscopic equipment but is presently being phased out of many hospitals because of the safety aspects, as toxicity of fumes causes lung, eye, and skin irritation to health workers. These risks can be reduced by proper ventilation, good work practices, and use of personal protective equipment.

References

1. Weinberger MW. Cystoscopy for the practising gynecologist. Clin Obstet Gynecol 1998; 41(3): 764–76.
2. Bagley DH, Huffman JL, Lyon ES. Cystourethroscopy. In: Bagley DH, Huffman JL, Lyon ES, eds. Urologic Endoscopy: A Manual and Atlas. Boston, MA: Little Brown, 1985: 77–97.
3. Cundiff GW. Instrumentation for cystourethroscopy. In: Cundiff GW, Bent AE, eds. Endoscopic Diagnosis of the Female Lower Urinary Tract. Philadelphia, PA: WB Saunders, 1999: 9–16.
4. Bent AE. Endoscopic photography of bladder and urethra. In: Cundiff GW, Bent AE, eds. Endoscopic Diagnosis of the Female Lower Urinary Tract. Philadelphia, PA: WB Saunders, 1999: 83–91.
5. Hulka JF, Reich H. hight: optics and television. In: Hulka JF, Reich H, eds. Textbook of haporoscopy, 2nd edn. Philadelphia: WB Samders, 1994: 9–22.
6. Matin EC. Ureteric injury in gyrecologic surgery. J Urol 1953; 70: 51–7.
7. Gilmour DT, Dwyer PL, Carey MP. Lower urinary tract injury during gynaecological surgery and its detection by intraoperative cystoscopy. Obstet Gynecol 1999; 94; 883–9.
8. Conger K, Beecham CT, Horrax TN. Ureteral injury in pelvic surgery: current thought on incidence, pathogenesis, prophylaxis and treatment. Obstet Gynecol 1954; 3: 343–57.
9. Bagley DH, Huffman JL, Lyon ES. Irrigation. In: Bagley DH, Huffman JL, Lyon ES, eds. Urologic Endoscopy: A Manual and Atlas. Boston: Little Brown, 1985: 265–9.
10. Dwyer and Garland. Instrumentation and catheterization: risks and remedies. In Starton SL, Dwyer PL, eds. Urinary Tract Infection in the Female. 2000: 278–80.
11. Apell RA, Flynn JT, Paris AN, Blandy JP. Occult bacterial colonization of bladder tumours. J Urol 1980; 124: 345–6.
12. Christensen MM, Madsen PO. Antimicrobial prophylaxis in transurethral surgery. Urology 1990; 3(Suppl); 11–14.
13. Victorian Drug Usage Advisory Committee 1998. Therapeutic Guidelines: antibiotics, 10th edn. Melbourne: Therapeutic Guidelines Ltd, 1998: 302.

4

Cystourethroscopy: technique, indications, and complications

Tan Poh Kok and Peter L Dwyer

Introduction

Endoscopic examination of the urethra and the bladder should perhaps be considered as separate procedures when using rigid endoscopic equipment, as different sheaths and scopes are needed for adequate inspection. Careful endoscopic evaluation of the urethra is as important as that of the bladder, if pathology is not to be overlooked or misdiagnosed. As described in Chapter 3, examination of the urethra requires a 0° or 30° scope to fully visualize the lumen and a non-fenestrated sheath with a straight tip to distend the urethra (Figures 4.1). Irrigation through the cystourethroscope using a fenestrated sheath will not distend the female urethra as the fluid will leak around the instrument. The bladder should be viewed by using a 70° scope with fenestrated sheath. Flexible fibercystoscopes allow examination of the urethra and the bladder using the same instrument which can be rotated 270° to completely see within the bladder.

Preoperative preparation

Cystourethroscopy can be performed under general anesthesia or in an outpatient setting with topical or local anesthesia. Topical agents, such as 2% Xylocaine (lidocaine), gel help relieve discomfort but may cause reddening of the urethra, making it difficult to assess the degree of inflammation. The choice of irrigation fluid is made based on the type of cystoscopic procedure to be carried out. For simple diagnostic cystoscopy, 1 L of water or saline is usually sufficient. Electrically conductive fluid (normal saline) cannot be used if endoscopic fulguration is necessary.

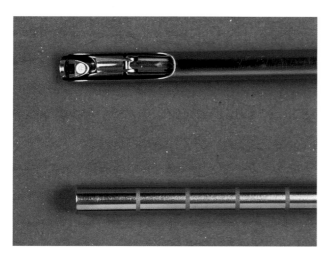

Figure 4.1
Fenestrated sheath with 70° scope (above) and Sasche sheath (below).

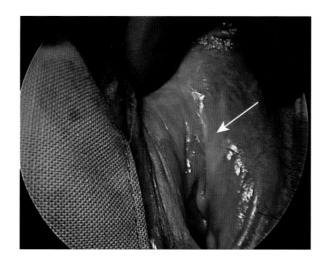

Figure 4.2
Stenosis of the external urethral meatus (arrow) in a woman with voiding difficulty.

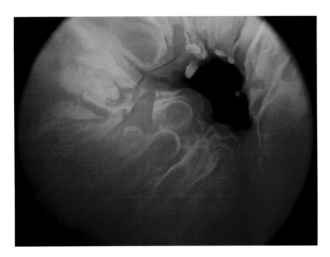

Figure 4.3
Urethroscopy using a 0° scope and Sasche sheath showing an inflamed urethra with inflammatory polyps and bladder neck in the distance.

Inspection of the urethral meatus

The patient is put in the lithotomy position and her bladder is emptied. The urogenital area is cleansed with an antiseptic solution. The urethral meatus should be inspected directly for position and the presence of pathology, and adequacy of the urethral lumen for cystoscopy should be assessed. The mean urethral caliber in the adult female is 22 Fr, with 95% of patients between 18 and 30 Fr.[1] If the meatus is adequate, the procedure can continue with the introduction of the cystoscope. Meatus stenosis is relatively rare in women but can occur (Figure 4.2 and also see Chapter 6). In women with urethral strictures, the length of the narrowed segment should be estimated and dilation then performed. A urethrogram or urethroscopy with a smaller instrument may be necessary if the extent of the narrowing cannot be determined (see Chapter 6).

Introduction of the cystourethroscope and urethroscopy

To avoid any mucosal trauma, the cystourethroscope should have an atraumatic rounded tip such as the closed or visual obturator. The cystourethroscope may be passed either under direct visualization or in a blind manner, although the former is considered the preferred technique. Direct vision insertion clarifies the position of the cystourethroscope (0° scope and Sasche sheath) in the urethral lumen and permits inspection of the urethral mucosa

to detect inflammation and lesions such as diverticula, polyps, or fronds (see Figure 4.2) (see Chapter 6) prior to any trauma induced by the instrument. In the normal urethra the submucosal vasculature is well developed and prominent with good urethral tone, unlike the pale, flat mucosa in a patulous urethra seen in elderly postmenopausal women or post irradiation. In the normal functioning urethra seen by urethroscopy in the conscious patient, the urethra closes during pelvic muscle contraction and the bladder neck remains closed with coughing or Valsalva maneuvers as compared to the rigid fibrotic urethra seen in intrinsic stress dysfunction (ISD) stress incontinence which opens readily during urethral filling and remains open even with pelvic muscle contraction. Any obstruction such as a stricture or foreign body can also be seen during direct introduction. The instrument may be passed blindly when a visual obturator is not available. This should be done with a closed obturator to minimize mucosal injury which would otherwise be more likely to occur when attempting to insert the telescope with the relatively sharp unprotected sheath along the urethra.

During direct introduction, the center of the urethral lumen should be kept in the center of the visual field as the endoscope is advanced. If the urethra is patulous (intrinsic sphincter dysfunction) or the bladder poorly compliant, irrigation through the cystourethroscope may not distend the bladder as the fluid leaks through the urethral meatus around the instrument. Distention can be achieved by using digital pressure to partially occlude the urethra against the back of the pubic symphysis with the forefinger and the thumb. During blind insertion, the urethral meatus is visualized and the tip of the obturator is placed against the meatus and advanced in a cephalic and slightly anterior direction towards the umbilicus. The obturator should advance about 3–4 cm before it is removed and the telescope is inserted into the sheath.

The introduction of the cystourethroscope must always be performed in the gentlest manner whether the patient is awake or anesthetized. The instrument must never be forced into the bladder as it will only result in pain, bleeding, and a false passage, which further hinder the procedure. The key factors for successful introduction of the cystourethroscope are a well-lubricated instrument, adequate lumen, and a good understanding of the urethral anatomy.

Cystoscopy

As the cystoscope enters the bladder, the vesical neck is observed during bladder filling by placing the endoscope in the proximal urethra. In outpatient cystoscopy using lidocaine gel only, the patient is asked to report the first sensation of fluid entering the bladder, the desire to urinate, and fullness. A post-void residual urine estimation can be performed if the patient has micturated prior to cystoscopy to

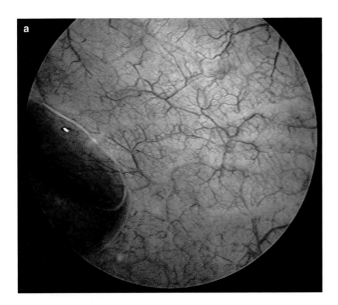

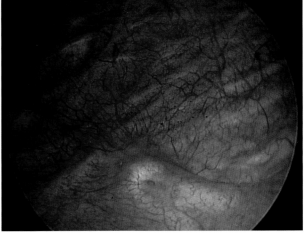

Figure 4.5
Right ureteric orifice with prominent interureteric ridge.

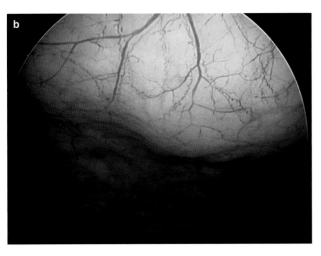

Figure 4.4 (a,b)
(a) Bladder dome with gas bubble. (b) Indentation of anterior bladder wall by symphysis pubis.

avoid bladder overdistention; the irrigating fluid is turned off when the patient feels full (mild discomfort). Once into the bladder, the urethroscope is replaced with the 70° telescope. The bladder is systematically inspected.

The first landmark when performing cystoscopy is the bladder neck (see Figure 4.1b). This is the reference point of the entry into the bladder. When the patient is in the dorsal lithotomy or sitting position, the next landmark is the air bubble within the bladder, which identifies the bladder dome (Figure 4.4a). Inferior to the air bubble on the interior of the anterior bladder wall there is frequently an indentation or protrusion, which is the back of the symphysis pubis (Figure 4.4b). This can be mistaken for an external mass by the inexperienced. The bladder trigone and ureteral orifices (Figure 4.5) are then inspected. The interureteric ridge, which lies posterior to the bladder neck

between the two ureteric orifices, is a useful landmark for ureteric identification. The ureteric orifices can be found by positing the cystoscope at 30° from the perpendicular.

The ureteric orifices appear as a slit or small cleft in the bladder mucosa about 1–2 cm lateral to the midline bilaterally. A characteristic vascular pattern is often seen around the orifices. Prominent submucosal vessels are usually seen medial, inferior, and lateral to the orifice, leaving a relatively avascular arc distal to the os. Orifices should be watched until urine efflux is seen. Urinary efflux is accompanied by lateral contraction (peristalsis) of the ureteral musculature and opening of the orifice. Urine exits the ureter as a jet of darker-colored fluid (Figure 4.6a,b), causing turbulence in the distending medium. When obscured by inflammation or other lesions, the ureteric orifices can be identified by administering a colored dye which is excreted in the urine after intravenous injection. Indigo carmine, which can be seen as a blue jet from the orifices (Figure 4.7), has been used for this purpose. The position and the configuration of each orifice should be observed. This can be viewed with a 30° or 70° telescope. The position of the ureteric orifices may be altered by congenital factors or as a result of surgery (Figure 4.8a,b), inflammation, or tumor. Variation on the shape of the ureteric orifice can be seen from slit-like to a rounded golf-hole shape (Figure 4.9) and is usually without functional significance.

After the trigone, the bladder floor posterior to the interureteric ridge is examined. Foreign bodies, stones, and blood clots (Figure 4.10) are commonly located in this dependent location. The bladder base may be difficult to visualize in women with large cystocele or when a diverticulum is present (Figure 4.11); elevation of the

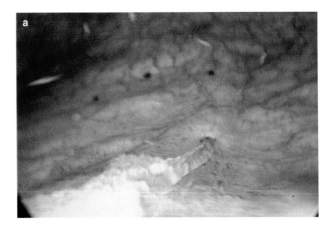

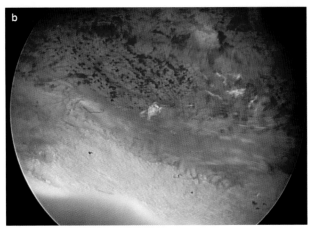

Figure 4.6
(a) Left ureteric orifice with efflux of urine. (b) Urine jet from RUO containing stringy particulate material; also note squamous metaplasia of trigone.

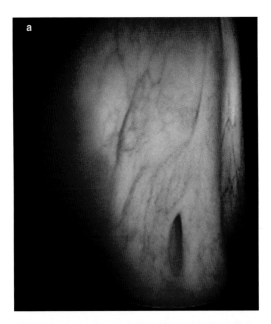

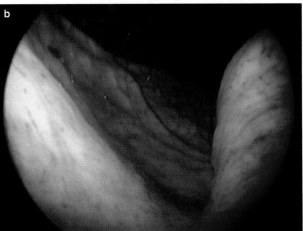

Figure 4.8
(a) Left ureteric orifice pulled superiorly by a Burch colposuspension suture. (b) Left ureteric orifice is difficult to see as the bladder base is distorted by anterior colporrhaphy.

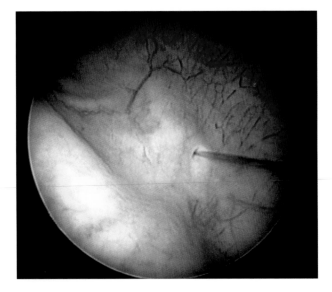

Figure 4.7
Right ureteric jet of indigo carmine.

anterior vaginal wall with a finger will improve vision. By sweeping the angular lens (70–90°) from the bladder dome to the vesical neck in a progressive clockwise manner and then moving from the posterior to the anterior surface, the remainder of the bladder is inspected systematically. Intravesical sutures from retropubic suspensions (e.g. Burch colposuspension) (Figure 4.12) and retropubic slings (Figure 4.13) will be found to perforate the bladder dome at 11 and 1 o'clock. The color, vascularity, and configuration of the bladder mucosa, should be described. Mucosal lesions, including papillary or sessile

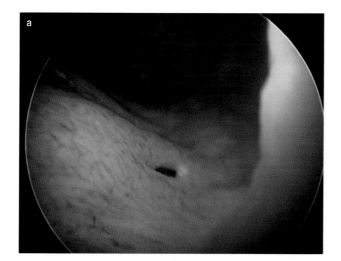

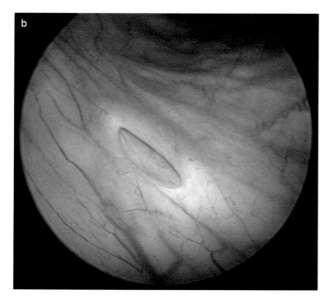

Figure 4.9
(a) Normal left ureteric orifice. (b) Round golf holed right ureteric orifice.

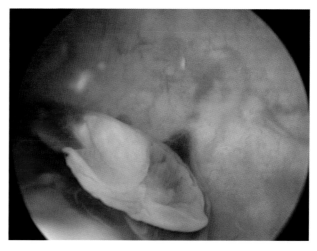

Figure 4.10
Organizing blood clot lying on base of bladder.

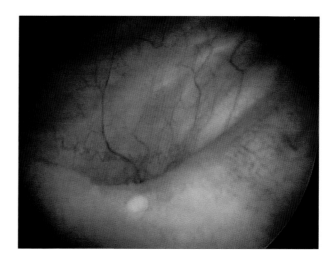

Figure 4.11
Bladder diverticulum posterior to the interureteric ridge.

epithelial growths and irregular or erythematous mucosa, should be biopsied for evaluation. Bladder wall trabeculations from muscular hypertrophy should be noted and may be indicative of obstruction, bladder overactivity, or the aging process. After bladder inspection, the endoscope is slowly withdrawn and the entire volume of urine and irrigation fluid within the bladder is drained.

Postoperative care

Minimal medical care is necessary after a simple cystoscopy. Patients, however, must be informed of potential hematuria, dysuria, and sometimes air in the urine during the first several voidings after cystourethroscopy. The possibilities of urinary tract infection (UTI) or retention must also be highlighted. The role of routine antibiotics prophylaxis after cystourethroscopy remains controversial.[2] Routine prophylactic antibiotics are currently not justified except for women who have a history of recurrent UTI, impaired bladder emptying, or have cardiac valvular disease and are at high risk for developing subacute bacterial endocarditis. Recommended antibiotics by the American Heart Association include penicillin/ampicillin plus gentamicin administered intravenously preoperatively and continued for a total of three doses.[3,4]

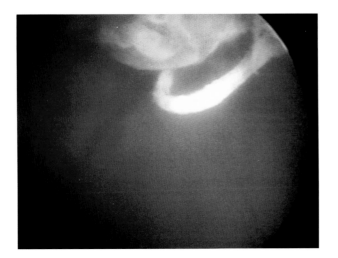

Figure 4.12
Intravesical Burch colposuspension suture at 1 o'clock surrounded by edematous mucosa found 1 year postoperatively in a woman with recurrent urinary infection and irritable bladder symptoms.

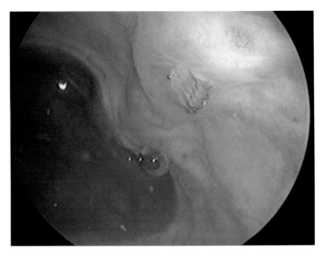

Figure 4.13
Intravaginoplasty sling (IVS) of polypropylene type peretrating the bladder mucosa at 1 o'clock found 2 years postoperatively in a woman with recurrent stress incontinence.

Indications and contraindications for cystourethroscopy

Cystourethroscopy is indicated in clinical situations (Table 4.1) where assessment of:

- structural anatomy and integrity of the lower urinary tract is required
- tissue is needed for histological assessment
- endoscopic access to upper urinary tract is required

Endoscopic examination of the urethra and bladder may reveal the cause of persistent or recurrent UTIs and voiding dysfunction. Routine cystourethroscopy to assess urinary incontinence is probably not justifiable. However, patients with persistent or atypical incontinence or recurrent incontinence after surgical repairs should undergo cystourethroscopy to rule out a urinary fistula. Some gynecologists have found cystourethroscopy useful in differentiating urethral hypermobility from intrinsic urethral sphincteric deficiency.[2] In patients with primary incontinence, endoscopy should be performed when other lower urinary tract abnormalities are suspected.

It is important to exclude lower urinary tract tumors (as well as upper tract tumors) in patients with hematuria or abnormal urinary cytology. Periodic endoscopic evaluation of the bladder for recurrences may be required in women following treatment of their bladder tumor.

The major contraindication to cystourethroscopy is known or suspected UTI. Cystitis should be treated before

Table 4.1   Indications for cystourethroscopy

Assessment of:

1. Persistent or recurrent urinary tract infections
2. Irritative voiding symptoms
3. Obstructive voiding symptoms
4. Atypical incontinence and fistula evaluation
5. Trauma to lower urinary tract
6. Urethral or bladder diverticulum
7. Foreign body

Histological evaluation:

1. Hematuria
2. Abnormal urine cytology
3. Interstitial cystitis
4. Staging for cervical cancer

Assessment of the lower and upper urinary tract during pelvic and urogynecological surgery to confirm:

1. Ureteral patency and function
2. Bladder and urethra integrity

cystoscopy, which otherwise may result in severe exacerbation of the infection, even with septicemia or bacteremia. Women with asymptomatic bacteriuria should be given prophylactic antibiotics during and after cystoscopy. Unstable medical conditions requiring urgent treatment are another contraindication to cystoscopy.

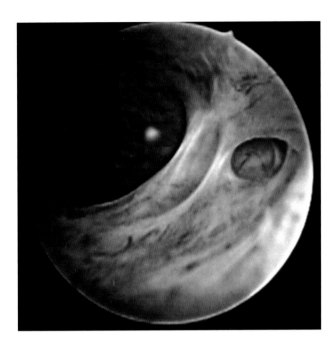

Figure 4.14
Urethroscopic photograph of scarred urethra from previous urethral diverticulectomy.

Indications for diagnostic cystourethroscopy

Recurrent urinary tract infection

Structural and functional abnormalities of the urinary tract in women with recurrent UTI are uncommon,[5] so cystoscopy is indicated only when a structural or functional abnormality is suspected. Women with previous urogenital surgery may have impaired bladder emptying, or suture erosion (Figure 4.12) or penetration into the lower urinary tract with calculus formation causing recurrent UTI. These women should have cystourethroscopy performed early, as delay in diagnosis can lead to morbidity for these patients and medicolegal problems for the clinician. Women with persistent hematuria following UTI resolution should also be investigated with cystourethroscopy to exclude urinary tract cancer.

Urinary incontinence and voiding dysfunction

The two primary functions of the lower urinary tract are to store urine efficiently and competently and to empty on command at an appropriate time and place. These functions are best assessed using urodynamic investigations. Storage phase disorders are evaluated using filling cystometry and using Valsalva or leak point pressures. During the voiding phase, function is evaluated using bladder pressure/urinary flow

study (uroflowmetry) and measurement of residual urine volume. Poor urinary flow may be caused by an outlet obstruction (e.g. urethral stricture) resulting in high voiding pressure and low urinary flow; or by poor detrusor function from denervation or damage of the bladder musculature.

Although there is no need for routine cystourethroscopy in the assessment in female incontinence, occasionally cystourethroscopy is required to exclude a structural cause for the incontinence. Urinary incontinence can be caused by a fistula, either congenital or occurring secondary to surgical or radiation injury (see Chapters 5 and 12). Cystourethroscopy rarely provides much information on lower urinary tract function, especially if performed when the patient is anesthetized. However, the urethra may appear patulous and scarred (Figure 4.14) in women with ISD stress incontinence, women with an overactive bladder, or chronic urinary retention may be detrusor muscle hypertrophy and trabeculation of the bladder wall (Figure 4.15).

Women with impaired bladder emptying should be considered for cystourethroscopy to exclude any structural cause such as urethral stricture (see Figure 4.2). If a stricture is found, treatment with urethral dilatation or urethrotomy may be appropriate. Obstruction following stress incontinence surgery is common and may be caused by a sling placed under excessive tension or a urethral suspension procedure where the bladder neck has been oversuspended. A urethral sound or dilator placed in the urethra may reveal abnormal urethral angulation or excessive mid-urethral or bladder neck kinking from the sling or sutures.

Evidence of outlet obstruction may be seen in the bladder with trabeculation of the bladder wall (Figure 4.15), with diverticular formation and ureteric reflux. Dilatation of the upper urinary tract and hydronephrosis may be also present on imaging.

Irritative bladder symptoms

Women with urinary frequency and urgency or pain who have a low voided volume on their urinary diary should have cystourethroscopy to determine the cause of their bladder hypersensitivity. Causes of bladder hypersensitivity are outlined in Table 4.2. Treatment of these symptoms will depend on the cause. Functional causes of detrusor overactivity and

Table 4.2   Causes of bladder hypersenstivity
Infective cystitis (UTI)
Non infective cystitis (e.g. cystitis cystica, granulomatus cystitis)
Drug induced cystitis
Calculus
Foreign bodies
Radiation cystitis
Tumor
Functional causes (e.g. overactive bladder)

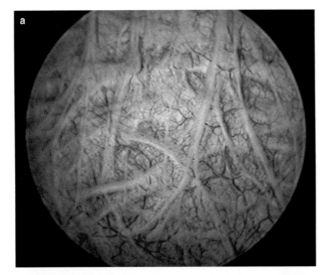

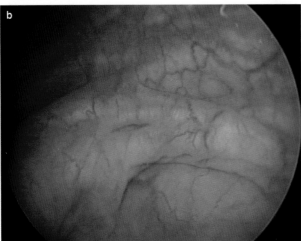

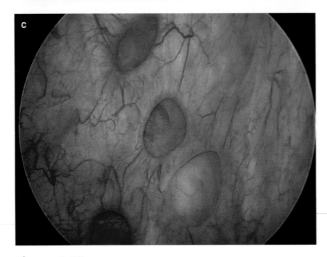

Figure 4.15
Moderate and severe bladder trabeculation.

hypersensitivity are usually treated with bladder retraining and anticholinergic medication in the first instance. Cystodistention is part of the diagnostic process in women with hypersensitive bladders, including interstitial cystitis.

Cystodistention also provides a short-term symptomatic relief in 20–30% of these patients (see Chapter 8).

Diagnostic findings in women with interstitial cystitis are generalized petechial hemorrhages, which often bleed in cascades from the actual bladder walls when the bladder is being emptied. During bladder filling, there may be mucosal tearing, fissuring, and ulceration (see Chapter 8).

Hematuria

The causes of hematuria are similar to those conditions causing bladder hypersensitivity (Table 4.2). Lower urinary tract cancer is the major concern in any woman with hematuria and the reason why early cystourethroscopic evaluation of the urinary tract is necessary. Other causes of hematuria need to be accurately diagnosed and treated. Along with endoscopy, urine microscopy and culture, urine cytology and imaging of the urinary tract by ultrasound or radiologically (computed tomography [CT] scan) may be appropriate. The diagnosis and treatment of urinary malignancy are discussed in Chapter 10.

Trauma to the lower urinary tract

Trauma to the urinary tract can occur as a result of an accident (e.g. motor car, sporting injury), iatrogenic (as a result of surgery), or rarely be self-inflicted. Cystourethroscopy plays an important role in the diagnosis and treatment of the injuries. Urinary tract injury should be considered especially in certain types of accidents (e.g. fractured pelvis; saddle injuries) and the appropriate investigations, including endoscopy, be performed.

In the case of surgical trauma, endoscopy also plays an important role in prevention. The upper and lower urinary tracts are always at risk during pelvic surgery, and cystourethroscopy following surgery will enable the surgeon to confirm the patency and bilateral function of the ureters and also the integrity of the lower urinary tract with no inadvertent injury from tearing, clamping, or inadvertent foreign body penetration (suture or synthetic mesh). Because of the importance of this area to gynecologists, prevention of upper and lower urinary tract injury is covered in Chapter 14.

Complications of cystourethroscopy

The most significant cause of morbidity after cystourethroscopy is infection, although the actual incidence of procedural infection is not well documented. The rate of bacteriuria after outpatient cystourethroscopy has been reported as 2.8–16.6%.[6,7] Its clinical significance is not clear because most patients have no or few symptoms and bacteriuria often resolves spontaneously. The risk of infection with

Table 4.3 Complications of cystourethroscopy

Urinary tract infection
Hematuria
Painful or urgent urination
Voiding difficulty
Injury to bladder/urethra

cystourethroscopy will vary with the time and complexity with endoscopic surgery. In a study of male patients, the incidence of UTI after transurethral section of a bladder tumor is 38% compared with 11% after transurethral prostate surgery and 5% after diagnostic cystoscopy.[8] When bacteriuria is present preoperatively, the risk of postoperative infection increases significantly, up to 60% in a study by Christensen and Madsen.[9] For immediate surgery in women with bacteriuria, gentamicin 5–7 mg/kg intravenously should be given. Alternatively, cefotetan or cefoxitin intravenously can be used as a single agent at the time of induction.[10]

Pyelonephritis, which is an uncommon complication, must be managed promptly with appropriate antibiotics.

The most frequent complication is urgency or burning sensation with urination, secondary to irritation of the bladder wall and urethra (Table 4.3). Patients with preoperative irritative voiding symptoms may have exacerbation of these symptoms. Short-term hematuria may also be experienced.

Bladder perforation can occur when the endoscope is not inserted under direct visualization or if coincidental procedures such as biopsy or tumor resection cause damage to the detrusor wall. Consideration should be given to urethral bladder drainage postoperatively if the patient is considered at risk. Difficulty passing the endoscope through the urethra can cause trauma or create false passages.

References

1. Weinberger MW. Cystoscopy for the practising gynecologist. Clin Obstet Gynecol 1998; 41(3): 764–76.
2. Cundiff GW. Perioperative evaluation of vesical and ureteral integrity. In Cundiff GW, Bent AE, eds. Endoscopic Diagnosis of the Female Lower Urinary Tract. Philadelphia, PA: WB Saunders, 1999: 59–66.
3. Antibiotic prophylaxis for surgery. Med Lett Drugs Ther 1979; 21: 76.
4. Kaplan EL Prevention of bacterial endocarditis. Circulation 1977; 56: 139–43a.
5. Dwyer PL, O'Reilly M. Recurrent urinary tract infection in women. Curr Opin Obstet Gynecol 2002: 14: 537–43.
6. Manson AL. Is antibiotic prophylaxis indicated after outpatient cystoscopy? J Urol 1988; 140: 316–17.
7. Richards B, Bastable JRG. Bacteriuria after outpatient cystoscopy. Br J Urol 1977; 49: 561–4.
8. Apell RA, Flynn JT, Paris AN, Blandy JP. Occult bacterial colonization of bladder tumours. J Urol 1980; 124: 345–6.
9. Christensen MM, Madsen PO. Antimicrobial prophylaxis in transurethral surgery. Urology 1990; 3(Suppl): 11–14.
10. Victorian Drug Usage Advisory Committee. Therapeutic Guidelines: Antibiotics, 10th edn. Melbourne: Therapeutic guidelines Ltd, 1998: 302.

5

Congenital urinary tract anomalies

Peter L Dwyer

Introduction

The urinary and genital tracts are closely related functionally and anatomically and have a common embryological development with interaction between the two ductal systems necessary for normal growth. Congenital abnormalities of the urinary system are often associated with abnormalities in the genital tract. Thompson and Lynn[1] found that 35% of females with unilateral renal agenesis have partial or complete duplication of the genital tract. In another study renal agenesis was present in 43% of women with uterus didelphys (Figure 5.1) and 10% of patients with genital tract abnormalities had an abnormal or ectopic kidney.[2]

Congenital abnormalities of the urinary tract usually present to pediatricians or pediatric urologists as childhood urinary disorders of urinary incontinence and urinary tract infection, or failure to thrive. However congenital anomalies can present later in life to gynecologists and urologists with late-onset symptoms or as an ongoing management problem of a previously diagnosed congenital condition. Ectopic ureters in females are frequently not diagnosed until adult life, with pregnancy or childbirth precipitating urinary incontinence (see Cases 1 and 2). The author also knows of two cases of ectopic ureters misdiagnosed as stress incontinence that were only correctly diagnosed following an unsuccessful Burch colposuspension.

Congenital anomalies may present with symptoms of urinary incontinence, urinary tract infection, an abdominal or pelvic mass (hydronephrotic or pelvic kidney), vaginal discharge, or other urogynecological symptoms. These abnormalities may be asymptomatic and found during routine examination or cystourethroscopy in the adolescent or adult woman. Therefore it is important that clinicians working in the area of female pelvic floor dysfunction are familiar with the embryology of the urinary and genital tracts and have an excellent knowledge of congenital malformations of the urogenital system, their diagnosis and treatment. Cystourethroscopic evaluation of the lower urinary tract plays an important role in the management of these congenital anomalies. Case studies are presented to

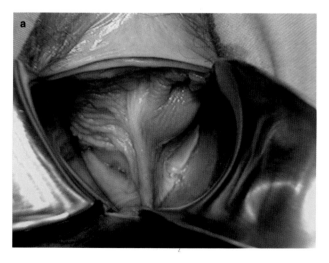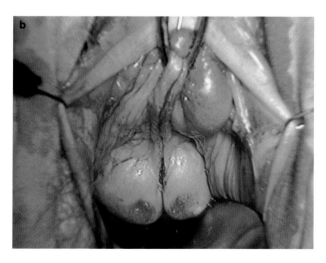

Figure 5.1
(a) Uterus didelphys with midline vaginal septum, and (b) with septum excised revealing two cervices.

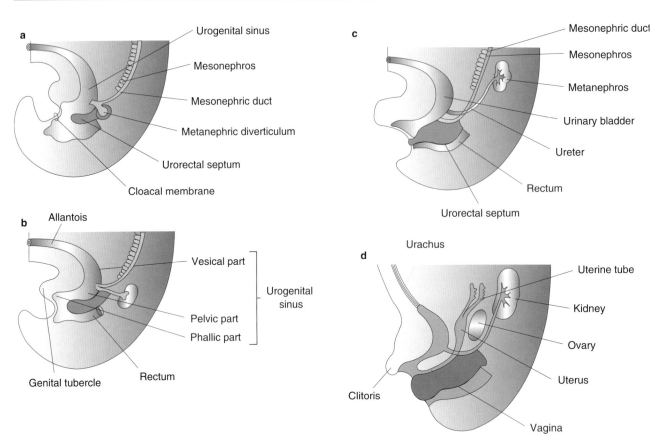

Figure 5.2
From the 6th to the 12th week of embryological development the urorectal septum divides the cloaca into the urogenital sinus and definitive rectum. A pair of ureteric buds grows upwards from the distal mesonephric duct near its insertion into the cloaca to become the renal pelvis, calyces, and collecting ducts and induce the overlying sacral intermediate mesoderm (metanephros) to develop into the primitive kidney.

demonstrate some of the clinical and endoscopic findings to be found in women with congenital urinary anomalies.

Embryology

The urinary and genital systems in the female are structurally and functionally separate, unlike in the male, although in both sexes the embryological development is closely associated. In the embryo, two pairs of genital tracts develop: the mesonephric ducts (wolffian ducts) become the male urogenital system and the paramesonephric ducts (müllerian ducts) become the female reproductive system.

The urogenital systems develop from the intermediate mesoderm, which extends along the dorsal body cavity in the embryo by the 5th week following fertilization and forms the urogenital ridge and mesonephric ducts. A pair of ureteric buds grows upwards from the distal mesonephric duct near its insertion into the cloaca to become the renal pelvis, calyces, and collecting ducts and induce the overlying sacral intermediate mesoderm (metanephros) to develop into the primitive kidney (Figure 5.2). Absence of the developing ureteric buds results in renal agenesis. The

trigone of the bladder is derived from the caudal ends of the mesonephric ducts (Figure 5.3).

By the 6th week the urogenital septum divides the cloaca into a ventral urogenital sinus and a dorsal rectum. The upper part of the urogenital sinus forms the bladder, which is continuous with the allantois, which obliterates to form the urachus (medium umbilical ligament) connecting the apex of the bladder to the umbilicus (see Figure 5.2). The epithelium of the bladder is derived from the endoderm of the urogenital sinus, while the epithelium of the terminal part of the urethra is derived from surface ectoderm. The paramesonephric ducts develop as an ingrowth of coelomic epithelium anterolateral to the mesonephric ducts and give rise to the fallopian tubes and uterus, while the epithelium of the vagina is derived from the endoderm of the urogenital sinus and the vaginal fibromuscular wall from the surrounding mesenchyme.

The primordial germ cells migrate from the yolk sac along the dorsal mesentery of the hindgut to the gonadal ridges and primitive gonads present on the medial side of the mesonephros. These cells give rise to oogonia in the ovaries and spermatogonia in the testes. Testosterone produced by the fetal testes induces male development by stimulating the mesonephric ducts to form male genital ducts, while müllerian

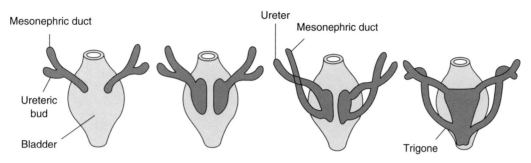

Figure 5.3
The development of the dorsal aspect of the vesicourethral canal, showing the relationship between the ureters, mesonephric ducts, and the trigone. The trigone of the bladder and posterior proximal urethra are derived from the caudal ends of the mesonephric ducts.

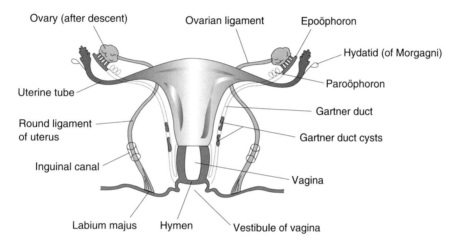

Figure 5.4
The female genital tract and its relationship to vestigial remnants of the mesonephric duct. The mesonephric duct disappears but may persist as Gartner's duct cysts between the layers of the broad ligament or in the anterior lateral wall of the vagina and give rise to the epoöphoron and paroöphoron, which can become enlarged to form a paraovarian cyst.

inhibiting substance produced by the female primordial gonads causes regression of the paramesonephric ducts.

In the female, at 5 weeks' gestation, buds grow from the urethra into the surrounding mesenchyme to form paraurethral glands (of Skene), which is the female equivalent of the prostate in the male at the site of entry of the mesonephric ducts (wolffian ducts). Bilateral outgrowths of the urogenital sinus form the greater vestibular glands of Bartholin. The mesonephric duct disappears but may persist as vestigial remnants such as Gartner's duct cysts (between the layers of the broad ligament or in the anterior lateral wall of the vagina) and give rise to the epoöphoron and paroöphoron, which can become enlarged to form a paraovarian cyst (Figure 5.4).

The external genitalia do not develop definite male or female characteristics until the 12th week under the influence of testosterone or estrogen hormones. In the female, the primordial phallus forms the clitoris in the second trimester. The urogenital folds become the labia minora and only fuse posteriorly to form the perineum. The labiosacral swellings remain unfused to form the labia majora.

Congenital abnormalities of the kidneys and ureters

The kidney may fail to develop on one or both sides. Unilateral renal agenesis occurs in 1 in 1000 newborn infants and is frequently associated with ipsilateral genital abnormalities; the left side is more often affected than the right.[3] Renal function is usually normal as there is compensatory hyperplasia of the other kidney.

One or both kidneys may be in an abnormal shape or position. A kidney may fail to ascend and rotate medially, remaining in the pelvis (pelvic kidney) and may present to the clinician as a pelvic mass. When the lower poles of the kidneys are fused (horseshoe kidney), normal ascent may be prevented. If ascension occurs, both kidneys may be fused and present on the one side. The incidence of pelvic kidney is 1 in 800 and horseshoe kidney is 1 in 6000.

Premature bifurcation of the ureteric bud can result in two or more ureters, with typically the lowest branch draining

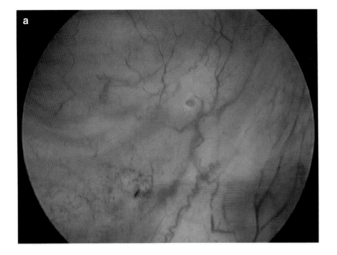

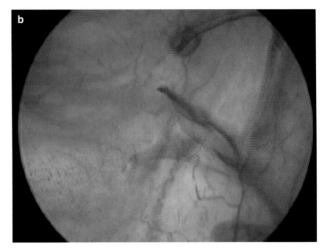

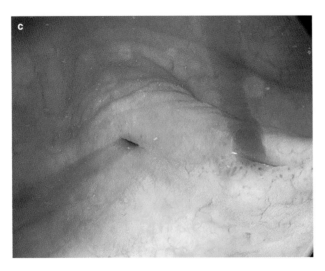

Figure 5.5
Indigo carmine jets from the lower (a) and upper ureteric orifice (b) in a woman with duplication of the left ureter (a,b) and right ureteric (c).

most of the normally functioning kidney. Duplication of the ureters results from division of the metanephric diverticulum and may be partial (bifid ureter) or complete (double ureter). The incidence of ureteral duplication is 0.5–1 per 100.[4] Bifid ureters descend from the kidney and join with only one ureter opening into the bladder; double kidneys can open separately into the bladder (Figure 5.5), urethra, or genital tract. The caudal ureteric bud becomes the ureter to the lower pole of the kidney and is incorporated into the bladder wall at the superior lateral aspect of the trigone. The cranial bud becomes an ectopic ureter and is carried inferiorly to its final connection with the distal mesonephric duct or definitive urogenital sinus, inserting into the bladder, urethra, vagina, uterus, or vestibule. Weigert (1877) and Meyer (1946) described how the final location of the ectopic ureter into the lower urinary tract is along a line (the ectopic pathway) coursing mediosuperior from the normally situated ureteric orifice along the inferolateral border of the trigone to the internal urethral meatus (vesical ectopia), posterolateral urethra (Figure 5.6), and ipsilateral vaginal introitus.[4] Some

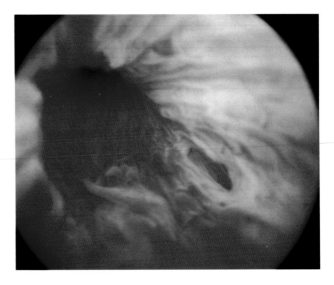

Figure 5.6
Urethroscopic picture of left ectopic ureter entering proximal urethra.

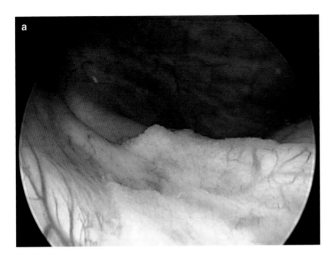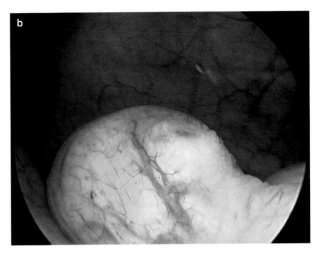

Figure 5.7(a,b)
Cystoscopic view of right-sided ureterocele in a woman with moderate squamous metaplasia of the trigone before (a) and after (b) ureteric contraction.

clinicians only define ureters as ectopic if they drain extravesically into the urethra or genital tract. If vesical ectopia is excluded, approximately one-third of ectopic ureters terminate into the urethra, one-third the vestibule, slightly less into the vagina, and 5% into the cervix or uterus.[5] Schulman[6] stated the more distal the insertion, the greater the degree of renal hypodysplasia. A congenital ureterocele is a ballooning of the submucosal ureter (Figure 5.7), usually of the upper pole ectopic ureter of a duplex system, and is frequently associated with ureteric obstruction.

Ectopic ureters may be associated with a single or duplex system. Women with duplex ureter systems where the ureters are functionally normal are asymptomatic and are usually detected after childhood. Urinary incontinence occurs when the ectopic ureter inserts into either the lower urinary tract below the urethral sphincter or the genital tract. Urinary leakage similar to other fistulae is continuous but is also associated with normal voiding. Vaginal and vestibular ectopias may be derived from the insertion of ectopic ureters into persisting Gartner's ducts and present as a congenital urethrovaginal fistula (Case 1). Extraurethral urinary leakage may be seen in the vagina or an ectopic opening may be seen in the vaginal or vestibular areas. An abdominal mass may be palpable if the kidney is hydronephrotic, although severe abnormalities are usually detected in childhood.

Gartner's duct abnormalities have been reported in the literature to be associated with a single ectopic ureter and unilateral renal agenesis.[7,8] Sheih et al[9] documented 20 school-aged girls with unilateral renal agenesis and Gartner's duct cysts in a mass screening program looking for occult renal abnormalities; one-half had coexisting müllerian abnormalities. There are also a number of case reports in the literature of Gartner's duct cysts associated with vesicovaginal and urethrovaginal fistula.[10–12] Gotoh and Koyanagi[13] proposed that ureteric ectopia with

Gartner's duct cyst are caused by failure of separation of the ureteric bud from the mesonephric duct, which leads to persistence of Gartner's duct, frequently with cystic dilation. The ectopic ureter may drain into Gartner's duct (Case 1) or the urethra (Case 2); abnormal development of the ureter subsequently causes maldevelopment or absence of the ipsilateral kidney. Abnormal mesonephric duct development is frequently associated with a corresponding fusion anomaly of the paramesonephric ductal system with uterus didelphys (double uterus and cervix) with midline vaginal septum (Cases 1 and 3).

Imaging of the upper and lower urinary tracts is essential, either radiologically with an intravenous pyelogram and voiding cystourethrogram or by ultrasound. These investigations may reveal unilateral or bilateral duplication of the upper urinary tract. Ureteric ectopia usually involves the cranial ureteric bud passing to the upper renal pole, which is usually dysplastic and poorly functioning. Contrast material may be present in the vagina in the pre-void radiograph. Renal scintigraphy using technetium-labeled dimercaptosuccinic acid (DMSA) can be used to detect salvageable functional renal tissue. DMSA is secreted by the tubules and measures renal function rather than renal blood flow. In the majority of cases cystourethroscopy will establish the insertion point of the ectopic ureter into the urethra (see Figure 5.6) and any other congenital abnormalities that may be present such as urethral diverticulum (see Figure 5.9), urethrovaginal fistula, and ectopic ureterocele.

Treatment of the ectopic ureter depends on the function of the ipsilateral and contralateral kidney. Urological referral may be necessary for surgery to remove a non-functional hydronephrotic kidney or in some cases to implant a ureter in the presence of functional renal tissue, which can be performed as an open or laparoscopic procedure.[14] In Cases 1 and 2, Gartner's duct cyst and fistula repair was successfully

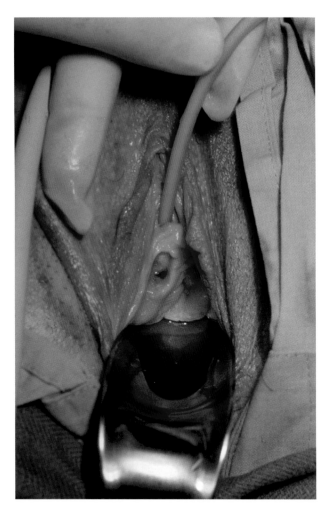

Figure 5.8
Ostium of ectopic ureter inferolateral to external urethral meatus, with indwelling Foley catheter (Case 1).

performed transvaginally with a layered closure of the urethrovaginal fistula with Martius graft reinforcement. In Case 1 the lower ectopic ureter was also removed vaginally. In Case 2 the refluxing ectopic ureter may have been the cause of the woman's recurrent urinary tract infections, which were controlled by prophylactic antibiotics. Reflux of urine and urinary tract infection can occur due to a poorly developed submucosal flap valve in ectopic ureters (see Figures 5.6 and 5.15). Reflux occurs in urethral ectopia only during micturition. In the literature, surgical correction of Gartner's duct cyst with ectopic ureter and associated renal genesis with or without fistula has been performed abdominally with excision of the dysplastic kidney or ureteric reimplantation, and abdominal removal of the Gartner's duct cyst with repair of any associated urinary fistula. With this approach the bladder and urethra frequently need major reconstruction with reimplantation of the other ureter.[15,16] The transvaginal approach with the removal of Gartner's duct cyst and fistula repair does appear to be a safe and effective alternative approach, at least in postpubertal females where vaginal access is available.[12] In

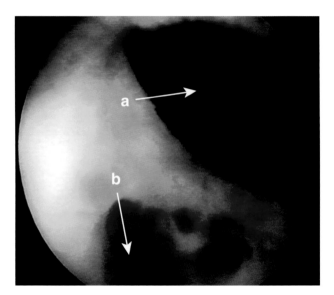

Figure 5.9
Cystoscopic photograph of bladder neck (a) and large posterior urethral diverticulum (b). The surrounding urethral wall is transparently thin.

Case 1 the lower ectopic ureter was removed vaginally, which would seem to be preferable to the abdominal approach in women with no functional kidney.

Case 1

A 32-year-old woman with known uterus didelphys, vaginal septum, and absent right kidney presented with urinary stress incontinence that was present during childhood but became more severe following her first pregnancy and uncomplicated vaginal delivery 4 years earlier. On examination, a fistulous opening was seen near the right of the external urethral meatus (see Figure 5.8). Ultrasound examination confirmed duplication of the uterus and cervix with bilateral normal ovaries. No kidney was visualized in the right renal fossa; the left kidney was 12 cm in length with no evidence of pelvicalyceal dilatation. Intravenous pyelography (IVP) showed rapid excretion from a normal left single renal pelvis and computed tomography (CT) was unable to locate any renal tissue on the right and confirmed the presence of mild left renal hypertrophy.

On urodynamic assessment no detrusor overactivity was present, the bladder capacity was 420 ml, and leakage occurred from the external urethral meatus and fistulous orifice during coughing.

Laparoscopy and hysteroscopy confirmed duplication of the uterus and cervix, the uterine cavities were normal in appearance, and the fallopian tubes were patent. On cystourethroscopy the right hemitrigone was absent; a fistulous opening surrounded by thin transparent mucosa was present on the posterior proximal urethra opening into a

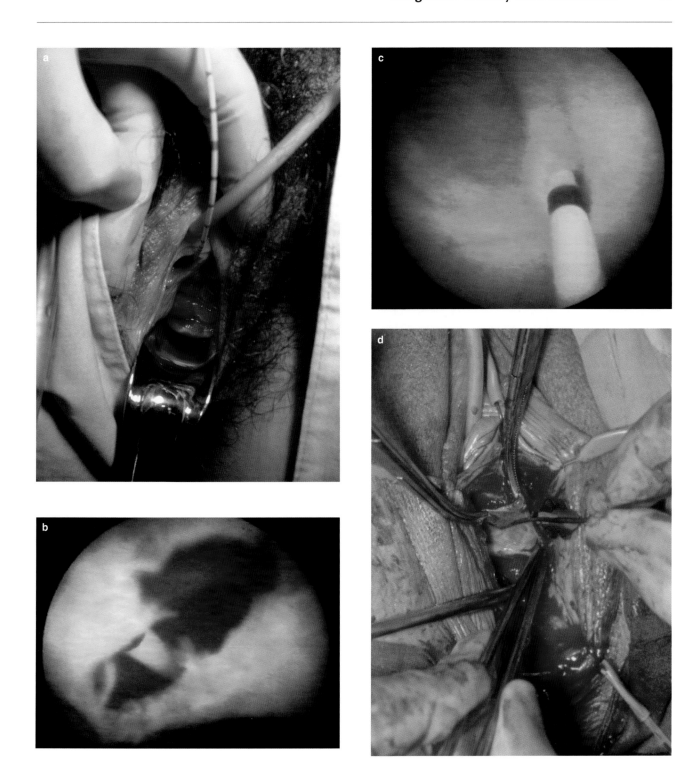

Figure 5.10
A 5 Fr ureteric catheter was passed through the ectopic vestibular opening (a), through the cystic space
(b), into a right ectopic ureter (c). Vaginal dissection with partial excision of the urethrovaginal fistula and
wall of Gartner's duct cyst (d). A lacrimal probe is passed through a diverticular communication into the urethra.

3 cm cystic space (Figure 5.9). A ureteric catheter was passed through the ectopic vestibular opening, through the cystic space, into a right ectopic ureter (Figure 5.10). Contrast medium was injected, showing a blind-ending 15 cm right ureter and a 4 × 3 × 2 cm cystic space in communication with urethra and vestibule (Figures 5.11 and 5.12).

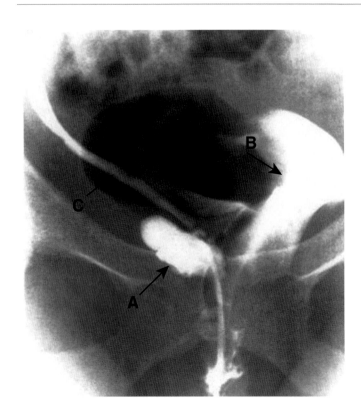

Figure 5.11
Anterior-posterior radiological view of retrograde
catheterization following injection of contrast medium
into right ectopic ureter showing 15 cm right ureter
(C) and a 4 × 3 × 2 cm cystic space (A) in communication
with urethra and vestibule. The bladder is situated
superiorly (B).

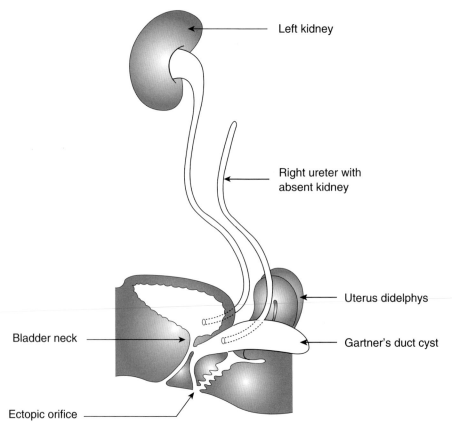

Figure 5.12
Lateral view of Case 1, showing urogenital abnormality.

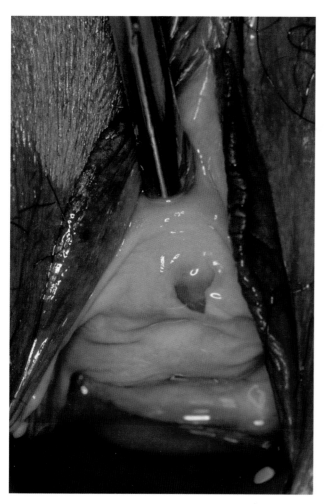

Figure 5.13
Fistulous opening of ectopic ureter leaking urine inferior to external urethral meatus with Hegar dilator (Case 2).

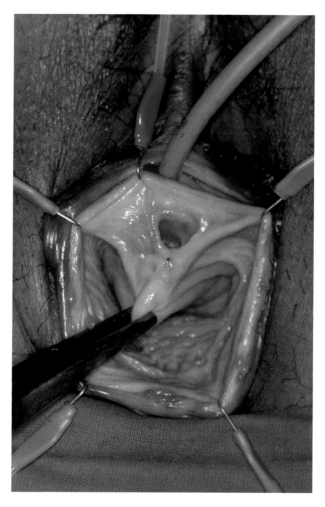

Figure 5.14
Operative view of Case 2 further demonstrating left ectopic ureter held open by a Brantley Scott retractor.

Surgery was declined by the patient at that time, as she desired a further pregnancy. The following year she became pregnant again and had a normal vaginal delivery. Her incontinence deteriorated further, with constant urinary leakage requiring the use of 10 pads a day. Six months following delivery, surgical repair was performed transvaginally, the Gartner's duct cyst was excised with the proximal ectopic ureter (Figure 5.10c), and a layered repair of the urethra was performed and reinforced with a Martius labial graft. Histology of the excised Gartner's duct cyst showed a fibromuscular wall with a few non-specific glands seen within an inflamed stroma and a denuded epithelium. The woman's continence was restored and she remained symptom-free over a 6-year follow-up.

Case 2

A 54-year-old Korean woman who migrated to Australia was referred with urinary incontinence and a urethrovaginal

fistula. History taking was difficult because of poor English; she had a long history of urinary stress incontinence, which was worse over the last 4 years. She had five previous pregnancies in Seoul: three were difficult vaginal forceps deliveries and the last two were elective cesarean sections. She also had a history of recurrent urinary tract infection. On examination; there was a fistulous opening 2 cm above the external meatus on the anterior vaginal wall. There was marked leakage through the fistula with coughing (Figures 5.13 and 5.14).

Urodynamic studies were performed; no detrusor overactivity was present, the bladder capacity was 450 ml, there was no demonstrable urethral stress incontinence, but leakage occurred through the vaginal fistulous ostium with coughing. Bladder emptying was normal.

Cystourethroscopy confirmed the presence of a urethrovaginal fistula which was surgically repaired vaginally with layered closure and a Martius graft. The left ureteric orifice was found to be absent. Following surgery, the woman's urinary incontinence was cured, but she continued to have

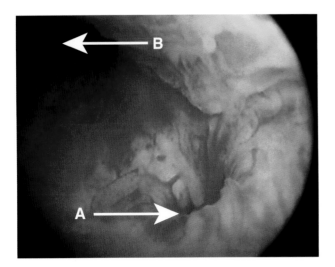

Figure 5.15
Urethroscopic view of refluxing left ectopic ureter (A) entering proximal urethra inferior to bladder neck (B).

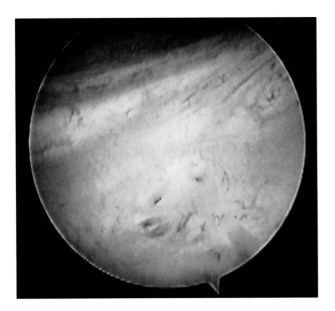

Figure 5.16
Absent left ureteric orifice and left hemitrigone.

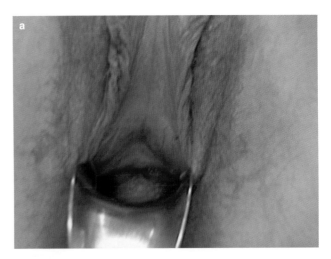

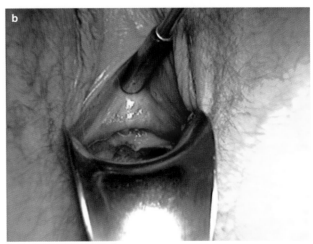

Figure 5.17
(a) The external urethral meatus is not present in its normal midline position on the vestibule between the clitoris and vaginal opening but (b) can be seen entering onto the lower anterior vaginal wall.

urinary tract infections. Abdominal ultrasonography and CT showed an absent left kidney and hypertrophic right kidney; on voiding cystourethrogram, there was reflux of contrast medium up a left ectopic ureter, which entered the proximal urethra. Cystourethroscopy confirmed the presence of the left urethral ectopic ostium (Figure 5.15), the lef hemitrigone and ureteric orifice was absent, and small pit marks were present where the ureteric orifice was normally situated (Figure 5.16). The right ureteric orifice was normally situated and functioning. This fistula was initially thought to be caused by obstetric trauma, but the lack of vaginal and perifistular fibrosis in the presence of a urethral ectopic ureter and renal agenesis make a congenital etiology likely. The woman's

recurrent urinary tract infections were successfully treated with prophylactic antibiotics and she declined any further surgery for her ectopic ureter.

Severe congenital urethral abnormalities such as common urogenital sinus syndrome, where there is a single opening for the urethra and vagina, are usually detected in childhood. Less severe anomalies may present in adult females as abnormally sited urethra usually associated with other urogenital anomalies (ectopic urethra).

Case 3

A 20-year-old woman with multiple congenital urogenital abnormalities presents with intermittent urinary retention. Corrective surgery was performed in early childhood to treat

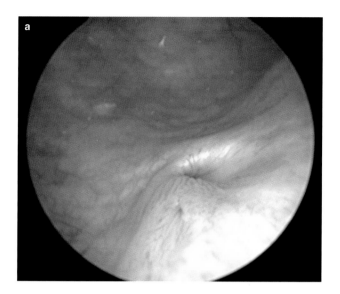 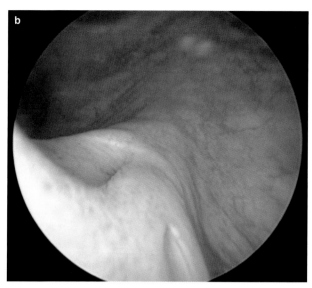

Figure 5.18
Duplex ureteric orifices on left (a) and right (b) side of an abnormally shaped trigone.

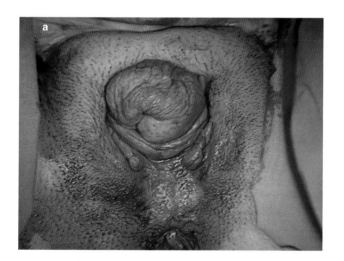 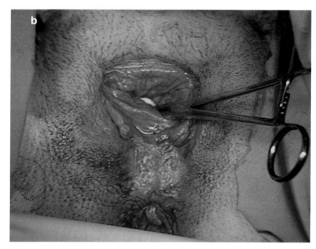

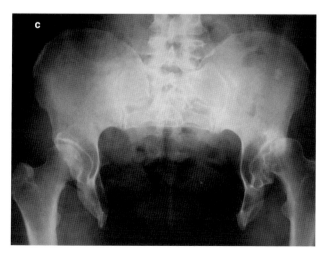

Figure 5.19
A 48 year old woman with complete vaginal eversion and congenital bladder extrophy. Recontruction and a urinary diversion was performed in early childhood Uterovaginal prolapse developed in her 30's and a total abdominal hysterectomy and adominal colposacropexy, and then transvaginal bilateral sacrospinous colpopexy were performed without success. In a and b the prolapse is displayed out and reduced with a sponge forceps; note the poorly developed labia majora and minora which occurs with defective median embryological development. (c) Anterior-posterior radiological view of the pelvis showing gross pubic diastasis and absence of symphysis pubis. The vaginal eversion was treated surgically with an extraperitoneal uterosacral suspension and polypropylene mesh reinforcement.

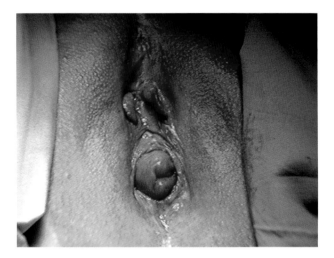

Figure 5.20
A 23-year-old nulliparous woman with uterovaginal prolapse and congenital vesicae ectopia. The labia minora, majora, and clitoris are underdeveloped.

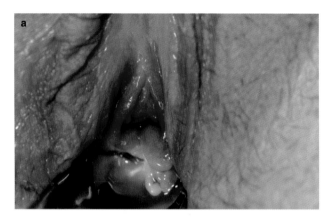

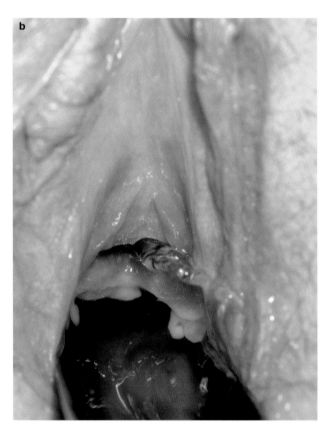

Figure 5.21
(a) A 22-year-old nulliparous woman with known history of uterus didelphys and vaginal septum presented with severe stress urinary incontinence. The external urethral meatus is patulous and open with the bladder neck visible on external inspection. (b) Urine leakage can be seen when traction is placed on the posterior vaginal wall with a Sims speculum.

hydrometrocolpos caused by a distal vaginal septum with obstruction. On examination the external urethral meatus was in an abnormal position with urethral entry into the lower anterior vaginal wall (Figure 5.17) instead of normal midline entry in the vestibule between the clitoris and vaginal opening. CT imaging shows a hypodysplastic left kidney and hydronephrotic right kidney. The woman's renal function tests show mild impairment; she has good urinary control. Her voiding dysfunction and urinary retention was improved following urethral dilation under general anesthesia.

Extrophic abnormalities of the lower urinary tract occur in 1 in 50 000 live female births[17] and represent a spectrum of embryological developmental disorders of median mesenchymal migration, including bladder extrophy, epispadias, and cloacal extrophy. Bladder extrophy is caused by incomplete median closure of the lower abdomen and pelvis and is a result of failure of mesenchymal cell migration ventrally between ectoderm and endoderm during the 4th week of fetal development. Poor muscle and connective tissue development of the anterior abdominal wall and pelvis result in exposure and protrusion of the posterior wall of the bladder, pubic diastasis with underdevelopment of the symphysis pubis (Figure 5.19). The urethra is completely epispadiac and the clitoris is bifid. There is also absent or underdevelopment of the labia minora and majora (Figure 5.20).

In the past, effective reconstruction was considered too difficult, so the urinary flow was diverted into an ilio-conduit with external drainage. More recently, bladder extrophy is repaired in the neonatal period with reconstruction of the abdominal wall bladder and urethra. Females with bladder extrophy can present in adult life with severe uterovaginal prolapse caused by absence of pelvic floor musculature and ligamentous support and

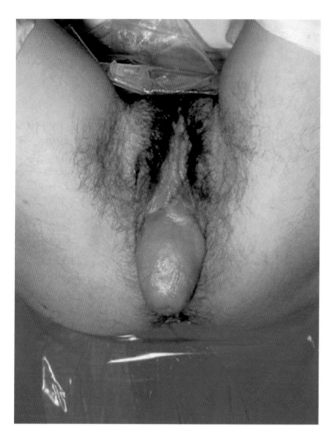

Figure 5.22
25-year-old nulliparous woman with spina bifida and complete uterovaginal prolapse. She had an ilioconduit urinary diversion for poor urinary control during childhood.

Table 5.1 Congenital causes of urinary incontinence

Ureteric ectopia
Common sinuse sydrome
Congenital short urethra
Extrophic anomalies:
   Bladder extrophy
   Epispadias
Neurological abnormalities:
   Spina bifida
   Sacral agenesis
   Tethered cord syrdrome

have a wide open anterior vagina caused by deficient midline development of the clitoris, labial minora and majora. Repair of the prolapse with vulvovaginal reconstruction may be necessary.

Less severe forms of extrophy can occur with female epispadias with the urethra split dorsally up to the bladder neck leading to incompetence and continual urethral leakage. In the congenital short urethra, the urethral folds fail to fuse in the midline; the urethral length is shortened (1–2 cm). Urethral sphincter function is at the level of the bladder neck, which may provide sufficient urinary control to escape detection during childhood. Urinary incontinence may deteriorate later in pregnancy and childbirth when the bladder neck becomes incompetent.

Case 4

A 22-year-old nulliparous women with a known history of uterus didelphys and vaginal septum presented with severe stress urinary incontinence. She had previously had a diagnostic laparoscopy and excision of the vaginal septum. On examination, the external urethral meatus is patulous and open. There was marked urinary on bladder compression or on gentle traction on the posterior vaginal wall (Figure 5.21). There was marked urinary leakage on bladder compression or on gentle fraction on the posterior vaginal wall. On cystoscopy, the trigone was absent and the ureteric orifices were abnormally sited at 3 and 9 o'clock above the bladder neck. There was only a small section of bladder neck providing any urinary control.

Surgical treatment is performed transvaginally with elongation and reconstruction of the urethra (as in Figure 5.21) but can be performed abdominally using tubulized trigone and bladder neck plication.

Congenital spinal conditions such as myelomeningocele and spina bifida, sacral agenesis, and tethered cord syndrome can result in a neuropathic bladder and congenital urinary incontinence. These neurological deficits can also cause pelvic floor denervation and result in early-onset uterovaginal prolapse in young nulliparous women (Figure 5.22).

References

1. Thompson DT, Lynn HB. Genital anomalies associated with solitary kidney. Mayo Clin Proc 1966; 41: 538.
2. Semmens JP. Congenital anomalies of female genital tract. Functional classification based on review of 56 personal cases and 500 reported cases. Obstet Gynecol 1962; 19: 328–52.
3. Doroshow LW, Abeshouse BS. Congenital unilateral solitary kidney: report of 37 cases and a review of the literature. Urol Surv 1961; 11: 219–29.
4. Stephens FD. Congenital Malformations of the Urinary Tract. New York: Praeger Publishers, 1983.
5. Ellerker AG. The extravesical ectopic ureter. Br J Surg 1958; 45: 344–53.
6. Schulman CC. The single ectopic ureter. Eur Urol 1976; 2: 64–9.
7. Shibata T, Nonomura K, Kakizaki H et al. A case of unique communication between blind-ending ectopic ureter and ipsilateral hematocolpometra in uterus didelphys. J Urol 1995; 153: 1208–10.

8. Acien P, Susarte F, Romero J et al. Complex genital malformation: ectopic ureter ending in a supposed mesonephric duct with renal agenesis and ipsilateral blind hemivagina. Eur J Obstet Gynecol Reprod Biol 2004; 117: 105–8.

9. Sheih CP, Li YW, Liao YJ et al. Diagnosing the combination of renal dysgenesis, Gartner's duct cyst and ipsilateral mullerian duct obstruction. J Urol 1998; 159: 217–21.

10. Sanuma H, Nakai H, Shishido S et al. Congenital vesicovaginal fistula. Int J Urol 2000; 7: 195–8.

11. Koyangi T, Takamatsu T, Kaneta T, Terashima M, Tsuji M. A spontaneous vesico-ectopic ureterovaginal fistula in a girl. J Urol 1977; 118: 871–2.

12. Dwyer PL, Rosamilia A. Congenital urogenital anomalies that are associated with persistence of Gartner's duct; a review. Am J Obstet Gynecol 2006; 195(2): 354–9.

13. Gotoh T, Koyanagi T. Clinicopathological and embryological considerations of single ectopic ureters in Gartner's duct cyst; a unique subtype of single vaginal ectopia. J Urol 1987; 137: 969–72.

14. Wang DS, Bird VG, Cooper CS, Austin JC, Winfield HN. Laparoscopic upper pole heminephrectomy for ectopic ureter; initial experience. Can J Urol 2004; 11: 2141–5.

15. Albers P, Foster RS, Bihrle R, Adams MC, Keating MA. Ectopic ureters and ureteroceles in adults. Urology 1994; 45(5): 870–4.

16. Sumfest JM, Burns MW, Mitchell ME. Pseudoureterocele; potential for misdiagnosis of an ectopic ureter as a ureterocele. Br J Urol 1995; 75: 401–5.

17. Lattimer JK, Smith MJK. Extrophy closure: A follow up of 70 cases. J Urol 1966; 95: 356.

6

Urethral and periurethral conditions

Peter L Dwyer

Introduction

Endoscopic evaluation of the urethra is an important diagnostic tool in the evaluation of urethral and periurethral pathology. These conditions may present to the clinician as pain which may be constant, intermittent, or associated with voiding (dysuria) or sexual intercourse (dyspareunia). Other presentations may be urethral or vaginal discharge; hematuria; or as a periurethral mass. Stress incontinence may be present if there is interference with the normal urethral sphincter mechanism. Treatment of many of these conditions is surgical, with the vaginal approach usually the simplest and preferred option. With the advent of minimally invasive mid-urethral slings, visualization of both bladder and urethra are necessary to exclude potential injury to the urinary tract and urethroscopy may be necessary to deal with any intraurethral injury (Figure 6.1). Injury to the urethra during stress incontinence surgery and how it is treated are discussed in more detail in Chapter 13.

Endoscopy of the urethra for the diagnosis and treatment of urethral and periurethral disorders is important for both gynecologists and urologists who require the appropriate skills and knowledge. In this chapter urethral and periurethral conditions are reviewed with particular emphasis on the use of urethroscopy in management.

Evaluation

Endoscopic evaluation is only one of a number of diagnostic tools available to the clinician for the evaluation of urethral and periurethral pathology. Careful evaluation of the presenting symptoms and examination finding is equally important in reaching a diagnosis. Inspection of the external urethral meatus (EUM) and anterior vaginal wall and palpation of the urethra and adjacent areas for masses by digital compression against the back of the symphysis should be performed. Other investigations that may be of value are a urinary diary, uroflowmetry, and cystometry with measurement

of post-void residual urine volume, urethral swabs, and urinary microscopy and culture. Imaging techniques may include abdominal and vaginal ultrasound, micturating cystourethrograms and double balloon urography, computed tomography (CT), and magnetic resonance imaging (MRI).

The technique of urethroscopy is discussed in Chapter 4. Urethroscopy plays a major role in the diagnosis of intraurethral and periurethral pathology and is of value in assessing some elements of urethral function. Complete visualization of the urethra will require the use of a urethroscope with Sasche sheath which has a straight distal tip to allow distention of the urethra. Urethroscopy can be performed with the patient anesthetized for complete visualization of the urethra with any intraurethral surgery that may be appropriate. Dynamic urethroscopy, a concept pioneered by Jack Robertson, is performed with the woman awake and responding to verbal requests such as cough, Valsalva, or contract the pelvic floor muscles. In the normal functioning urethra, the urethra closes during pelvic muscle contraction, and the bladder neck remains closed with coughing or Valsalva maneuvers unlike the rigid fibrotic urethra seen in intrinsic sphincter dysfunction (ISD) stress incontinence which opens readily during urethral filling and remains open even with pelvic muscle contraction.

Periurethral masses

Periurethral vaginal masses, which may be found by clinicians on routine gynecological examination or at the time of cystourethroscopy, are frequently associated with urinary or genital symptoms. Cystourethroscopy plays an important role in the diagnosis of periurethral masses, primarily to exclude a urethral diverticulum (UD) and other intraurethral causes (e.g. tumors). Urethral cancer can present as hematuria or an anterior vagina wall swelling or mass (see Figure 10.15), and requires urgent diagnosis and treatment. Urethral cancers will be covered in Chapter 10. Injury to the urinary tract can occur in the surgical

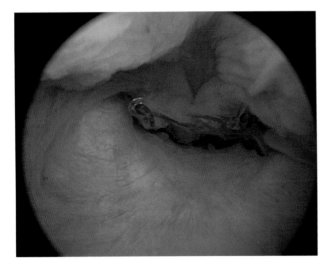

Figure 6.1
Urethroscopic picture of tension-free vaginal tape (TVT) sling (blue) inadvertently placed through proximal urethra. This patient presented with postoperative voiding difficulty and urinary tract infection.

Table 6.1   Differential diagnosis of periurethral and anterior vaginal wall masses

Urethral diverticulum
Simple vaginal cysts
Embryological cystic remnants of Gartner's duct
Skene's gland cysts or abscess
Leiomyoma
Ectopic urethrocele
Vaginal wall inclusion cyst
Müllerian cyst
Mesonephric cyst (Gartner's cyst)
Urothelial cyst
Periurethral injections for stress incontinence
Endometriosis
Vaginal wall abscess, e.g. infected urethral sling
Nephrogenic adenoma
Benign and malignant conditions, including carcinoma
    and sarcoma of the urogenital tracts

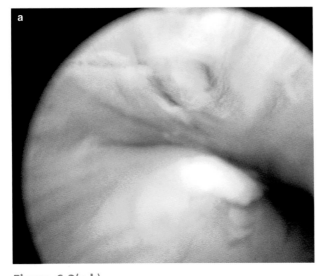
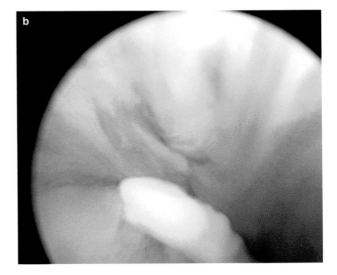

Figure 6.2(a,b)
Urethral diverticulum oozing purulent material through midline posterior opening.

management of periurethral conditions, so that endoscopic inspection following surgery should be performed. Any damage caused should be repaired to prevent the risk of postoperative complications such as urethral stricture or urethrovaginal fistula, difficult problems which are not uncommon after urethral and periurethral surgery.

The differential diagnosis of periurethral and anterior vaginal wall masses is shown in Table 6.1. Urethral prolapse and urethral caruncle usually present more as a protrusion from the EUM and should not be confused with other anterior vaginal wall masses.

Urethral diverticulum

A urethral diverticulum is a cystic outpouching of the urethra that is frequently asymptomatic or causing minimal urinary symptoms until ductal obstruction and infection occurs and an abscess develops (Figure 6.2). Presenting symptoms may be a vaginal mass or urinary incontinence, including stress incontinence and, less commonly, post-micturition dribbling. Urethral pain may occur during voiding or during sexual intercourse and the patient may complain of urinary frequency,

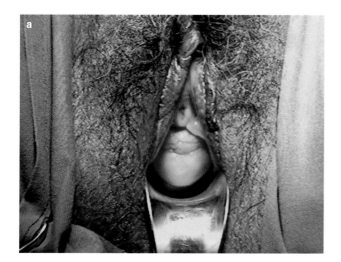
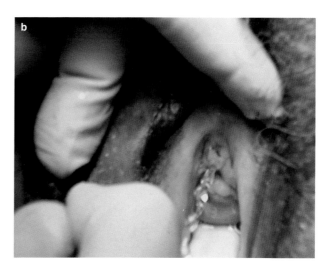

Figure 6.3(a,b)
Large non-infected urethral diverticulum, which when compressed against the back of the symphysis causes urethral leakage of urine.

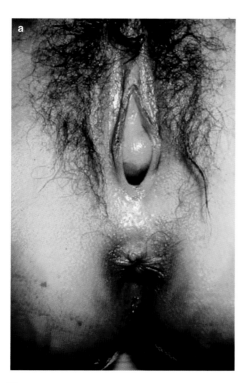
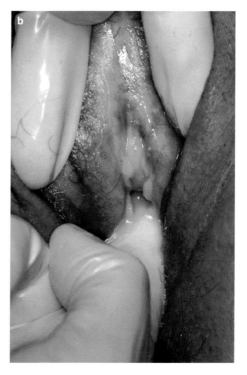

Figure 6.4(a,b)
Urethral diverticulum, which when compressed causes a purulent urethral discharge.

urgency, or voiding difficulty. The incidence of UD in women has been estimated to be between 1% and 5% and most commonly presents between the ages of 30 and 50 years old.[1]

On examination, there may be a tender or non-tender periurethral mass in up to 90% of cases,[2] which on compression between the vaginal examining finger and the back of the pubic symphysis may result in urethral urine leakage (Figure 6.3) or a purulent urethral discharge (Figure 6.4). A urethral diverticulum may also be the cause of recurrent urinary tract infection, estimated in one study[2] to occur in 40% of cases. Urinary stasis and cellular debris within the diverticulum, together with urinary infection (Figure 6.5), may also predispose to calculus formation, which is reported to occur in 1–10% of cases.[3]

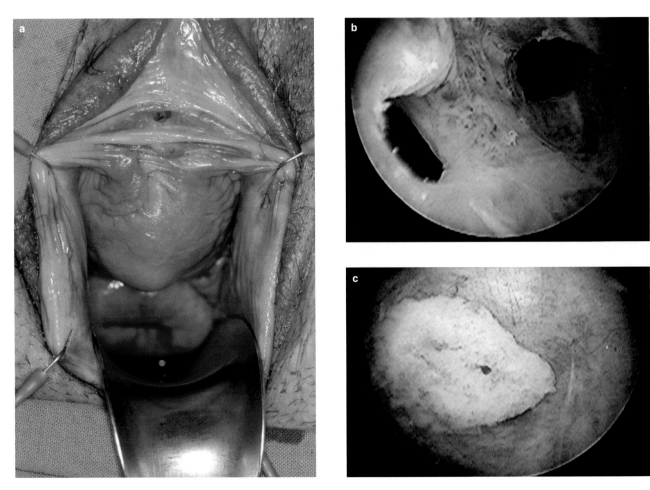

Figure 6.5(a–c)
Large urethral diverticulum is evident on vaginal examination. On urethroscopy there is a large diverticulum orifice (b) present inferiorly and to the left of the bladder neck. The urethroscope was passed into the diverticulum and there was cellular debris at its base (c).

Adenocarcinoma (Figure 6.6) and, less commonly, transitional carcinoma have been associated with urethral diverticulum.

Cystourethroscopic assessment and etiology

Urethroscopy can play an important role in diagnosing urethral diverticulum by the detection of a diverticulum orifice (Figure 6.7a), which may extrude purulent material (if infected) when compressed (Figure 6.7b). Urethroscopy has been reported to be able to visualize a urethral defect or the diverticular ostium in up to 60%[4] of UD, although with modern endoscopic equipment in experienced hands we believe the diagnostic rate using urethroscopy is higher. However, the diverticular orifice may not be visible if blocked or surrounded by inflammation.

Cystoscopy and complete visualization of the bladder is necessary to diagnose other causes for the patient's urinary symptoms and/or paraurethral mass. Urethral diverticula have been classified by Leng and McGuire[5] into either narrow-necked diverticula, which are the commonest variety and are prone to obstruction and infection (Figure 6.7a), or wide-necked open shallow diverticula (Figure 6.8), which occur following urethral surgery, typically either a urethrovaginal fistula repair or excision of a urethral diverticulum. However, the orifice can vary in size, shape, and position, which is probably a reflection of a multifactorial etiology of urethral diverticulum. The orifice of the diverticulum can vary from pinhole small to large, and be in the midline posterior (Figure 6.7a) or lateral (Figure 6.5b), and enter the proximal (Figure 6.9) or distal urethra. A proximal or mid-urethral diverticulum is more frequently associated with disturbance of the urethral sphincter mechanism and

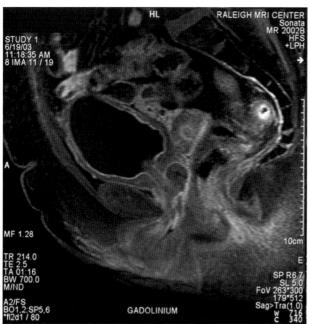

Figure 6.6
MRI showing an intradiverticular filling defect which was a urethral adenocarcinoma. This was missed by the other imaging modalities of ultrasound and CT scanning. (Courtesy of R Foster.[8])

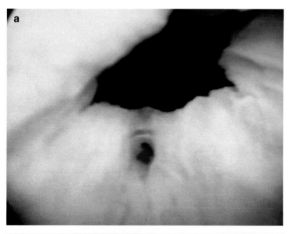

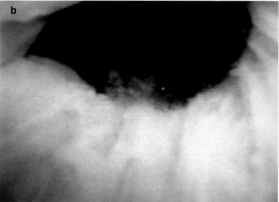

Figure 6.7
Midline UD orifice (a) seen on urethroscopy with a puff of purulent material extruded when compressed (b).

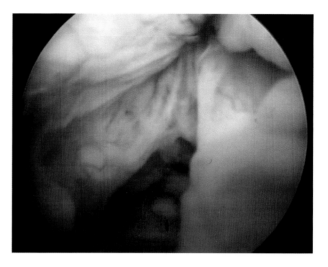

Figure 6.8
Wide-necked open shallow urethral diverticulum in a woman with previous urethral diverticulum repair, urethrovaginal fistula, and transvaginal repair with Martius graft.

stress incontinence. Congenital diverticula have also been reported to arise from the anterior urethra as a result of failed urethral duplication[6] but have not been seen by this author.

The etiology of urethral diverticulum is not well understood and in most cases open to conjecture. However, urethral diverticulum can broadly be classified into congenital and acquired. Congenital causes are thought to be rare. In a case where the urethral diverticulum is associated with a Gartner's duct cyst and other urogenital abnormalities (Figure 6.10), the congenital etiology is beyond doubt. However, there may be other congenital urethral diverticulum where this causation is less obvious but a congenital etiology is suspected because of the symmetrical midline position of the diverticular orifice (see Figure 6.7a) or the transitional cell mucosa and fibromuscular wall of the diverticulum. Infection and abscess formation occur secondary to stasis of urine and the accumulation of cellular debris in the diverticulum, which makes for a potent inoculum. It is generally believed that most cases of urethral diverticulum are acquired secondary to infection of one of the mucinous paraurethral glands (Figure 6.11) which results in abscess formation and then rupture into the urethra.[7] Infection in a paraurethral cyst is another possible cause of acquired UD. The open wide-necked diverticula that occur following urethrovaginal fistula repair (see Figure 6.8) or urethral diverticulum surgery (Figure 6.12) are secondary to weakness in the fibromuscular wall of the urethra. This defect is caused by either inadequate repair or, more likely, breakdown of the repair site secondary to infection with resultant weakness

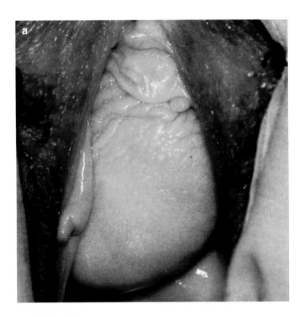

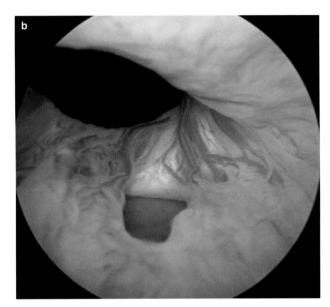

Figure 6.9(a,b)
Large urethral diverticulum with posterior midline diverticular orifice.

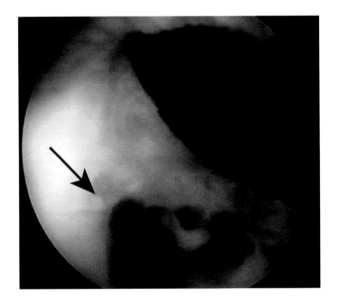

Figure 6.10
Congenital UD (arrow) with Gartner's duct cyst; bladder neck above.

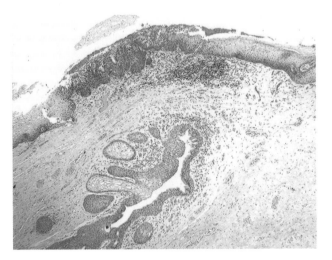

Figure 6.11
Histology of cross section through distal urethra showing mucinous paraurethral glands that open into the urethra. The keratinized stratified squamous epithelium of the distal urethra changes to non-keratinized stratified squamous epithelium seen above these glands more proximally.

in the urethral wall followed by herniation of the urethral mucosa.

Other investigations

Radiological imaging with a micturating cystourethrogram or retrograde positive pressure urethrogram using a

Trattner double-balloon catheter (Figure 6.13) will also confirm the diagnosis of UD, reveal the number and location of the diverticulum, and the presence of any filling defects which may be suggestive of a calculus or tumor. Newer imaging modalities such as MRI (see Figure 6.6; Figure 6.14) and CT scans have the potential to improve the clarity of the imaging and improve diagnostic accuracy, especially in women with complex diverticulum where

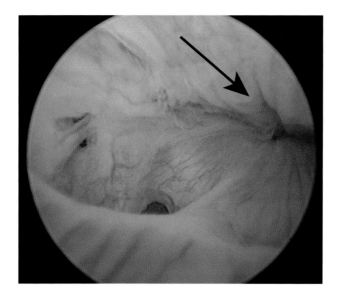

Figure 6.12
Recurrent shallow UD seen with urethroscopy 4 months following transvaginal excison. Arrow to closed bladder neck above.

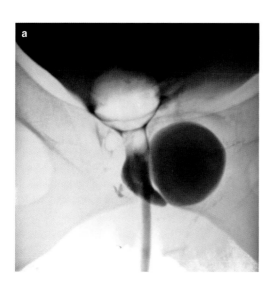

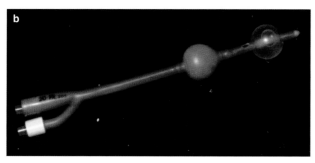

Figure 6.13
(a) Positive pressure retrograde urethrography using a (b) Trattner double-balloon catheter. The distended balloons can be seen above and below a horseshoe shaped mid-urethral diverticulum.

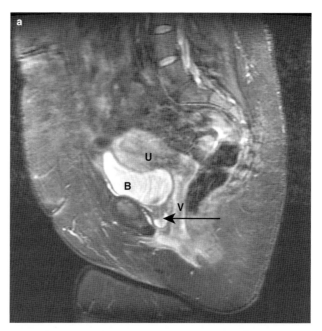

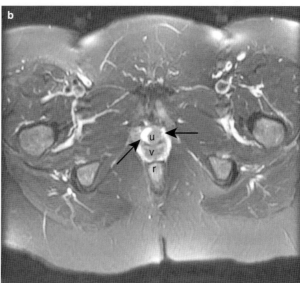

Figure 6.14
A sagittal T2-weighted MRI image of the pelvis with arrow to the diverticulum: V, vagina, U, uterus and B, bladder. (b) Axial MRI image labeled with arrows to the diverticulum, which extends in a horseshoe shape around the urethra: u, urethra, v, vagina, r, rectum.

previous surgery has failed.[8] Vaginal ultrasound is readily available and provides good imaging at low cost (6.15a–d) and is safe to use in pregnancy (Figure 6.16).[9] Over 50% of women with urethral diverticulum have urinary symptoms such as incontinence or voiding difficulty; in these cases, urodynamic studies to assess bladder and urethral function preoperatively are appropriate.[3] Urinary problems such as

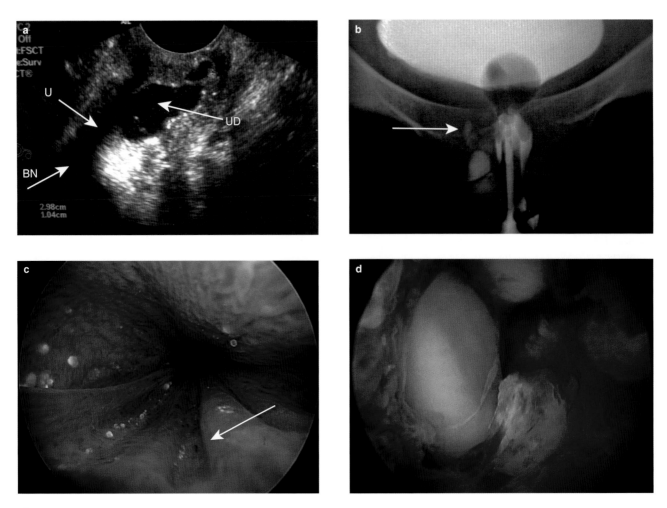

Figure 6.15
This 56 year old woman presented with urinary frequency, recurrent UTI, occasional stress and urge incontinence, and postmicturition dribbling. On examination there was a 3cm paraurethral mass. (a) Perineal ultrasound revealed a right-sided irregular cystic structure 3cm in maximal diameter. (b) A cystourethrogram usinga Trattner catheter confirmed the diagnosis of urethral diverticulum and the presence of radio-opaque calculi (arrow). (c) On urethroscopy there was a small midline posterior diverticular orifice found (arrow). (d) when the diverticulum was opened the presence of calculi was confirmed. U, urethra; BN, bladder neck; UD, uerthral diverticulum.

incontinence and voiding dysfunction can also occur de novo postoperatively following excision and repair of the diverticulum.

Symptomatic urethral diverticulum should be treated surgically with transvaginal excision of the diverticulum through a midline or inverted U incision. Some authors[8] suggest injection of methylene blue either directly in the diverticulum or indirectly with positive pressure urethral infusion to more clearly outline the urethral orifice and diverticulum. Wide lateral vaginal dissection is required to allow a multilayered closure of the urethra and periurethral fascia using 4/0 Vicryl interrupted sutures can be performed without tension (Figure 6.17). This dissection is relatively bloodless and straightforward to

surgeons used to vaginal surgery. However, meticulous care needs to be taken, particularly with urethral closure, as infection is frequently present if complications of ure-throvaginal fistula or recurrent diverticulum are to be avoided. A Martius fat pad graft can be used if the repair site appears tenuous, although this is rarely necessary. The size of the urethral diverticulum can vary in size from less then a centimeter to a large diverticulum greater than 10 cm in diameter which extends laterally around the urethra and bladder base and up into the retropubic space. In our experience transvaginal excision is possible and preferable even with large diverticulum extending into the retropubic space although wide mobilization of the bladder is required.

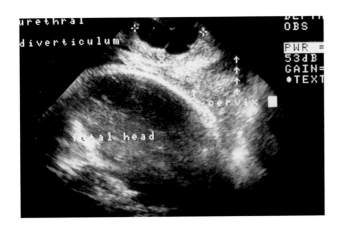

Figure 6.16
Multilocular UD detected on ultrasound imaging during late pregnancy.

Spence and Duckett described a simpler procedure to treating distal UD.[10] The urethra is opened from the external urethral meatus to the mouth of the diverticulum; the edges of the urethra and infected diverticular wall are sutured to create an enlarged spatulated external urethral meatus (EUM).[10] However, in this time of mirrors and increased self-awareness, cosmetic results are important, particularly in the young, and should be discussed with the patient preoperatively. In addition, this procedure is unsuitable for proximal or mid-urethral diverticulum and will result in incontinence secondary to disruption of the normal continence mechanism.

In the author's experience, postoperative stress incontinence is an uncommon problem following repair even if present preoperatively. The performance of stress incontinence procedures at the time of repair either with urethral suspension procedure or sling may impede urethral healing and cause sling erosion or voiding difficulty. If stress incontinence becomes a problem postoperatively, it can be treated with a minimally invasive sling procedure such as a tension-free vaginal tape (TVT). Other postoperative surgical complications reported in one study of 63 women[2] were urethrovaginal fistula (4%), stress incontinence (9%), recurrent urinary tract infection (UTI) (29%), urethral stricture (2%), and recurrent diverticulum (4%) (see Figure 6.12).

Skene's cyst or abscess

Skene's gland is a small group of mucinous glands which open through a single duct onto the left and right sides of the external urethral orifice and are the female equivalent of the prostatic ducts and glands. If these become blocked or infected, a cyst (Figure 6.18) or abscess can develop (Figure 6.19). The cyst is typically lined by transitional epithelium similar to a urothelial vaginal wall cyst. Presenting symptoms are a small painful paraurethral lump, dyspareunia, vaginal discharge, or a UTI. When symptomatic, surgical excision is indicated. Recurrence of an infected Skene's abscess can occur, so marsupialization of the abscess, as Spence and Duckett described, may be necessary.[10]

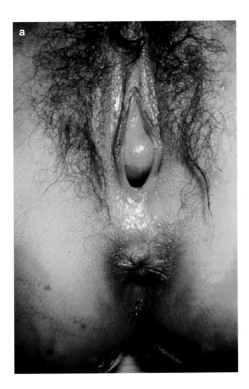

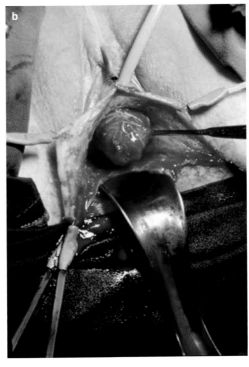

Figure 6.17(a,b)
UD before and after wide surgical dissection and prior to excision and multilayer closure of urethral wall and fascia.

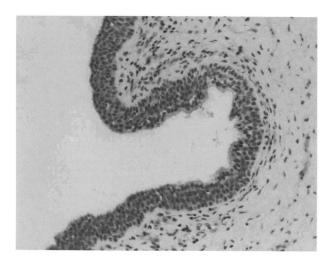

Figure 6.18
Histology of Skene's duct cyst. Fibromuscular tissue contains a cyst predominantly lined by transitional-type epithelium with occasional focal squamous metaplasia. There is a mild and patchy infiltrate of acute and chronic inflammatory cells.

Other periurethral masses

Leiomyoma may present as anterior vaginal wall masses (Figure 6.20(a)) and are smooth, round, solid, and non-tender. They may originate from the urethra, bladder, or vaginal wall. It is important to distinguish between urethral leiomyomas, which arise from urethral smooth muscle, and paraurethral leiomyomas, which arise from smooth muscle in the anterior vaginal wall or vesicovaginal septum.[11] Treatment is by local transvaginal excision if possible. Urethral leiomyomas are more likely to present with urinary symptoms such as incontinence or voiding difficulty, and may protrude through the urethral meatus. They are more fixed on vaginal examination and urethral entry, and reconstruction is more likely during surgical excision than with paraurethral leiomyoma, which shell out without lower urinary tract injury (see Figure 6.20(a–g). Malignant change in the leiomyoma is rare.

Periurethral and anterior vaginal wall cysts can have a number of possible causes, which can be diagnosed on their clinical and surgical features, and histological findings.[12] Epithelial inclusion cysts are common and occur as a result of traumatic or surgical implantation of the vaginal wall into the underlying tissues. This may occur by accident (e.g. during childbirth), although some surgeons have implanted the vaginal wall on purpose, using it as a graft in the treatment of stress incontinence and vaginal prolapse. The fluid of inclusion cysts is frequently turbid or sebaceous and the cyst is lined by stratified squamous epithelium (Figure 6.21(a–c)). Other cysts have an embryological origin, being derived from

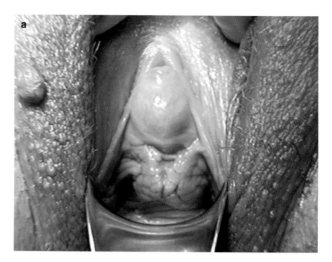

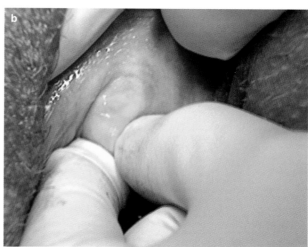

Figure 6.19
(a) Infected Skene duct cyst at external urethral meatus and (b) pus extruding from external urethral meatus with cyst compression.

the paramesonephric (müllerian) or mesonephric duct. Cysts of müllerian origin are the next most common cause of anterior wall cysts. They are usually unilocular and contain mucus (Figure 6.22a, b). The epithelium of these cysts is ciliated cuboidal or columnar mucinous secretory cells (Figure 6.22c, d), resembling the endocervix, fallopian tube, or endometrium. Urothelial cysts are lined by epithelium resembling the urinary tract, either transitional or stratified columnar, and are similar to Skene's duct cyst. Urothelial cysts are usually small and present mainly around the distal urethra. Mesonephric cysts (Gartner's duct) are rare and are lined by non-mucus-producing cuboidal or low columnar epithelium. Although uncommon, they can be associated with other congenital urogenital abnormalities and connect with the urethra or bladder, so that misdiagnosis and surgical excision has resulted in a urinary fistula (see Chapter 5).

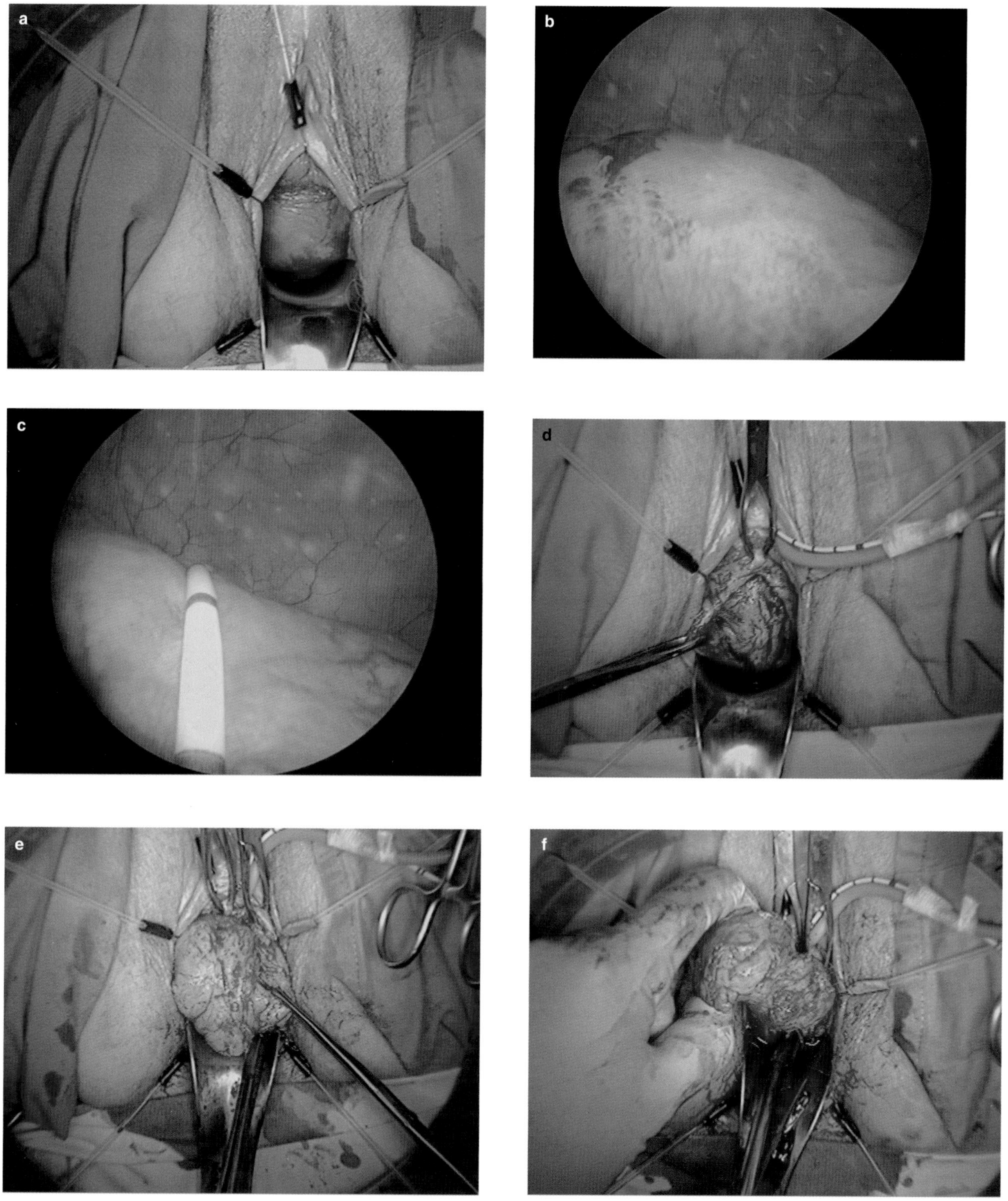
a
b
c
d
e
f

Figure 6.20(a–g) (Continued)

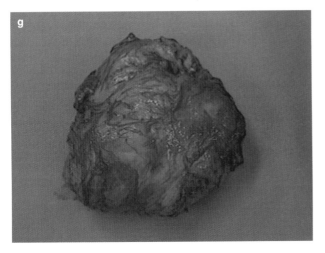

Figure 6.20(a–g)
(a–d) Leiomyoma of the anterior vaginal wall. A 56-year-old woman who presented with a 6 cm asymptomatic anterior vaginal wall mass which was detected initially on a pelvic ultrasound. On examination, the mass was firm and distended the anterior vaginal wall (a). CT scan of the pelvis showed a solid well circumscribed solid mass in the vagina, indenting the posterior wall of the bladder. Cystourethroscopy confirmed a mass indenting the posterior bladder wall and trigone (b). A left ureteric catheter was passed to protect the ureter during surgical excision (c). A midline anterior vaginal wall incision was performed and the fibroid was shelled out with sharpened and blunt dissection (d–g). A cystoscopy was repeated and confirmed that no ureteric or bladder injury occurred during dissection. The vaginal defect was closed in layers. Histopathology confirmed leiomyoma of the anterior vaginal wall.

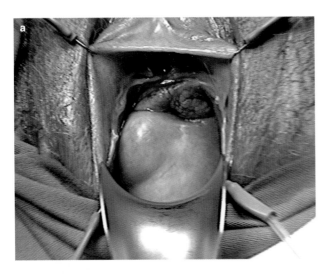

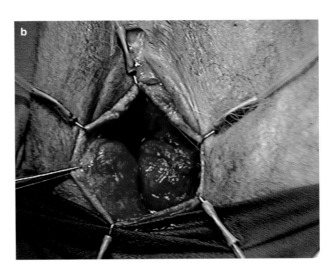

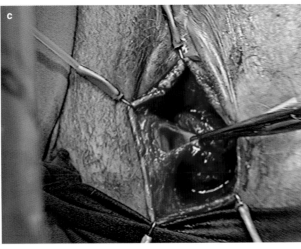

Figure 6.21 (a–c)
Right paraurethral cyst, which, on dissection was a vaginal inclusion cyst containing sebaceous material in a woman who had a previous vaginal repair with inlaid vaginal skin graft. Note how the cyst is adherent to the vaginal wall.

Nephrogenic adenoma derives its name from its histological resemblance to primitive renal tubular structure with irregular branching tubules set in an edematous stroma (Figure 6.24). This is a form of immature urothelial metaplasia and is frequently associated with chronic irritation, urinary infection, or diverticula. Clinical presentation may be acute or chronic cystitis with hematuria, frequency, and dysuria, or as a paraurethral or paravesical mass. On

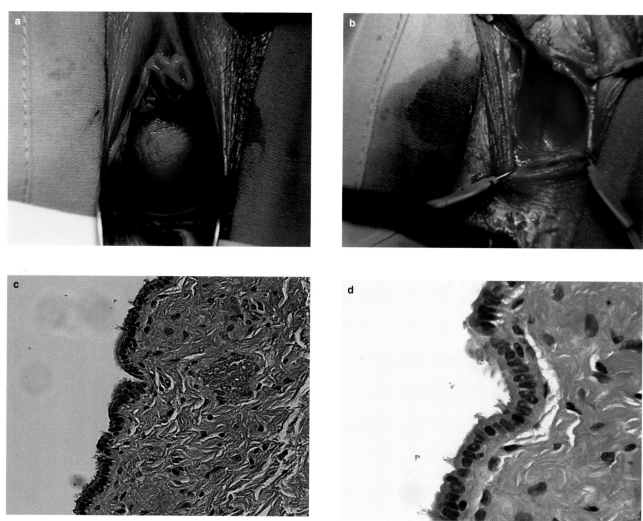

Figure 6.22
Right anteriolateral paraurethral müllerian cyst (a) which when opened at the time of vaginal surgery was unilocular and contained mucus (b). (c) and (d), histology of low and high resolution of the cyst wall show a lining of ciliated columnar epithelium similar to epithelium found in the fallopian tube or endocervix.

cystoscopy, the lesions may be papillary, polypoidal, or sessile with raised yellow plaques. The papillary component can be mistaken for a transitional cell carcinoma but can be differentiated on histology by the presence of a single layer of cytologically normal cuboidal cells lining the stalks with a lack of any nuclear anaplasia. Nephrogenic adenoma is not associated with malignancy but can reoccur (Figure 6.23).

Infection and abscess formation can occur in the anterior compartment secondary to the introduction of synthetic graft material for the treatment of stress incontinence or vaginal prolapse. Clinically, this may present as a tender anterior vaginal wall mass (Figure 6.24a), vaginal discharge and bleeding, or irritable bladder symptoms and incontinence. On cystoscopy, the bladder wall adjacent to the inflammatory condition is edematous and inflamed (Figure 6.24b).

Other intraurethral pathology
Urethral injury, strictures, and adhesions

Any injury to the urethra may result in intraurethral adhesions and urethral fibrosis with stricture formation. This can result in a poorly functioning urethra that is unable to maintain normal sphincteric closure (ISD stress incontinence) or is unable to relax and open during voiding; or both. Urethral injury can result from infection, intraurethral and periurethral surgery, urethral instrumentation including forceful catheterization (Figure 6.25), radiation (Figure 6.26), and repeated overdilatation of the urethra. Injury to the female urethra can also occur as a result of

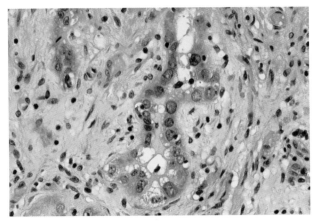

Figure 6.23
Nephrogenic adenoma of the urethra in a 42-year-old woman who presented with vaginal pain, dysuria and a tender 3 cm paraurethral swelling. Histopathology showed irregular tubules set in an edematous stroma containing occasional polymorphs. The tubule is lined by cells with regular nuclei. H and E × 40.

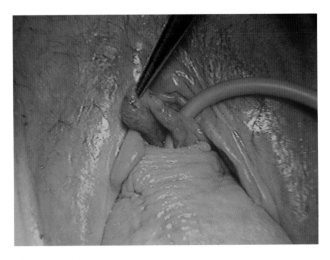

Figure 6.25
Urethral catheter injury resulting in urethrovaginal fistula.

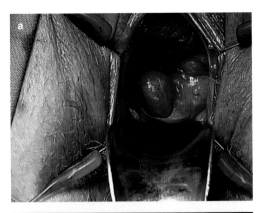

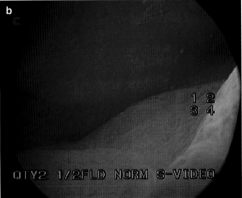

Figure 6.24 (a,b)
(a) Inflammatory vaginal polyp secondary to infected synthetic mesh used in vaginal suspension operation (b) Cystoscopy in a woman with infected intravaginal sling (IVS) multifilament sling and pelvic abscess presenting 3 years following insertion, with pelvic pain, vaginal discharge, and severe urinary incontinence. On cystoscopy, the left bladder base was grossly edematous and a left ureteric orifice (LUO) could not be seen, palency was confirmed by injection of indigo carmine. The infected sling was removed through an abdominovaginal approach and all infected tissue was removed.

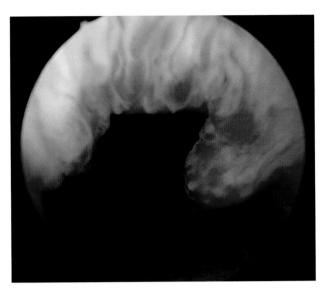

Figure 6.26
Inflammatory urethral polyp at the bladder neck in a woman who had radiation for cancer of the cervix.

direct trauma from a saddle-type injury and indirectly as a result of a pelvic fracture injury, frequently resulting from a motor car accident. This can result in rupture of the urethra in the acute phase and, more long term, cause disruption to urethral structure and function (Figure 6.27a,b). If either the bony supports (namely, the symphysis pubis or pubic rami) are fractured or the pubourethral ligaments or urethra are damaged, the sphincter mechanism can become incontinent with stress incontinence developing. Surgical repair may involve reconstruction of the urethra or resupporting the urethra with a mid-urethral sling, or both.

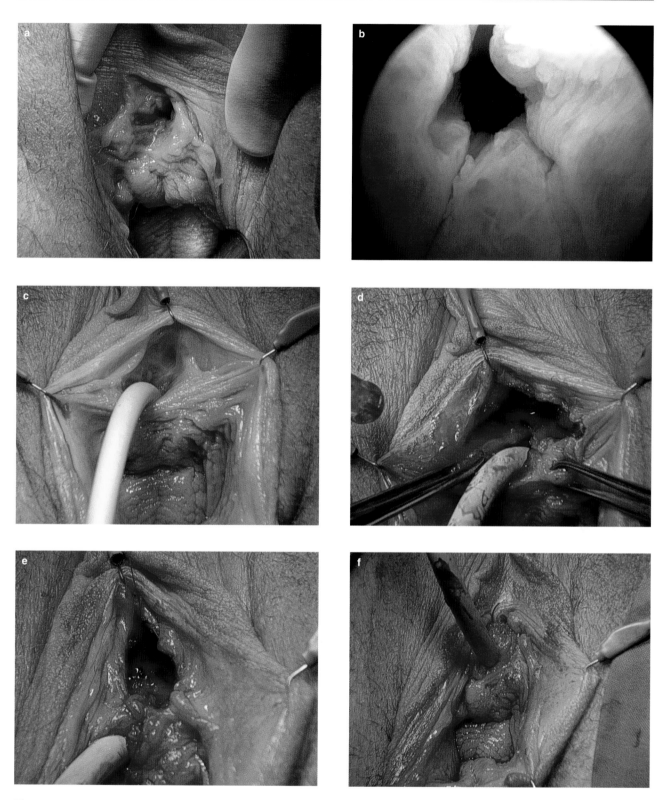

Figure 6.27

A 39-year-old woman who suffered diastasis of the symphysis pubis, avulsion with rupture of the distal urethra at the age of 30 years. (a) On examination, the external urethral meatus was gaping with a significant anterior wall defect and the bladder neck visible. (b) Open patulous bladder neck on urethroscopy. (c) Urethral catheter in situ revealing anterior wall defect. (d–f) Incision anterior to EUM opening the preurethral space and the anterior urethral wall reconstructed. The preurethral space was closed with reattachment of the pubourethral ligament.

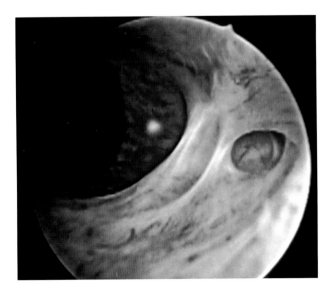

Figure 6.28
Urethral scarring resulting from surgery for a UD.

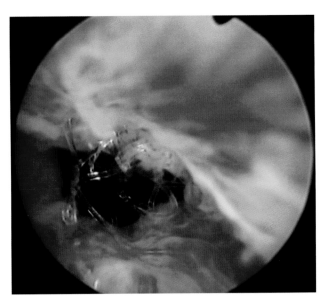

Figure 6.29
Urethral penetration by polypropylene fibers from a TVT suburethral sling.

Case 1

A 39-year-old woman who suffered diastasis of the symphysis pubis, avulsion with rupture of the distal urethra at the age of 30 years in a motor car accident. This was repaired following the accident, although she continued to have symptoms of stress incontinence. Her incontinence became much worse during her first pregnancy. When she presented after the pregnancy, the EUM was gaping with a significant anterior wall defect (Figure 6.27a) and the bladder neck visible. On urethroscopy, the lower urethra was functionally absent, with a patulous and open urethra and bladder neck (Figure 6.27b) and whitish appearance of stratified squamous epithelium. The preurethral space was opened (Figure 6.27c) and the anterior urethral wall reconstructed. The preurethral space was closed with reattachment of the pubourethral ligament (Figure 6.27d–f). A mid-urethral sling may also be needed to support the urethra and restore urethral sphincter competence.

Impaired bladder emptying is common in women, present in 13% of all women sent for urodynamics assessment in our clinic with previous stress incontinence and prolapse surgery, the second most common cause after neuropathic disorders.[13] Symptoms of impaired bladder emptying are poor urinary stream, intermittent flow, hesitancy, and incomplete bladder emptying. These symptoms can be unreliable in the diagnosis of voiding dysfunction, so that an objective assessment with urodynamics and pressure flow studies is appropriate before a diagnosis of obstructed voiding can be made.

A urethral stricture is a narrowing of the urethra which can be congenital or acquired. Congenital abnormalities of the urethra can cause narrowing and voiding difficulty and these have been covered in Chapter 5 (see Figure 5.17a). Excision of a UD with inappropriate urethral repair can result in urethral scarring and narrowing (Figure 6.28). The urethra can also be injured during removal of other periurethral cysts or tumors where it is inadvertently opened or in the performance of stress incontinence procedures when the sling has been placed through the urethral wall (Figures 6.29 and 6.30) (see Chapter 11).

Outlet obstruction can be treated surgically when symptoms are severe and objectively confirmed. Urethral strictures can be incised and/or dilated, and any foreign body obstruction endoscopically removed. Urethral dilatation up to Hegar size 14 or 30 Fr can be safely performed and is usually successful (Figure 6.31), although further dilatations may be necessary over time as voiding symptoms tend to reoccur. The use of the urethrotome to make a posterior urethral incision is unnecessary in the female and has a significant risk of postoperative stress incontinence or fistula formation. If the cause of the voiding is a stress incontinence procedure with oversuspension of the bladder neck at colposuspension or an excessively tight sling, removal of the suspension sutures or division of the sling may be required by the vaginal or retropubic approach.

Urethral meatal stenosis is uncommon in women but can occur secondary to infection, or in association with atrophic or dysplastic conditions of the vulva and vagina. These vulval conditions may be associated with pruritus

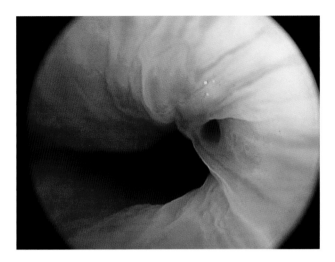

Figure 6.30
Urethral scarring following placement and removal of transobturator TVTO (Gynecare J and J) sling.

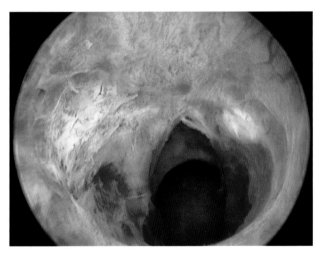

Figure 6.31
Urethroscopy following urethral dilatation up to Hegar size 14 in a woman who developed a mid-urethral stricture following a vaginal repair and urethral catheterization.

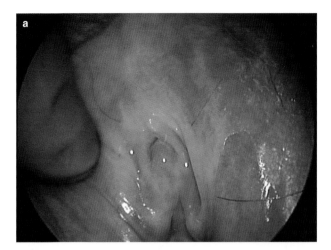

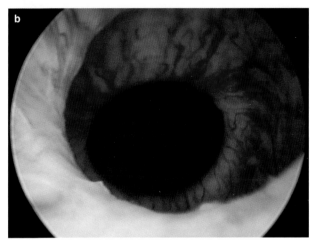

Figure 6.32
Meatal stenosis of the external urethral meatus (EUM) in a 50-year-old woman with lichen planus of the vulva. She presented with symptoms of voiding difficulty and vulval pruritus. The external urethral meatus was narrowed (a) and it was not possible to pass a 5 Fr urethral catheter. Once the EUM was dilated the remaining urethra was normal (b). Her symptoms of voiding difficulty resolved following urethral dilation and cystourethroscopy under general anesthesia.

and introital narrowing and labial adhesions. Symptoms are poor urinary flow and urinary hesitancy, and on examination the external urethral meatus is stenosed (Figure 6.32), making it difficult to pass even a small-diameter catheter without pain. Meatal dilatation with treatment of the underlying cause is usually effective.

Labial agglutination and adhesions normally occurs in the elderly but can also affect young children and is thought to be caused by atrophic changes secondary to estrogen deprivation.[14] This can be of varying degrees but when severe can result in complete closure of the introitus, leaving only a pinhole opening for urine to pass through (Figure 6.33). Presenting symptoms are voiding difficulty and intermittent dribbling incontinence with urine collecting

in a distended vagina. Local application of estrogen cream results in introital opening normalization, which needs to continue long term to prevent reagglutination. These women are not sexually active. In long-standing cases or when conservative treatment has been unsuccessful, surgical separation of the labia is required.

Urethral mucosal polyps, prolapse, and urethral caruncle

Urethral polyps and mucosal fronds are common and are seen in the upper half of the urethra and at the bladder neck. They are a mucosal inflammatory response to chronic

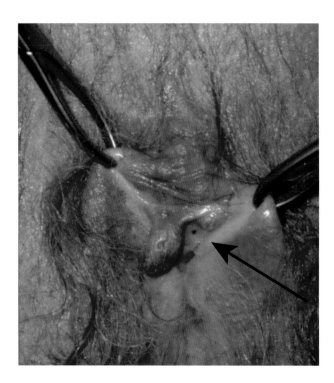

Figure 6.33
Photograph of a 78-year-old woman with fused labia minora and pinhole introital opening (arrow) to allow passage of urine. The vagina was dilated and distended with urine on ultrasonic imaging. The introitus was opened by gentle digital manipulation under general anesthetic.

irritation caused by a recurrent urinary tract infection (Figure 6.34a), catheter usage (Figure 6.34b), and radiation (see Figure 6.26). Polyps may be polypoid (Figure 6.24c,d), and sessile (Figure 6.34d) and are usually asymptomatic. It has been suggested[15] that there is an association with subsequent malignancy, although there is no evidence to support this theory. No treatment is necessary except normal measures to prevent further predisposing factors such as a UTI. Similarly, inclusion cysts are normal variants and may be present in the urethra or bladder, and are usually of no significance (Figure 6.35a,b).

Urethral mucosal prolapse is seen in children and older postmenopausal women, suggesting a possible hormonal etiology. Urethral prolapse of a minor degree is a common finding in elderly women and is usually asymptomatic; referral by primary care physicians of these patients is usually for a 'polyp' seen during routine Papanicolaou (Pap) smears screening. Asymptomatic small urethral prolapses can be treated conservatively with estrogen cream (Figure 6.36). Large urethral prolapses may present with pain, dysuria, postmenopausal bleeding, voiding difficulties, and a purple meatal mass (Figure 6.37). Treatment is usually surgical with excision of the prolapse mucosa and mucosal resuturing using 4/0 Vicryl. Small prolapses are frequently misdiagnosed as urethral caruncles. These small chronic granulomatous lesions of unknown etiology present on the posterior lip of the external urethral meatus. They may present as a urethral lump and cause dysuria and bleeding (Figure 6.38), and on examination are pedunculated erythematous lesions that bleed on contact. Histologically, they have epithelial hyperplasia and/or fibrocapillary proliferation with a dense

polymorph and lympocyte inflammatory response. Excision and histopathological examination are necessary to exclude the possibility of alignancy.[16]

Urethritis and the urethral syndrome

The symptom complex of pain, usually in the urethral or vaginal area, associated with urinary frequency and urgency where there is no urinary infection or other diagnosable cause is termed the urethral syndrome. Women presenting with these symptoms are a common and difficult referral to gynecologists and urologists. Urinary tract infection has usually been excluded prior to referral, but this may often not be clear because of early and liberal use of antibiotics in women with symptoms of cystitis. Therefore, repeated urine examination with microscopy and culture to exclude bacteriuria may be necessary. The presence of an infection should be suspected if there is persistent pyuria (>8 leukocytes/ml urine). Urinary tract infection has traditionally been defined by $>10^5$ bacteria per ml of freshly voided midstream urine. This definition has been found too insensitive, with up to 50% of clinical infection undiagnosed.[17] Therefore, a lower bacteriuria rate of 10^3 organisms has been accepted to indicate infection in women with symptoms (Infectious Diseases Society of America Consensus definition).[18] Asymptomatic bacteriuria is defined on the basis of two consecutive, clean-voided urine specimens with more than 10^5 organisms per ml.

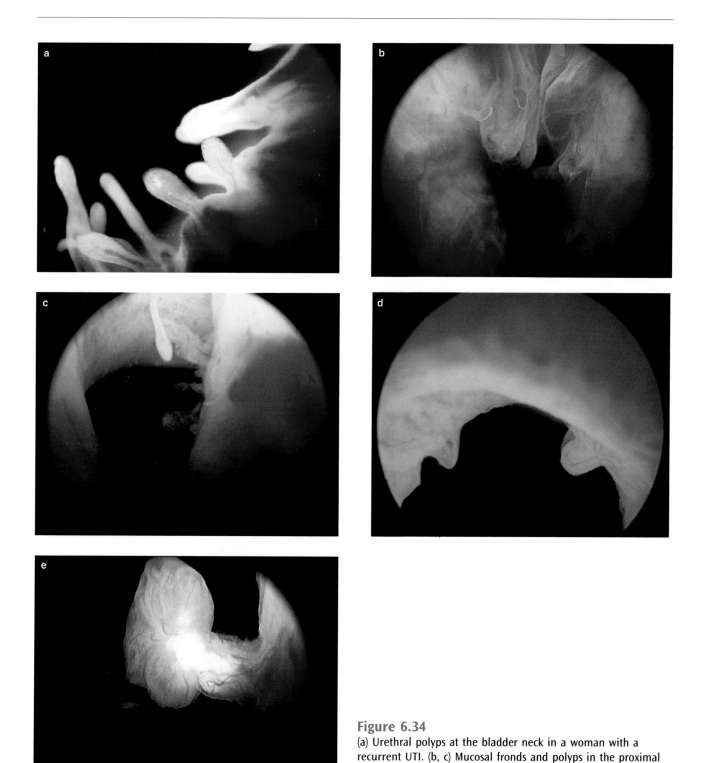

Figure 6.34
(a) Urethral polyps at the bladder neck in a woman with a recurrent UTI. (b, c) Mucosal fronds and polyps in the proximal urethra. (d) Sessile polyps at the bladder neck. (e) Pedunculated polyp in the proximal urethra.

The presence of pyuria in women without significant bacteriuria may indicate an infective etiology such as *Chlamydia trachomatis, Mycoplasma,* or some other fastidious organism, especially if the woman is sexually active. Urethral swabs for culture of *Chlamydia* and *Neisseria gonorrhoeae* should be performed. Latham and Stamm[19] suggested a trial of doxycycline with sulfamethoxazole–trimethoprim in women with sterile

pyuria. Women with long-standing symptoms (>6 months) of urethral pain and/or frequency and urgency are unlikely to have an infective cause. Clinical irritant (soaps, douches, spermicidals) or systemic disease (Reiter's syndrome) should also be excluded as a cause of symptoms. Reiter's syndrome consists of urethritis, conjunctivitis, and arthritis and is associated with infections, usually *Chlamydia trachomatis.* Women with

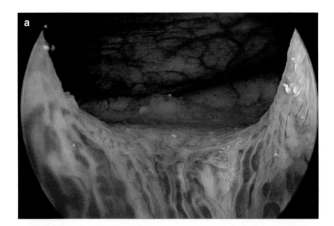

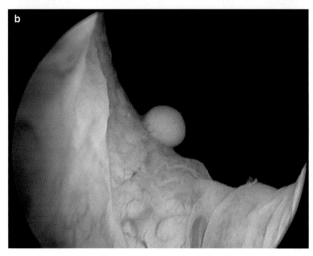

Figure 6.35
(a) An open bladder neck with inclusion cysts and squamous metaplasia of the trigone. (b) Small inclusion cyst at the bladder neck.

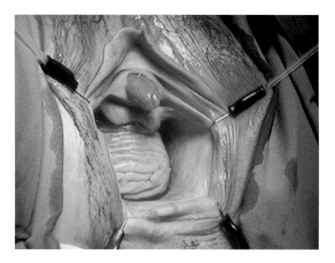

Figure 6.36
Asymptomatic prolapse of the posterior urethral mucosa in an elderly woman with vaginal prolapse.

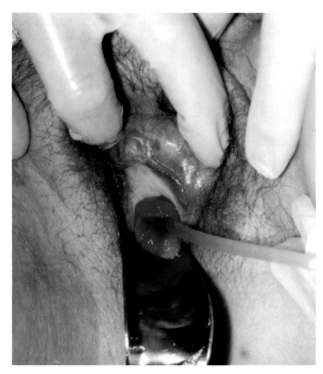

Figure 6.37
Large circumferential urethral mucosal prolapse in a woman with vaginal bleeding and voiding difficulty.

interstitial cystitis also frequently have urethral pain and pain referred to the vaginal vulva and rectum. This pattern is indicative that a field change occurs in women with chronic pelvic pain syndrome and that there is considerable overlap in the pain distributions in these areas.

Cystourethroscopy is an important investigational tool in the assessment and diagnosis of patients with chronic pelvic pain, especially in the presence of irritable bladder symptoms. The diagnosis of the urethral syndrome is essentially one of exclusion of urogenital infection and non-infective causes of urethritis (Figure 6.38) such as urethral diverticulum, strictures, tumors, trauma, and foreign bodies. Bladder pathology should also be excluded as a cause of the urinary symptoms. Other appropriate investigations are a urinary diary, urine microscopy, culture, and cytology, and imaging by ultrasound or a CT scan of the lower urinary tract and pelvis.

Treatment of pelvic pain syndromes, particularly in relation to the urethral syndrome, should be conservative and supportive, and includes behavioral modification with bladder retraining, neuromodulation techniques such as transcutaneous electrical nerve stimulation (TENS) or sacral nerve stimulation, and nortriptyline and gabapentin for neuropathic pain. In a recent randomized double-blind

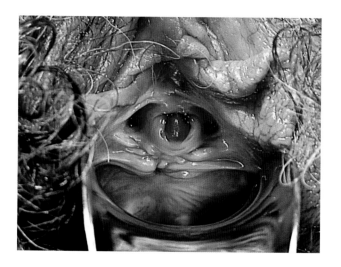

Figure 6.38
Urethral caruncle in a woman with dysuria and urethral tenderness.

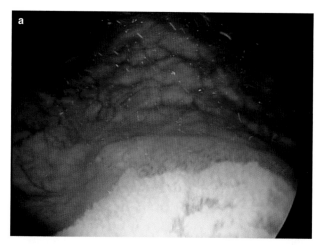

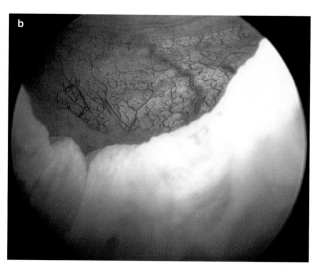

Figure 6.40
Cystourethroscopic view of normal squamous epithelium on the trigone, commonly referred to as squamous metaplasia (a) and of the proximal urethra (b).

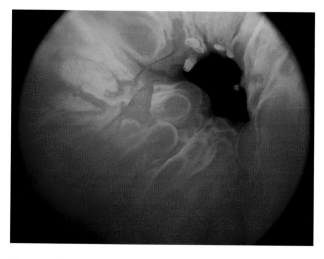

Figure 6.39
Acute urethritis with urethral polyps in a woman with a urinary tract infection.

study for the treatment of post-herpetic neuralgia of 70 patients over 9 weeks, the visual analog score (VAS) and pain scores were significantly reduced in both groups. Patients showed significant improvement in sleep scores with nortriptyline (46%) and gabapentin (52%). Both drugs were equally efficacious, but gabapentin was better tolerated.[20] Urethral dilatation and cystodistention have been found to be of some value in these patients, but the benefits are often temporary.[21]

Traditionally, labels of 'trigonitis and urethrotrigonitis' and 'squamous metaplasia' have been given to the cobblestone or granular appearance of the trigone (Figure 6.40 a) and bladder

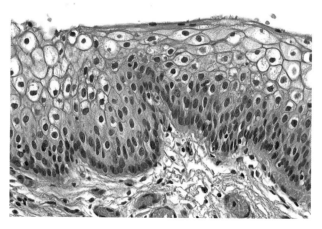

Figure 6.41
Histology of stratified squamous metaplasia on the trigone.

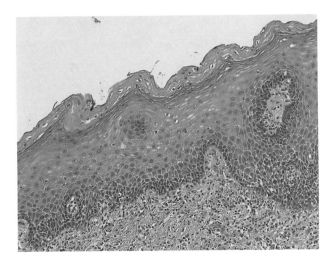

Figure 6.42
Histology of vaginal wall showing keratinized stratified squamous epithelium.

neck (Figure 6.40b) which is a normal variant in healthy mature women (see Chapter 2) and, histologically, is squamous epithelium (Figure 6.40).[22] These areas in the past have been resected and coagulated for supposed 'trigonitis' but it is a normal cystoscopic finding in women without irritative bladder symptoms.[23] The squamous epithelium of the urethra and trigone is from the same embryological source as the vagina: namely, the urogenital sinus. The epithelium at the EUM is keratinized stratified squamous epithelium and is continuous with the skin of the vestibule and the vagina (see Figure 6.42) (see Chapter 2).

References

1. Leach GE, Bavendam TG. Female urethral diverticula. Urology 1987; 30: 407–15.
2. Ganabathi K, Leach GE, Zimmern PE, Dimochowski RR. Experience with the management of urethral diverticulum in 63 women. J Urol 1994; 152: 1445–52.
3. Blander DS, Zimmern PE. Diagnosis and management of female urethral diverticulum and urethrovaginal fistula. In: Stanton SL, Zimmern PE, eds. Female Pelvic Reconstructive Surgery. London: Springer-Verlag, 2003.
4. Saito S. Usefulness of diagnosis by the urethroscopy under anesthesia and effect of transurethral electrocoagulation in symptomatic female urethral diverticula. J Endourol 2000; 14: 455–7.
5. Leng WW, McGuire EJ. Management of female urethral diverticula: a new classification. J Urol 1998; 160: 1297–300.
6. Silk MR, Lebowitz JM. Anterior urethral diverticulum. J Urol 1969; 101: 66–7.
7. Routh A. Urethral diverticulum. Br Med J 1890; 1, 361.
8. Foster RT, Amundsen CL, Webster GD. The utility of magnetic resonance imaging for diagnosis and surgical planning before transvaginal periurethral diverticulectomy in women. Int Urogynecol J Pelvic Floor Dysfunct 2007; 18: 315–19.
9. Moran PA, Carey M, Dwyer PL. Urethral diverticula in pregnancy. Aust NZ J Obstet Gynaecol 1998; 38: 102–6.
10. Spence HM, Duckett JW. Diverticulum of the female urethra. J Urol 1970; 104: 432–7.
11. Ozel B, Ballard C. Urethral and paraurethral leiomyomas in the female patient. Int Urogynecol J Pelvic Floor Dysfunct 2006; 17: 93–5.
12. Deppisch LM. Cysts of the vagina: classification and clinical correlations. Obstet Gynecol 1975; 45: 632–7.
13. Dwyer PL, Desmedt E. Impaired bladder emptying in women. Aust NZ J Obstet Gynaecol 1994; 34: 73–8.
14. Ong N, Dwyer PL. Labial fusion causing voiding difficulty and urinary incontinence. Aust NZ J Obstet Gynaecol 1999; 39: 391–3.
15. Herr HW. In: Walsh PC, Recik AB, Vaughan EW, Wein AJ, eds. Campbells Urology, 7th edn. Philadelphia, PA: WB Saunders, 1997: 3407–8.
16. Cimentepe E, Bayrak O, Unsal A et al. Urethral adenocarcinoma mimicking urethral caruncle. Int J Urogynecol J Pelvic Floor Dysfunct 2004; 38: 521–2.
17. Stamm WE, Counts GW, Running KR et al. Diagnosis of coliform infection in acutely dyuric women. N Engl J Med 1982; 307: 463–8.
18. Hooton TM. Recurrent urinary tract infection in women. Int J Antimicrobial Agents 2001; 17: 259–68.
19. Latham H, Stamm WE. Urethral syndrome in women. Urol Clin North Am 1984; 11: 95–101.
20. Chandra K, Shafiq N, Pandhi P, Gupta S, Malhotra S. Gabapentin versus nortriptyline in post-herpetic neuralgia patients: a randomized double blind clinical trial – the GONIP Trial. Int J Clin Pharmacol Ther 2006; 44: 358–63.
21. Rutherford AJ, Hinshaw K, Essenhigh DM, Neal DE. Urethral dilation compared with cystoscopy alone in women with recurrent frequency and urgency. Br J Urol 1988; 61: 500–4.
22. Wiener DP, Koss LG, Sablay B, Freed SZ. The prevalence and significance of Brunn's nests, cystitis cystica and squamous metaplasia in normal bladders. J Urol 1979; 122: 317–21.
23. Schaeffer AJ. Infections of the urinary tract. In: Walsh PC, ed. Campbell's Urology, Vol 1. Philadelphia, PA: WB Saunders; 1997: 596.

7

Infective and non-infective cystitis

Anna Rosamilia and Peter L Dwyer

Introduction

Women with infective and non-infective cystitis have similar clinical presentations of frequency, urgency, and dysuria or bladder pain. Cystourethroscopy is an important tool in the diagnosis and management of patients with irritable bladder symptoms. On occasion, biopsy and histological review will be required to complete the diagnosis. However, infection should be excluded by urine analysis with microscopy and culture and treated if possible before performing any endoscopic assessment of the urinary tract. Cystoscopy should not be performed in the presence of overt infection but should be delayed until the infection has been treated by antibiotics. In one study women with preoperative bacteriuria had a 60% incidence of bacteremia and a 10% risk of septicemia.[1] Prophylactic antibiotics should be given with cystoscopy in women with a past history of recurrent urinary tract infection (UTI) or at higher risk of UTI following urinary instrumentation: e.g. diabetes, women with a structural or functional urinary tract abnormality. The use of prophylatic artibiotics during cystoscopy is discussed in Chapter 4.

In this chapter we discuss infective and non-infective causes of bladder inflammation, and the role of cystourethroscopy in their diagnosis and management. In Chapter 8, we review the clinical syndrome that includes interstitial cystitis and painful bladder syndrome, more recently named bladder pain syndrome.

Infective cystitis (urinary tract infection)

It has been estimated that urinary tract infection or acute cystitis occurs in at least 10% of women in any given year, with more than half of all women having at least one infection in their lifetime.[2] In the majority of cases infection resolves either spontaneously or after antibiotic treatment; however, some women will have sporadic recurrences, with 25–50% having a further urinary infection within 1 year. Up to 5% have recurrent urinary tract infections.[3]

Escherichia coli is the commonest bacteria in urinary tract infection, causing 75–90% of all UTI, followed by *Staphylococcus saprophyticus* in 5–15% of cases, and then other enterococci such as *Klebsiella* spp. and *Proteus mirabilis*.[4]

In young women, the most important risk factor is a history of frequent or recent sexual activity.[5] In healthy postmenopausal women, estrogen deficiency may contribute, as may diabetes,[6] and there is an association of UTI with the presence of a cystocele and urinary incontinence.[7] In elderly institutionalized women, the risk increases with age and debility, especially where there is voiding dysfunction, vaginal prolapse, urinary or fecal incontinence.[8–10]

A 3-day course of trimethoprim will eradicate urinary pathogens within 7 days of starting treatment in 94% of women.[11] The prevalence of resistance to trimethoprim–sulfamethoxazole is up to 18% in some areas of the United States. However, it has been shown that overall cure rates of 80% or more can still be achieved with this antibiotic even when the prevalence of resistance reaches 30%.[12] A 3-day course of a fluoroquinolone such as norfloxacin would be the second-line agent. Nitrofurantoin also has a role to play but is less active against enterococci other than *E. coli* and is inactive against *Proteus*.

Recurrent infective cystitis

Recurrent infective cystitis refers to a symptomatic UTI following the clinical resolution of a previous UTI. Overall, between 20 and 40% of women will develop recurrent UTIs, but it is not known how frequently these recurrences would occur.[13] It is estimated that 10–15% of women over 60 years old have frequent recurrences. Continuous or postcoital low-dose antibiotic prophylaxis is effective in preventing recurrent UTI.[3]

Gynecological examination to exclude significant pelvic organ prolapse, pelvic masses, atrophic change, external

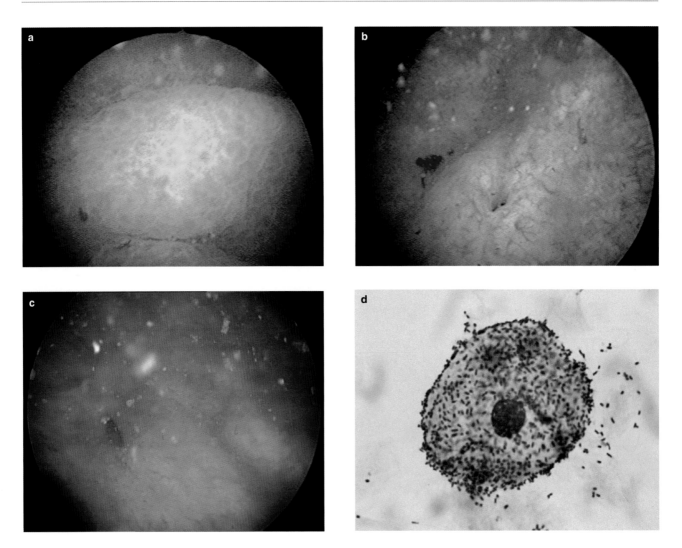

Figure 7.1
(a) Urinary tract infection with edematous inflamed bladder mucosa. (b,c) Increasing cloudy urine from exfoliated urothelium and bacteria (in b, the left ureteric orifice can be seen with a jet of indigo carmine). (d.) Exfoliated superficial urothelial cell with attached and phagocytosed bacteria from a woman with acute bacterial cystitis.

urethral stenosis, or diverticulum should be performed, as these conditions may predispose or be associated with recurrent UTI. Imaging with plain X-ray, renal ultrasound, or a computed tomography (CT) scan may be indicated in recurrent cases or where there is failure of symptom and bacteriological resolution in order to rule out upper tract abnormalities such as calculi or obstruction. Recurrent *Proteus* UTIs are often associated with calculi.[14]

Endoscopy is rarely helpful in acute uncomplicated UTI, but it is indicated in cases where symptoms persist, recur frequently, where no infection is found in the presence of pyuria, or where microscopic hematuria persists after appropriate treatment. Flexible or rigid cystoscopy can be performed under local or general anesthesia, but, if possible, should not be performed until the UTI is treated. This is performed in order to exclude underlying causes such as calculi (Figure 7.2),

foreign body such as suture (Figure 7.3), tumors, and other structural abnormalities that can predispose to infection. The typical cystoscopic finding in acute cystitis is inflamed, reddened, and edematous mucosa (Figure 7.1a); the urine is cloudy from exfoliated urothelium, which obscures good visualization (Figure 7.1b,c). In acute bacterial cystitis there is initially microbe invasion of the superficial cells of the urothelium, which triggers release of cytokines and chemokines, and causes bladder cell exfoliation making the urine turbid. Both are important host reactions to infection. The cytokines and chemokines initiate and regulate the inflammatory response, leading to neutrophil migration into the urothelium microscopically, and causing an inflamed edematous mucosa and irritable bladder symptoms. The urothelial cells attach and then phagocytose invading bacteria, and are then exfoliated and excreted in the urine (Figure 7.1d).

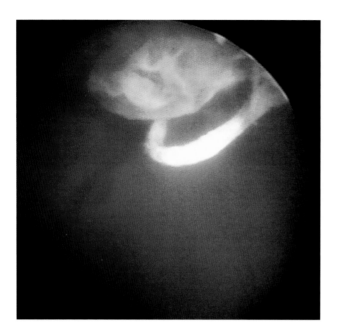

Figure 7.2
A non-absorbable suture surrounded by inflamed mucosa penetrating bladder dome found on cystoscopy in a woman with recurrent UTI 2 years after Burch colposuspension.

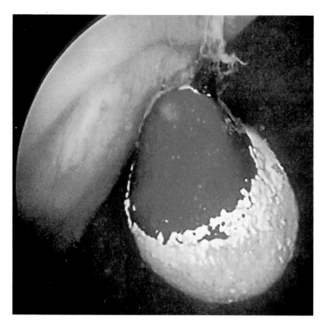

Figure 7.3
Calculus attached to non-absorbable Burch colposuspension suture at 11 o'clock inside bladder neck in a woman with bladder pain, frequency, and recurrent urinary tract infection.

The presence of sterile pyuria, especially in developing countries, would warrant investigation for taberculosis. Early morning urine collections for Lowenstein–Jensen culture, upper tract imaging, and cystoscopy should be performed during cystourethroscopy. The classic appearance at cystoscopy is an ulcer; biopsy will confirm the diagnosis. Tuberculous cystitis invariably occurs in association with upper tract tuberculous changes that are evident on investigation with CT or magnetic resonance imaging (MRI).[14]

The diagnosis of schistomiasis also requires upper tract imaging and the cystoscopic appearance is one of a 'sandy patch'.[14]

Cystitis cystica and cystitis glandularis

This describes the formation of cystic spaces within von Brunn's nests (aggregates of normal urothelium found in the lamina propria). They are usually located in the trigone or anterior bladder wall.[15] Cystoscopically, the appearance is of rounded clear or yellow 1–5 mm submucosal cysts (Figure 7.4), histologically, these are spaces lined by urothelium or cuboidal cells (Figure 7.5). Cystitis glandularis is the histological term given when there are columnar cells lining the spaces within von Brunn's nests (Figure 7.6); cystitis glandularis of the intestinal type relates to goblet cells and mucin production. The diffuse form is called intestinal metaplasia and is often associated with

chronic calculi or chronic catheterization; if extensive, it is a risk factor for adenocarcinoma. Up to the stage of intestinal metaplasia, these aforementioned changes are very common and considered normal variants.

Follicular cystitis

This appearance can be seen in association with bladder cancer and recurrent urinary tract infections. Cystoscopically, the bladder mucosa appears studded with tiny nodules of pink, gray, or white tissue. The lamina propria has lymphoid follicles with germinal centers.[16]

Papillary-polypoidal and bullous cystitis

These are reactive changes most often seen with an indwelling catheter; in some series, they are seen in 80% of catheterized patients.[17] Inflammation of the lamina propria, often with edema, leads to formation of inflammatory papillae. They usually occur on the dome or posterior wall and cystoscopically can resemble a papillary tumor. If very edematous and broad based, the term 'polypoid cystitis' is used[16] and if these formations are wide rather than tall the term 'bullous cystitis' is used. The urothelium overlying any abnormality in the lamina propria may be papillary and the term 'papillary hyperplasia' is used.[16]

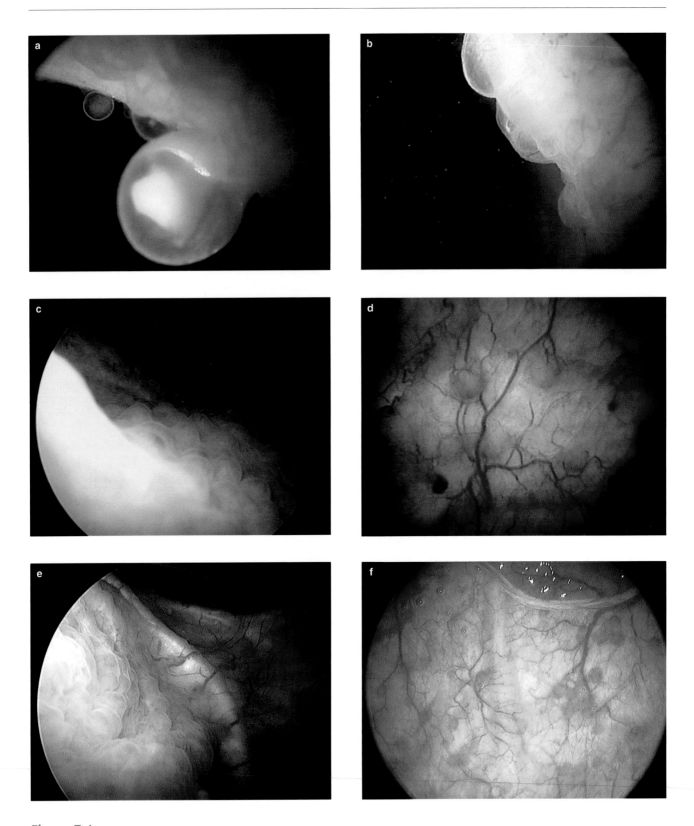

Figure 7.4
Cystoscopic appearance of cystitis cystica with rounded clear or yellow 1–5 mm submucosal cysts which when marked gives the bladder mucosa a cobblestone appearance.

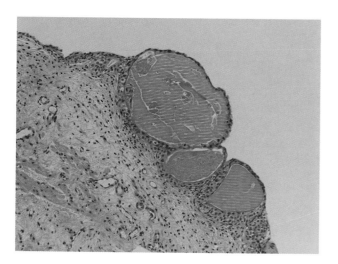

Figure 7.5
Histological specimen of cystitis cystica with small cystic von Brunn's nests containing eosinophilic acellular debris surrounded by urothelium.

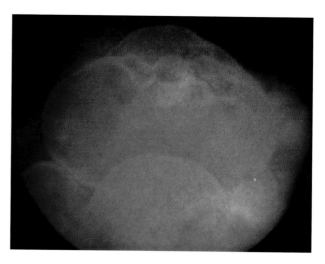

Figure 7.6
Cystitis glandularis. (Courtesy of R Millard.)

Encrusted cystitis

In the presence of chronic infection the urothelium is denuded, and debris, calcium salts, and a purulent exudate settle on the surface. The lesions can be single or multiple on cystoscopy. On microscopy, fibrin and inflammatory cells with calcified necrotic debris is seen and this process of encrustation can occur over a tumor.[18]

Eosinophilic cystitis

Eosinophilic cystitis is a rare condition now thought to affect adult women and men equally. The cause is unclear but it is associated with allergy, bladder tumor or trauma, parasitic infections, and cytotoxic therapy. The pathogenesis is probably an antigen–antibody reaction. The clinical presentation is with cystitis symptoms and often proteinuria, pyuria, and microscopic or gross hematuria. Eosinophiluria occurs in 10–30% but is not specific to this condition and blood eosinophilia occurs in one-third to one-half of cases. Cystoscopically, the appearance is of reddened polypoidal velvety lesions and mucosal edema; the bladder capacity may be reduced. Biopsy is necessary to establish the diagnosis and generally this shows the most intense inflammation predominantly with eosinophils and edema in the lamina propria in addition to a variable degree of fibrosis of the detrusor muscle. The management involves transurethral resection of the lesion, removal of any known (e.g. allergenic) cause, nonsteroidal anti-inflammatories, or corticosteroids.[19]

Granulomatous cystitis

Granulomatous cystitis is characterized by necrotic, foreign body or epitheloid granulomas, or diffuse histiocytic inflammation. It may occur following surgery (bladder biopsy or resection) or be secondary to intravesical BCG (bacille Calmette-Guérin) instillation or bacterial infection; tuberculous cystitis needs to be excluded.[16]

Malacoplakia

Malacoplakia or soft plaque is a rare chronic granulomatous disease more common in women. The patient may be asymptomatic or present with hematuria, frequency, urgency, dysuria, or pain. At cystoscopy, the typical appearance is multiple raised discrete plaques, usually < 2 cm with a central umbilicus, or less commonly, larger, firm, thickened, and granular nodules may be present with or without necrosis. They may appear as filling defects on contrast bladder imaging. The classic pathology shows sheets of cells with eosinophilic granular cytoplasm containing intracytoplasic inclusions, which are known as Michaelis–Gutmann bodies. Usually it is a benign and self-limited condition and is associated with UTI. It has a good response to prolonged treatment with fluoroquinolones.[20]

Radiation cystitis

Radiation cystitis of variable severity may be an early or late complication in patients undergoing radiotherapy for female genital tract or urinary tract cancer. Hemorrhagic cystitis after pelvic radiotherapy for bladder and cervical carcinoma occurs in 7–9% of patients and is related to the type of regimen used and the dose–time–volume relationship. A single dose greater than 20 000 to 25 000 rads or a complete course of 5000–6000 rads carries a definite risk of late subacute reaction. Biological factors are also important;

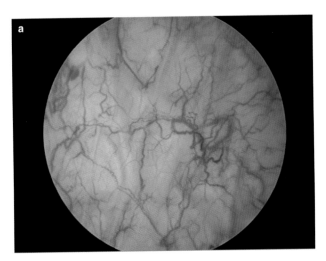

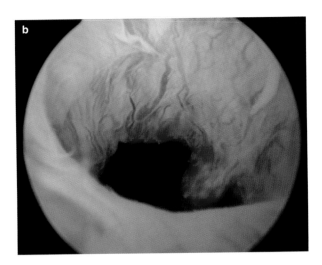

Figure 7.7
A 56-year-old woman presented with urinary frequency, urgency, and stress incontinence 3 years following hysterectomy with postoperative irradiation for adenocarcinoma of the cervix. On cystourethroscopy, the bladder mucosa was pale with an irregular vascularity (a); similar mucosal changes were seen in the urethra, with a polyp at the bladder neck (b).

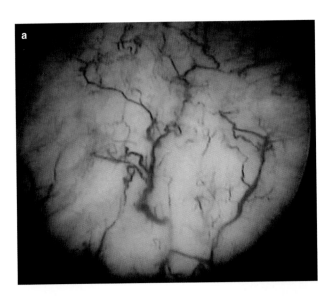

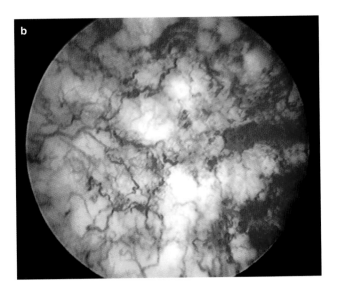

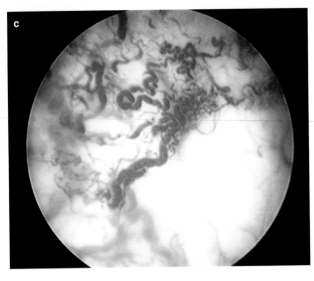

Figure 7.8
Chronic post-radiation changes with atrophic pale mucosa with central telangiectasis.

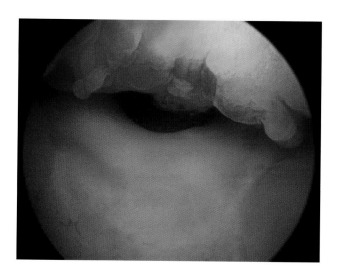

Figure 7.9
Large radiation-induced vesicovaginal fistula with pale atrophic bladder mucosa posteriorly and bullous edema anteriorly.

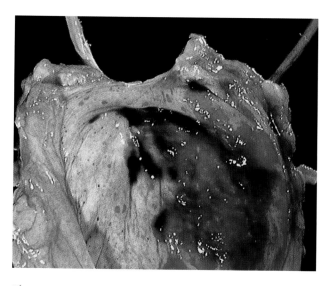

Figure 7.10
Cyclophosphamide hemorrhagic cystitis. (Courtesy of R Millard.)

the type of pre-existing carcinoma, post-operation irradiation, infection, previous radiotherapy, and racial differences increase susceptibility.[21]

Clinically, radiotherapy complications can be divided into acute (less than 6 months), subacute (6 months to 2 years), or chronic (2–5 years). Acute radiation cystitis presents with dysuria, urgency, frequency, and nocturia 4–6 weeks after radiotherapy. Usually the symptoms improve 2–6 weeks after the completion of radiotherapy. Bladder perforation, fistulas, or ureteritis may also occur. The cystoscopic appearance is of diffuse hyperemia with occasional petechiae; in

severe cases, partial desquamation with or without superficial ulceration may occur. Subacute cystitis is heralded by painless hematuria indicating chronic radiation cystitis with trigonal ulcers; its recurrence and severity are not always related to the occurrence of the acute symptoms previously or the radiation dose. Healing of ulcers may take weeks to months. The cystoscopic appearance is of areas of atrophic pale mucosa with central telangiectasis, bleeding ulcers, bladder wall necrosis, bullous edema, and tortuous blood vessels (Figures 7.7 and 7.8).

Chronic radiation cystitis may result in a contracted fibrotic bladder,[22] which develops insidiously and can be progressive, especially if infection, prior radionecrosis, surgery, or extensive carcinoma is present. Symptoms may include urinary frequency, nocturia, urinary incontinence, and hematuria, depending on radiation damage to bladder or urethra or both. The cystourethroscopic appearance is of pale mucosal atrophy, chronic vascular changes with telangiectasia, and fistula formation (Figures 7.8 and 7.9).

Drug-induced cystitis

The term 'drug-induced cystitis', as compared with 'drug-associated cystitis', is used where the causality has been proven by assessment of a large number of patients or by rechallenging with the same drug. This diagnosis requires a high index of suspicion and careful drug history. The time interval between drug administration and the onset of symptoms can be quite variable, ranging up to many years. Confirmation of the diagnosis occurs when the symptoms and the cystoscopic appearance resolve on drug withdrawal and recur on drug rechallenge. The latter is unlikely to occur in the clinical setting.

The majority of reports to the Australian Adverse Drug Reactions Advisory Committee were due to tiaprofenic acid (Surgam). Tiaprofenic acid was described as a cause of cystitis in 1991 by Ahmed and Davison[23] and resulted in major surgery in at least 17 patients because the drug was not suspected or known; there is one reported fatality.[24] In 1997, Henley et al found 108 reported cases in the UK; the mean duration of drug treatment prior to the onset of symptoms was 14 months, with a range of 6 days to 4 years. In 10% there were residual symptoms and in some cases fibrosis.[25] Similar results were reported in Australia, with median time to symptom onset of 6 months and a range of 0.1–47 months and a median interval between presentation to doctor and drug cessation of 3 months. In half the patients, withdrawal of the drug resulted in symptom resolution within 2 weeks. Increasing age was a risk factor for the development of tiaprofenic acid-associated cystitis, with a three-fold greater risk for persons aged 70 years or greater compared with age less than 55 years.[26]

Sporadic cases of dysuria and cystitis have been described in association with a number of non-steroidal anti-inflammatory drugs.[27] Danazol has been associated with hemorrhagic cystitis in patients with hereditary angioneurotic edema. Tranilast, an anti-asthma drug, has been reported to cause eosinophilic cystitis.[28] Cyclophosphamide and ifosfamide can induce hemorrhagic cystitis in 2–40% of patients (Figure 7.10): the metabolite responsible for this is acrolein, which causes death of urothelial cells. Clinically, hemorrhagic cystitis occurs 3 weeks to 6 months after the commencement of therapy and can have a presentation which varies from asymptomatic hematuria to fulminating ulcerating inflammation with life-threatening hemorrhage.[29]

References

1. Christensen MM, Madsen PO. Antibiotic prophylaxis in transurethral surgery. Urology 1990; 35 (Suppl): 11–14.
2. Foxman B, Barlow R, D'Arcy H, Gillespie B, Sobel JD. Urinary tract infection: self-reported incidence and associated costs. Ann Epidemiol 2000; 10: 509–15.
3. Hooton TM. Recurrent urinary tract infection in women. Int J Antimicrob Agents 2001; 17: 259–68.
4. Ronald A. The etiology of urinary tract infection: traditional and emerging pathogens. Am J Med 2002; 113 (Suppl 1A): 14S–19S.
5. Scholes D, Hooton TM, Roberts PL, Stamm WE. Risk factors for recurrent urinary tract infection in young women. J Infect Dis 2000; 182: 1177–82.
6. Boyko EJ, Fihn SD, Scholes D et al. Diabetes and the risk of acute urinary tract infection among postmenopausal women. Diabetes Care 2002; 25: 1778–83.
7. Raz R, Gennesin Y, Wasser J et al. Recurrent urinary tract infections in postmenopausal women. Clin Infect Dis 2000; 30: 152–6.
8. Sourander LB. Urinary tract infection in the aged – an epidemiological study. Ann Med Intern Fenn Suppl 1966; 45: 7–55.
9. Brocklehurst JC, Dillane JB, Griffith L, Fry J. The prevalence and symptomatology of urinary infection in an aged population. Gerontol Clin 1968; 10: 242–53.
10. Powers JS, Billings FT, Behrendt D, Burger MC. Antecedent factors in urinary tract infections among nursing home patients. South Med J 1988; 81: 734–5.
11. Warren JW, Abrutyn E, Hebel JR, Schaeffer AJ, Stamm WE. Guidelines for antimicrobial treatment of uncomplicated acute bacterial cystitis and acute pyelonephritis in women. Clin Infect Dis 1999; 29: 745–58.
12. Gupta K, Hooton TM, Stamm WE. Increasing antimicrobial resistance and the management of uncomplicated community-acquired urinary tract infections. Ann Intern Med 2001; 135: 41–50.
13. Foxman B. Recurrent urinary tract infection: incidence and risk factors. Am J Public Health 1990; 80: 331–3.
14. Arnold EP. Investigation. In: Stanton SL, Dwyer PL, eds. Investigations in Urinary Tract Infection in the Female. London: Martin Dunitz, 2000: 35–57.
15. Ito N, Hirose M, Shirai T et al. Lesions of the urinary bladder epithelium in 125 autopsy cases. Acta Pathol Jpn 1981; 31: 545–57.
16. Young RH. Pseudoneoplastic lesions of the urinary bladder. Pathol Annu 1988; 23 (Pt 1): 67–104.
17. Ekelund P, Johansson SL. Polypoid cystitis: a catheter associated lesion of the human bladder. Acta Pathol Microbiol Scand [A] 1979; 87: 179–84.
18. Jameson RM. Phosphatic encrusted cystitis. Br J Clin Pract 1967; 21: 463–5.
19. Teegavarapu PS, Sahai A, Chandra A, Dasgupta P, Khan MS. Eosinophilic cystitis and its management. Int J Clin Pract 2005; 59: 356–60.
20. Velasquez LJG, Velez HA, Uribe AJF. Malakoplakia in urology: six cases report and review of the literature. Actas Urol Esp 2006; 30(6): 610–18.
21. de Vries CR, Freha FS. Hemorrhagic cystitis: a review. J Urol 1990; 143: 1–7.
22. Norkool DM, Hampson NB, Giggons RP, Weissman RM. Hyperbaric oxygen therapy for radiation-induced hemorrhagic cystitis. J Urol 1993; 150; 332–4.
23. Ahmed M, Davison OW. Severe cystitis associated with tiaprofenic acid. BMJ 1991; 303: 1376–9.
24. Bramble FJ, Morlet R. Drug-induced cystitis: the need for vigilance. Br J Urol 1997; 79: 3–7.
25. Henley MJ, Harriss D, Bishop MC. Cystitis associated with tiaprofenic acid (Surgam): a survey of British and Irish urologists. Br J Urol 1997; 79(4): 585–7.
26. Buchbinder R, Forbes A, Kobben F et al. Clinical features of tiaprofenic acid (surgam) associated cystitis and a study of risk factors for its development. J Clin Epidemiol 2000; 53(10): 1013–19.
27. O'Brien WM. Adverse reactions to non-steroidal anti-inflammatory drugs. Am J Med 1986; 80 (Suppl 4B): 70–80.
28. Okada H, Minayoshi K, Goto A. Two cases of eosinophilic cystitis induced by Tranilast. J Urol 1992; 147: 1366–8.
29. Relling MV, Schunk JE. Drug-induced hemorrhagic cystitis. Clin Pharm 1986; 5: 590–7.

8

Interstitial cystitis/painful bladder syndrome/bladder pain syndrome

Anna Rosamilia and Peter L Dwyer

Introduction

Interstitial cystitis (IC) is the term given to a symptom complex of bladder pain or discomfort with frequency and urgency in the absence of any other cause and in association with a characteristic cystoscopic appearance. The typical cystoscopic findings of IC are the appearance of a Hunner's ulcer, often with a markedly reduced bladder capacity,[1] and the presence of glomerulations or petechial hemorrhages during bladder emptying.[2] These two appearances were used to categorize patients as classic/severe or mild/early, respectively, and were also used in the NIDDK (National Institute of Diabetes and Digestive and Kidney Diseases) consensus research definition of IC.[3] More recently, it has been apparent that there is a group of patients with a similar symptom profile but normal cystoscopy and this condition has been described as painful bladder syndrome (PBS) by the International Continence Society.[4]

In 2006 the European Society for the Study on Interstitial Cystitis (ESSIC) proposed a more taxonomically correct term, bladder pain syndrome (BPS), and a classification system based on cystoscopic and biopsy features.

The symptoms associated with this condition are non-specific. The symptom of urinary frequency can be altered by reduction of fluid intake and the absolute value is not as helpful as volume voided, which can be obtained from a 24-hour urinary diary. Urgency is also a common complaint, by which is meant a constant desire to void, discomfort, or pressure. Classically, the pain is associated with bladder filling and relieved by emptying. However, it is accepted that pain can be felt in the suprapubic area, vagina, urethra, vulva, perineum, or rectum. Many patients present with persistent symptoms following prolonged courses of treatment with antibiotics for an initial proven or presumed urinary tract infection. In clinical practice, consistently small urine volumes associated with

pain or discomfort rather than incontinence is a distinguishing feature from overactive bladder (OAB). Also, women with PBS/IC respond differently to anticholinergic mediation. Women with OAB respond well to anticholinergic drugs, whereas PBS/IC patients are frequently made worse with increased pain and voiding difficulty.

The etiology of PBS/IC is still unknown. However, there is no evidence to suggest that this is caused by infection. It is perhaps a neuropathic condition, with the pathophysiological process being one of neurogenic inflammation, as women with PBS/IC have been demonstrated to have increased sensory nerve fiber proliferation, and increased sensory neuropeptide and inflammatory mediator expression. Vascular changes may also play a role in pathogenesis. Women with PBS/IC have decreased microvascular density in the suburothelium,[5] and bladder vascular perfusion has been shown to decrease during bladder filling in PBS/IC compared with the opposite in asymptomatic controls.[6] Other proposed causes of the condition are a defective glycosaminoglycan (GAG) mucous layer with altered urothelial permeability.

Therefore, as PBS/IC is a separate entity, clinically, etiologically, and cystoscopically, we felt it appropriate to give it a separate chapter from other inflammatory bladder conditions.

Diagnosis

In order to make a diagnosis, history, physical examination, and some specific laboratory testing needs to be performed. The important features on history relate to the nature of the pelvic pain and its relationship to bladder filling or emptying, previous urinary tract infections, pelvic surgery, radiation, drugs, and comorbidities. The physical examination aims to exclude other differential diagnoses, such as vulvodynia, endometriosis, and urethral or other bladder pathology, and should include some assessment of vulval, vaginal, urethral, bladder or pelvic floor muscle, uterine or adnexal tenderness. Pain mapping with a cotton bud could be performed if vulval tenderness is present.[7] The basic investigations include urine microscopy and culture, urine cytology, and a voiding diary. If persistent sterile pyuria is present, culture for tuberculosis and imaging of the upper tracts is appropriate. Other investigations which may be useful include vaginal microscopy and culture to exclude vaginitis and pelvic ultrasound and sometimes laparoscopy to exclude conditions such as endometriosis.

An assessment of voiding and storage function by urodynamic assessment can be performed. Urodynamic assessment would be more important in the presence of urinary incontinence. Decreased compliance is quite uncommon and has an association with more severe disease. In practice, urodynamics gives limited information. Usually, the only finding is that of reduced awake capacity, which could have been predicted by the urinary diary.[8]

The use of symptom questionnaires such as the O'Leary–Sant symptom score[9] and a pain score using a visual analog scale (VAS) or the pelvic pain and urgency/frequency (PUF) scale[10] is useful at baseline and to monitor treatment response.

In some centers a potassium sensitivity test is used. Parsons described the instillation of 40 ml of water followed by 40 ml of potassium chloride solution (40 mEq in 100 ml water) and, after each, the patient rates severe pain or urgency (0 to 5). A positive test occurs when there is a 2 or greater response for potassium as compared with water.[11]

The potassium sensitivity test has a positive predictive value of 80% for IC in a group of patients fulfilling NIDDK criteria and very few false positives in asymptomatic patients. However, it is positive in 25% of women with a diagnosis of 'detrusor instability', 100% of acute urinary tract infection and 85% of a gynecological population with pelvic pain, including those with initial diagnoses such as vulvodynia, endometriosis, and vaginitis.[10]

Cystoscopy

Hunner, a gynecologist from Johns Hopkins Hospital, was the first to clearly describe the condition of interstitial cystitis in two classical manuscripts published in 1915 and 1918.[12] In these papers he discussed the clinical presentation, diagnosis, etiology, pathology, and treatment. He also gave a very clear description of the findings using an early cystoscope pioneered by Kelly in the knee-chest position. However, many clinicians have criticized Hunner's description. In 1977, Walsh stated that, 'The ulcers Hunner originally described were secondary to optic deficiency of early cystoscopes.'[13] Messing and Stamey stated 'we believe that the synonymity of Hunner's ulcer with interstitial cystitis has done more to prevent recognition of this disease than any other single factor.'[2]

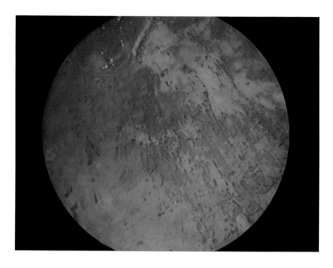

Figure 8.1
Hunner's ulcer. Whitish necrotic bladder mucosa and mucosal tearing surrounded by various degrees of erythematous bladder mucosa and petechial hemorrhages. See Hunner's descriptions in the text.

However Hunner's original descriptions of his cystoscopic findings[12] read well alongside cystoscopic pictures using modern endoscopic equipment:[1]

'The crucial test in cystoscopy is the finding of a small abrasion on the mucosa surface which, if not bleeding on discovery, will easily bleed on being touched.' (Figure 8.1)

'Occasionally the distention of the bladder by air as the patient assumes the knee-breast posture causes this area to split and a tiny stream of blood flows to the vertex.' (Figure 8.2)

'The ulcer is usually found in the vertex or free portion of the bladder.' (Figure 8.3)

'On cystoscopy one's attention is not infrequently first arrested by a glazed, dead, white appearance of a portion of the bladder mucosa.' (Figure 8.4)

'One may see a dead white scar area with a small congested area in the immediate neighbourhood and while one is examining this area the congestion becomes marked and may even begin to ooze blood.' (Figure 8.5)

In clinical practice today, cystoscopy is performed at some time in the work-up of most patients presenting with bladder pain, frequency, and urgency. The aim of cystoscopy is to exclude other conditions, positively diagnose interstitial cystitis, and record the extent of changes such as fissuring or ulceration, glomerulations, and bladder capacity, and to provide a therapeutic benefit by

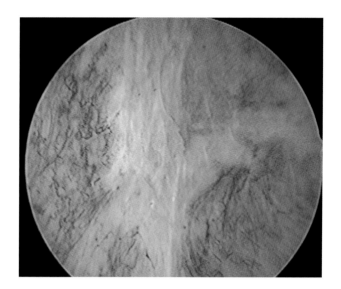

Figure 8.2
Hunner's ulcer. See Hunner's descriptions in the text.

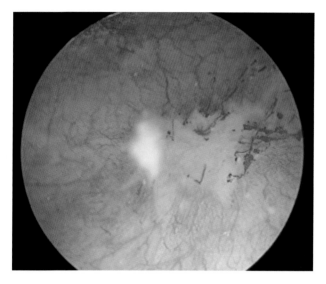

Figure 8.4
Hunner's ulcer. See Hunner's descriptions in the text.

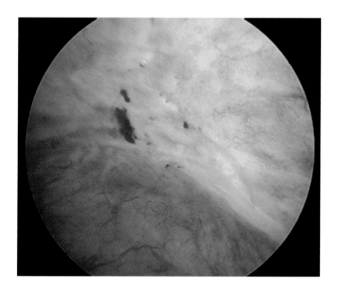

Figure 8.3
Hunner's ulcer. See Hunner's descriptions in the text.

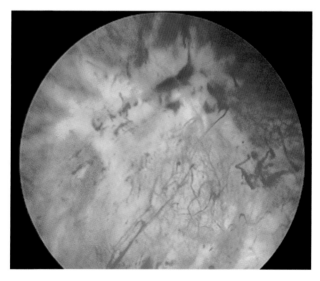

Figure 8.5
Hunner's ulcer. See Hunner's descriptions in the text.

hydrodistention.[4] Therefore, cystoscopy is usually be performed under anesthesia. The usual bladder discomfort experienced by these patients means that cystoscopy under local anesthesia gives limited information and is often counterproductive.

It is important to perform cystoscopy early in clinical situations of microscopic hematuria, abnormal cytology, sterile pyuria, or previous bladder or continence surgery where a foreign body may be present. A reasonable approach is that cystoscopy should be performed in the setting of severe symptoms or a lack of response to conservative therapies such as amitriptyline, simple analgesia, and physical therapies. It seems logical to perform cystoscopy before any intravesical therapy.

The anesthetist can often make the diagnosis of bladder pain syndrome by noting the discomfort during bladder hydrodistention which results in tachycardia and deep breathing. A rigid cystoscope is often used to allow for adequate biopsies. The filling medium ought to be glycine or water to allow for coagulation of biopsy sites if necessary

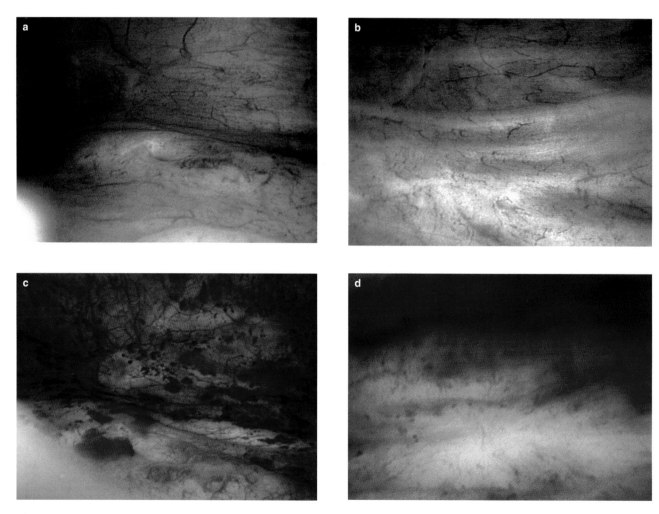

Figure 8.6
Cytoscopic photographs of a 25-year-old women with severe frequency, urgency, and bladder discomfort at the start of filling (a), at capacity of 400 m/s (b), during emptying (c), and towards the end of emptying when the urine is heavily bloodstained (d). Note the normality of the bladder mucosa during filling and widespread petechial hemorrhages during bladder emptying.

and should be placed 80–100 cm above the symphysis pubis with only gravity to aid filling. The bladder should be filled until the infusion fluid stops dripping, and sometimes the urethra needs to be occluded at the same time. The distention ought to be maintained for 2–3 minutes. Inspect the bladder during filling for fissuring, old scars, increased vascularity, and mucosal abnormalities, although in many cases the mucosa has a normal appearance. It is not until the bladder is emptied under vision that petechial hemorrhage (Figure 8.6) will be seen, usually in all quadrants except for the trigone (Figure 8.7). If pronounced, these hemorrhages can result in cascade bleeding (Figure 8.8) and a complete 'red-out' with gross terminal hematuria. On bladder refilling, visualization is more difficult, although 'splotchy' hemorrhages adjacent to bladder vessels can be seen (Figure 8.9).

The NIDDK criteria[3] stated that for a positive diagnosis of IC either glomerulations or a classic Hunner's ulcer were required in the presence of bladder pain or urgency. The glomerulations needed to be diffuse; at least 10 glomerlations per quadrant needed to be present in at least three quadrants.

The IC database group attempted to score the severity of glomerulations:[14]

- 0 = none or due to trauma
- 1 + = fewer than 3–5 per cystoscope field when held at 1 cm in focal areas only
- 2 + = either the above in a diffuse pattern or a greater density per scope field in a focal pattern
- 3 + = more than 5 glomerulations per cystoscope field over most of the bladder

The European group[5] have proposed the following classification for glomerulations at cystoscopy:

- grade 0 = normal mucosa
- grade I = petechiae in at least 2 quadrants
- grade II = large submucosal bleeding

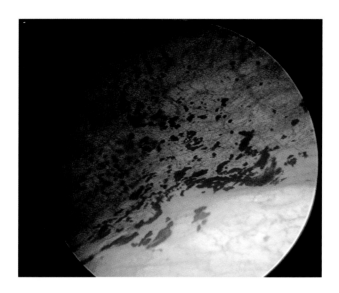

Figure 8.7
Right ureteric orifice and trigone in lower right corner with few petechial hemorrhages compared with petechial hemorrhages on surrounding lateral bladder wall.

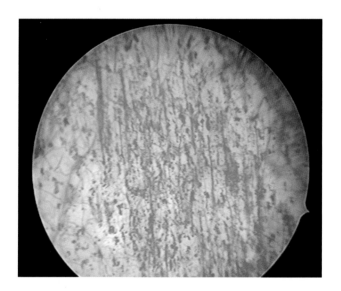

Figure 8.8
Petechial hemorrhages cascading from bladder dome.

- grade III = diffuse global mucosal bleeding
- grade IV = mucosal disruption with or without bleeding

The findings can be described and mapped in the anterior, posterior, lateral walls, and fundus, or dome. These changes can be recorded to dramatic effect with a series of images or a digital movie of the cystoscopic findings. Care needs to be taken in interpretation of artifacts: e.g. trauma

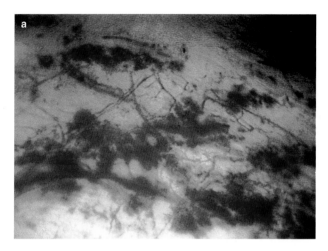

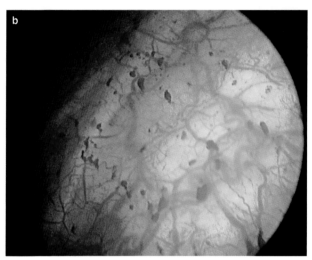

Figure 8.9(a,b)
Closer cystoscopic view of bladder vasculature and 'splotchy hemorrhages' post-bladder distention.

caused by introduction of the cystoscope and old biopsy sites (Figure 8.10). The volume of fluid emptied is measured as the cystoscopic capacity and the presence of terminal hematuria noted. This process can be repeated. If a biopsy is to be taken, the bladder should be filled only to one-third to one-half of the capacity in order to visualize the urothelium and allow the biopsy to be taken safely.

The cystoscopic findings most often associated with classical descriptions of IC are a Hunner's ulcer, described as patches of red mucosa exhibiting small vessels radiating to a central pale scar or fissure (Figure 8.11), and glomerulations, which are petechial hemorrhages (often with cascade bleeding) that can be seen during bladder emptying after hydrodistention (Figure 8.12). The cystoscopic capacity may often be reduced, in particular associated with ulceration or fissuring.[8]

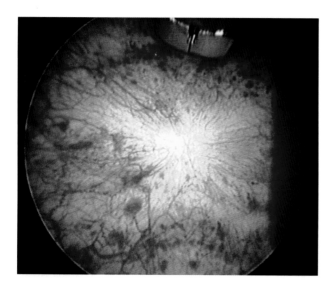

Figure 8.10
Old biopsy site with radiating fibrosis, which can be mistaken for Hunner's ulcer.

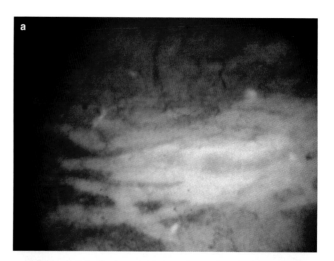

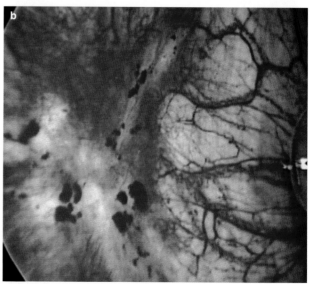

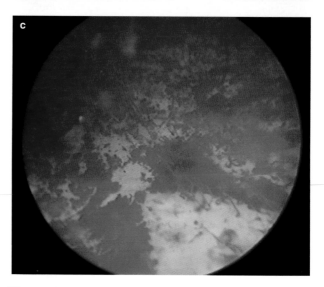

There are uncertainties about these cystoscopic features. The diagnosis of Hunner's ulcer varies between 6 and 50% in different series of IC patients.[8] Some of this discrepancy may be due to a real difference in the patient population, but some is due to the subjective nature of the diagnosis. Glomerulations are most likely a reflection of a chronically underdistended bladder and not specific to IC. Not all patients with symptoms of IC have glomerulations and not all patients with glomerulations have symptoms of PBS/IC.

There are a few papers that address the correlation between cytoscopic findings and symptoms or prognosis. The IC database had less stringent entry criteria compared with the NIDDK research definition, with 9% of patients having a normal cystoscopy.[15] In over 200 women a detailed symptom, urodynamic, and cystoscopic examination found an association between the presence of increased pain and a Hunner's patch (seen in 11%), and increased urgency with small (<400 ml) bladder capacity, which was seen in 6%. The study found no correlation between the severity of pain or urgency with the absence, presence, or density of glomerulations. Furthermore, a follow-up paper compared women whose cystoscopic appearance met NIDDK criteria and those who did not, and found a reduced median bladder capacity under anesthesia and increased daytime frequency and nocturia in the NIDDK group but no other differences.[16]

Bladder biopsy

There is much variation between papers that address IC and pathology, including the definition of what constitutes

Figure 8.11
(a,b) Hunner's ulcer. Mucosal tearing and ulceration surrounded by erythematous mucosa on the bladder dome at the end of bladder filling. (c) Widespread derse petechial bleeding except for the trigone in the lower right corner.

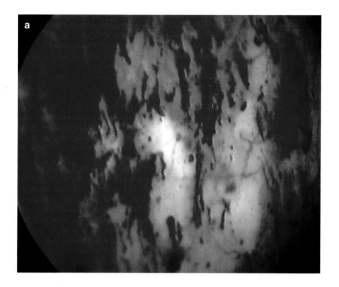

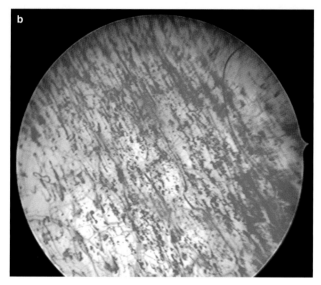

Figure 8.12(a,b)
Cascade bleeding from the bladder dome following cystodistention when the bladder is being emptied.

IC, how and where bladder biopsy is taken, how the biopsy is treated in terms of fixation and staining, which histological criteria are analyzed, differences in the inclusion of control subjects, and the type of control subject.[4] There is large international variation in the practice of bladder biopsy in IC, with Europe and Japan commonly performing biopsy. On the other hand, in the United States, the IC database study had an overall biopsy rate of 33% (range 9–64%).[15] The potential reasons to perform a biopsy in IC would be to confirm the diagnosis of IC, to exclude other conditions, if there were a prognostic or therapeutic value, and for research purposes. The potential benefit of these indications would have to be weighed up against complications and costs.

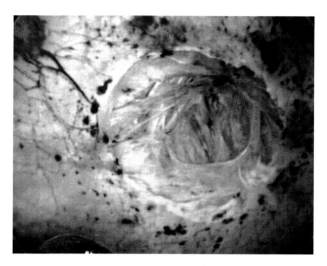

Figure 8.13
Cold-cup biopsy of bladder wall revealing underlying detrusor muscle.

The most common type of biopsy is a cold-cup biopsy from the most involved portion of the bladder. Even these biopsies may be quite deep and the bladder wall at times seems more friable (Figure 8.13), so we sometimes use postoperative short-term catheter drainage for deep biopsies. Also the post-cystoscopy insertion of intravesical bupivacaine local anesthesia may lower postoperative pain. The ESSIC group propose taking three biopsies, but there is not widespread consensus regarding the number of sites which ought to be sampled (www.essic).

Histopathology

The case for pathological confirmation of IC is strongest for the classic disease as defined by either a Hunner's ulcer or low anesthetic capacity. The most commonly reported histological changes in classic IC include epithelial ulceration or denudation, submucosal inflammation, granulation tissue formation, edema, congestion, hemorrhage, detrusor fibrosis, increased epithelial, submucosal, and detrusor mast cell number and activation, and increased neuronal staining (Figure 8.14a). Mast cells have been suggested to be important in the etiology of IC and a marker of severity, being increased more frequently in women with ulceration. They contain many granules (Figure 8.14b,c) which contain vasoactive and nociceptive chemicals; their increased presence in the detrusor muscle is thought to be of more significance than in the submucosa. Their significance in IC awaits further elucidation.

Early IC is generally characterized by normal or near-normal bladder capacity under anesthesia and glomerulations. Light microscopy findings range from mucosal

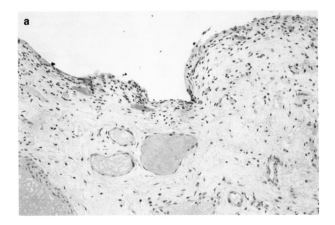

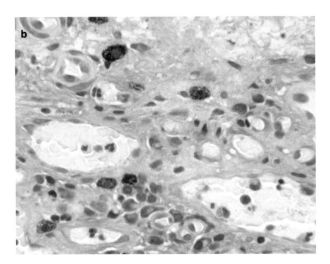

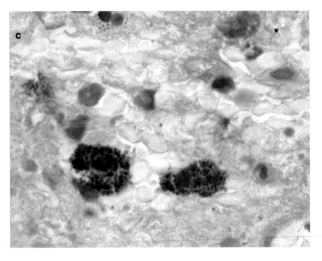

Figure 8.14
Histology of Hunner's ulcer. Loss of urothelium, submucosal inflammation with edema, congestion, and hemorrhage.
(b,c) Mast cells in the submucosa and detrusor muscle of a bladder biopsy of a woman with IC. Stain is with toluidine blue in low (b) and high (c) magnification of mast cells with many granules.

ruptures, submucosal hemorrhage, and mild inflammation in transurethral resection biopsies to normal histology in forceps biopsies approximately half the time. In other words, in the clinical setting of early IC, bladder forceps biopsy pathology may be normal and is not therefore useful as a confirmatory test.[4]

Therefore, the biopsy can be useful in confirming IC but usually in the clinical setting of severe disease. Urine cytology should be mandatory in the population at risk of malignancy but this would not include women under 40 years old. There is also the possibility of false-negative cytology, so that biopsy has an important role if malignancy is suspected. There are the rare occasions where other diagnoses such as eosinophilic cystitis are made. Biopsy remains an optional test in the diagnostic work-up of IC.

Management

General principles

Patient education, including an overview of management options, is the first step in management. Symptom reduction should be the goal of therapy as there is no evidence for disease progression. The natural history of the condition is that the symptoms often plateau or decrease to baseline level with varying flare-ups or fluctuations.

Information should be given that PBS/IC is a non-progressive, non-malignant condition and there are many treatment options, including expectant management. A large number of self-help strategies, natural therapies, and conservative and surgical options are available, which means that patients feel they have greater control and choice with regard to their own treatment path.

The Interstitial Cystitis Association (www.ichelp.org) and its affiliated international organizations are an important resource for patients, researchers, and clinicians[6] but can sometimes overwhelm the highly anxious patient.

Behavioral modification

A 1-day voiding chart gives both patient and clinician some objective measure of symptom severity and forms the basis of bladder re-education. Bladder training has been shown to increase voided volumes and improve frequency; however, the persistent sense of bladder fullness may still be a problem. Patients who experience pain more than frequency would be unlikely to tolerate bladder training as the sole intervention.

Physical therapy

Pelvic floor physical therapy is considered to have a place in the management of functional pelvic and perineal syndromes but there are no published randomized controlled trials (RCTs) to support this in IC. Biofeedback and soft tissue massage may aid in muscle relaxation of the pelvic floor. Some small uncontrolled series have reported success rates by varying techniques such as direct myofascial release, joint mobilization and home exercise program, transvaginal Theile massage, and electromyographic biofeedback. One of the few randomized placebo-controlled studies performed to assess this type of therapy in IC compared transdermal laser stimulation of the posterior tibial nerve to sham stimulation and found no difference between active and sham treatments.[17]

Dietary manipulation

A proportion of interstitial cystitis patients have symptom exacerbation related to the intake of specific foods and beverages and relief with the intake of urinary alkalinizers, increased water or milk. Most often, the exacerbating items are caffeinated, alcoholic, or citrus beverages or spicy foods.

Oral therapy

Interstitial cystitis/painful bladder syndrome is an extremely difficult condition in which to follow results of therapy. The disease tends to fluctuate in severity and up to 50% of patients experience temporary remissions unrelated to therapy for an average duration of 8 months.[18] Most therapies for IC have been associated with very promising initial results followed by either no or much reduced benefit when analyzed in a randomized placebo-controlled double-blind trial. It is crucial to take into account the placebo effect, which can be of the order of 30%.

During the 3rd International Consultation on Incontinence, the published literature with regard to treatment for interstitial cystitis was summarized based on the Oxford levels of evidence for specific treatment modalities for interstitial cystitis.[4] The four grades from the Oxford system are:

- grade A recommendation, which relies on level 1 evidence such as meta-analysis or good-quality RCTs
- grade B, which relies on level 2 (low-quality RCTs, good-quality cohort studies) or level 3 (case-control studies or case series) evidence
- grade C, based on majority or expert opinion
- grade D, where no recommendation is possible.[4]

All of the treatment options described below have grade B evidence apart from heparin, which is grade C.

Sodium pentosan polysulfate (Elmiron)

Sodium pentosan polysulfate (PPS) or Elmiron is a heparin analogue available in an oral formulation. The mechanism of action in IC is attributed to correction of a possible defect in the GAG layer, the ability to inhibit histamine release from mast cells, and a possible binding with inflammatory mediators in the urine. PPS has Food and Drug Administration (FDA) approval for the treatment of the pain of interstitial cystitis.

The studies for the FDA found 'more than slight improvement' in 28% with Elmiron treatment vs 13% with placebo.[19] This was followed by a study where 50% or more overall improvement was reported in 32% of the Elmiron group compared with 16% of the placebo group.[20] Elmiron is a well-tolerated medication and is efficacious in improving the pain of interstitial cystitis in up to one-third of patients, often requiring a 3–6-month treatment duration to see an effect.

Amitriptyline

Amitriptyline has become one of the most commonly used treatments for IC.[21] The only prospective, double-blind, placebo-controlled RCT of 50 patients showed a greater than 30% decrease in O'Leary–Sant symptom and problem scores at 4 months in 42% of the amitriptyline (up to 100 mg daily) vs 13% of the placebo group.[22] One-quarter of patients in a trial setting were unable to tolerate the sedation accompanying 75 mg amitriptyline daily.

Analgesics

Medications commonly used for chronic neuropathic pain syndromes can be used for IC, including antidepressants, anticonvulsants, non-steroidal anti-inflammatory drugs (NSAIDs), and antispasmodics. Opiates in this chronic pain state are most safely incorporated in the patient's treatment in the setting of a multidisciplinary pain clinic, which allows for regular reassessment.[23] Gabapentin has also been used in this setting, but no studies have been reported.

Intravesical therapy
Dimethyl sulfoxide

Until 1996, dimethyl sulfoxide (DMSO) was the only drug approved by the FDA for use in IC. It is a chemical solvent with anti-inflammatory, analgesic, muscle relaxant, mast cell inhibition, and collagen dissolution properties.[24] DMSO can be administered as single therapy or in combination with heparin, steroids, and a local anesthetic as a cocktail. The treatment regimens vary to suit the convenience of patient and therapist but once- or twice-weekly instillation for 8–12 treatments is commonly used. A response rate to DMSO of 50–90% has been reported,[25] with a relapse rate of up to 40%; however, three-quarters will respond to further DMSO. Adverse effects include a garlic-like breath odor and taste, and transient bladder irritability due to a chemical cystitis in 10% of patients. DMSO is cheap, has relatively few side effects, and self-instillation can be taught if required.

Heparin

Two clinical uncontrolled studies of intravesical heparin, 5000 units twice weekly, have been reported and show improvement in bladder symptoms.[26]

Surgery

Surgical options should be considered only when all conservative treatment has failed. The consequences of surgical intervention such as voiding dysfunction and the possibility of persistent pain and repeat surgery should be discussed. Surgical excision of ulcers is performed usually with short-term benefit only. Intravesical botulinum toxin for IC has been described, but information based on prospective randomized studies is not yet available.

Sacral neuromodulation consists of a two-stage procedure involving temporary or percutaneous sacral S3 or S4 root stimulation followed by permanent implantation in responders. Comiter reported a series of 17 of 25 patients with refractory IC with sustained effect on pain and frequency.[27] Peters and Konstandt reported a series of 21 IC patients: 20 patients reported moderate or marked improvement at 15 months follow-up with a one-third reduction in narcotic use.[28] Sacral nerve modulation is a promising surgical treatment for PBS/IC; however, more information is needed on long-term follow-up, adverse events, and reoperation rates. More recently described methods of neuromodulation, such as pudendal neuromodulation or paraurethral stimulation,[29] need to be assessed more fully.

Bladder augmentation or cystoplasty has been used for refractory IC/PBS for many years. First reports of ileocystoplasty were very good, but later publications were variable, with good results varying from 25% up to 100%.[30,31] Total cystectomy and urethrectomy is the ultimate option with simple or continent urinary diversion.[32]

References

1. Hunner GL. A rare type of bladder ulcer. Further notes with a report of eighteen cases. JAMA 1918; 70: 40.
2. Messing EM, Stamey TA. Interstitial cystitis, early diagnosis, pathology and treatment. Urology 1978; 12: 381–392.
3. Gillenwater JY, Wein AJ. Summary of the National Institute of Arthritis, Diabetes, Digestive and Kidney Diseases workshop on interstitial cystitis, National Institutes of Health, Bethesda, Maryland, August 28–29, 1987. J Urol 1988; 140: 203–6.
4. Hanno P, Baranowski A, Fall M et al. Painful bladder syndrome (including interstitial cystitis). In Abrams P, Cardozo L, Khoury S, Wein A, eds. 3rd International Consultation. on Incontinence. Health Publication, 2005.
5. Rosamilia A, Cann L, Scurry J, Rogers P, Dwyer PL. Bladder microvasculature and the effect of hydrodistention in interstitial cystis. Urology 2001; 57: 132.
6. Pontari MA, Hanno PM, Ruggieri MR. Comparison of bladder blood flow in patients with and without interstitial cystitis. J Urol 1999; 162: 330–4.
7. Nordling J, Anjum FH, Bade JJ et al. Primary evaluation of patients suspected of having interstitial cystitis. Eur Urol 2004; 45: 662–9.
8. Rosamilia A. Painful bladder syndrome/interstitial cystitis. Best Pract Res Clin Obstet Gynaecol 2005; 19: 843–9.
9. O'Leary MP, Sant GR, Fowler FJ Jr et al. The interstitial cystitis symptom index and problem index. Urology 1997; 49: 58–63.
10. Parsons CL, Dell J, Stanford EJ et al. Increased prevalence of interstitial cystitis: previously unrecognized urologic and gynecologic cases identified using a new symptom questionnaire and intravesical potassium sensitivity. Urology 2002; 60: 573–8.
11. Parsons C. Potassium sensitivity test. Tech Urol 1996; 2: 171.
12. Hunner GL. Elusive ulcer of the bladder: further notes on a rare type of bladder ulcer with a report of 25 cases. Am J Obstet 1918; 78: 374–95.
13. Walsh A. Interstitial cystitis. Observations on diagnosis and on treatment with anti-inflammatory drugs, particularly benzydamine. Eur Urol 1977; 3: 216–17.
14. Messing E, Pauk D, Schaeffer A et al. Associations among cystoscopic findings and symptoms and physical examination findings in women enrolled in the Interstitial Cystitis Data Base (ICDB) Study. Urology 1997; 49 (Suppl 5A): 81–5.
15. Tomaszewski JE, Landis J, Russack V et al. Biopsy features are associated with primary symptoms in interstitial cystitis: results from the interstitial cystitis database study. Urology 2001; 57: 67–81.
16. Erickson DR, Tomaszewski JE, Kunselman AR et al. Do the National Institute of Diabetes and Digestive and Kidney Diseases cystoscopic criteria associate with other clinical and objective features of interstitial cystitis? J Urol 2005; 173(1): 93–7.
17. O'Reilly BA, Dwyer PL, Hawthorne G et al. Transdermal posterior tibial nerve laser therapy is not effective in women with interstitial cystitis. J Urol 2004; 172(5 Pt 1): 1880–3.
18. Hanno PM, Landis JR, Matthews-Cook Y, Kusek J, Nyberg L Jr and The Interstitial Cystitis Database Study Group. The diagnosis of interstitial cystitis revisited: lessons learned from the National Institutes of Health Interstitial Cystitis Database Study. J Urol 1999; 161: 553–7.
19. Mulholland SG, Hanno P, Parsons CL et al. Pentosan polysulfate sodium for therapy of interstitial cystitis. A double-blind placebo-controlled clinical study. Urology 1990; 35: 552–8.
20. Rovner E, Propert KJ, Brensinger C et al. Treatments used in women with interstitial cystitis: the interstitial cystitis data base (ICDB) study experience. The Interstitial Cystitis Data Base Study Group. Urology 2000; 56: 940–5.

21. Parsons CL, Benson G, Childs SJ et al. A quantitatively controlled method to study prospectively interstitial cystitis and demonstrate the efficacy of pentosanpolysulfate. J Urol 1993; 150: 845–8.

22. van Ophoven A, Pokupic S, Heinecke A et al. A prospective, randomized, placebo controlled, double-blind study of amitriptyline for the treatment of interstitial cystitis. J Urol 2004; 172: 533–6.

23. Brookoff D. The causes and treatment of pain in interstitial cystitis. In: Sant GR, ed. Interstitial Cystitis. Philadelphia, PA: Lippincott-Raven, 1997: 177.

24. Sant GR, LaRock DR. Standard intravesical therapies for interstitial cystitis. Urol Clin North Am 1994; 21: 73–83.

25. Perez-Marrero R, Emerson LE, Feltis JT. A controlled study of dimethyl sulfoxide in interstitial cystitis. J Urol 1988; 140: 36–9.

26. Parsons CL, Housley T, Schmidt JD, Lebow D. Treatment of interstitial cystitis with intravesical heparin. Br J Urol 1994; 73: 504–7.

27. Comiter CV. Sacral neuromodulation for the symptomatic treatment of refractory interstitial cystitis: a prospective study. J Urol 2003; 169: 1369–73.

28. Peters KM, Konstandt D. Sacral neuromodulation decreases narcotic requirements in refractory interstitial cystitis. BJU Int 2004; 93(6): 777–9.

29. De Jong P, Radziszewski P, Dobronski P et al. Pelvic floor electrostimulation in patients with interstitial cystitis; a multicenter clinical investigation. Int Urogynecol J 2005; 16(Suppl 2) Abstract 51.

30. Nielsen KK, Kromann-Andersen B, Steven K et al. Failure of combined supratrigonal cystectomy and Mainz ileocecocystoplasty in intractable interstitial cystitis: is histology and mast cell count a reliable predictor for the outcome of surgery? J Urol 1990; 144: 255.

31. Webster GD, Maggio MI. The management of chronic interstitial cystitis by substitution cystoplasty. J Urol 1989; 141: 287–91.

32. Lotenfoe RR, Christie J, Parsons A et al. Absence of neuropathic pelvic pain and favorable psychological profile in the surgical selection of patients with disabling interstitial cystitis. J Urol 1995; 154: 2039–42.

9

Non-neoplastic abnormalities of the bladder

Peter L Dwyer

Introduction

In this chapter, non-neoplastic abnormalities of the bladder will be reviewed. Some of these conditions, such as bladder trabeculation, will be commonly seen during diagnostic cystoscopy, either as part of another procedure or in women with urinary symptoms; other conditions, such as ureteroceles and calculi, will be less often seen. Ureteroceles, is a ballooning of the distal ureter and not strictly a bladder abnormality, present to the cystoscopist as an intravesical distention at the ureteric orifice and, therefore, are a category placed in this chapter. All these conditions can be misdiagnosed or have inappropriate treatment that can cause significant ongoing morbidity for the patient and a loss of face and medicolegal problems for the doctor.

Lower urinary tract calculi

In most Western countries, primary bladder calculi are rare in women with normal lower urinary tracts, but they do occur in Pakistan, India, and the Middle Eastern countries where a low-protein, high-carbohydrate diet and chronic dehydration predispose to endemic stones.[1] Calculi in women in industrial countries occur predominantly as a result of structural or functional abnormality of the lower urinary tract.[1,2] Bladder calculi need a nidus to grow, and can develop as an encrustation on foreign bodies such as suture material (Figure 9.1), synthetic slings (Figure 9.2), and remnants of catheters. They also can occur secondary to stasis and infection, developing in bladder diverticulae (Figure 9.3), or in women with ureteroceles (Figure 9.4), outlet obstruction, and bladder trabeculation. Calculi have also been reported in women with vesicovaginal fistulae,[3] as a result of migration of an intrauterine device into the bladder,[4] and in women with severe vaginal prolapse[5] and outlet obstruction. Women who have undergone bladder surgery such as vesicovaginal fistula repair (see Figure 9.3) or bladder augmentation procedures are at increased risk of developing calculi even in the absence of intravesical

suture fragments or other foreign bodies. Less commonly, bladder calculi can originate in the kidney. Other possible inciting factors may be poor fluid intake, a diet with high protein, calcium, phosphate, or oxalate intake, and metabolic disorders resulting in increased calcium, cystine, and uric acid urinary excretion. Urinary tract infection (UTI) can occur as a result of calculi, although urinary infection can contribute to stone formation. Bacteria, particularly urea-splitting organisms such as *Proteus*, *Klebsiella*, *Serratia*, and *Enterobacter* spp., produce an alkaline urine which promotes stone formation (struvite or infection stone). *Proteus mirabilis* contains the enzyme 'urease', which breaks urea to ammonia and causes intense alkalinization of the urine, with precipitation of calcium, magnesium, ammonium, and phosphate salts and the subsequent formation of branched struvite renal stones.

The composition of bladder calculi is struvite or calcium oxalate, with or without phosphate, magnesium ammonium phosphate, uric acid, and cystine in order of prevalence.[1]

Urethral calculi are usually associated with urethral diverticulum or occasionally foreign bodies. Calculus formation is encouraged by the stasis of urine, and the build-up of cellular debris (Figure 9.5) and infection within the diverticulum. Treatment is surgical excision of the diverticulum with removal of the calculus.

Clinical presentation

Bladder calculi may be asymptomatic or cause dull bladder pain even in the absence of infection. Symptoms are urinary frequency, urgency, hematuria, and painful voiding (strangury) when the stone contacts the inflamed bladder wall at the end of micturition especially when the surface of the calculus is roughened and irregular (Figure 9.6). Recurrent UTI that responds poorly to conventional antibiotic therapy should alert the clinician to the possibility of a bladder stone. Women presenting with irritable bladder symptoms or recurrent infection, occurring for the first

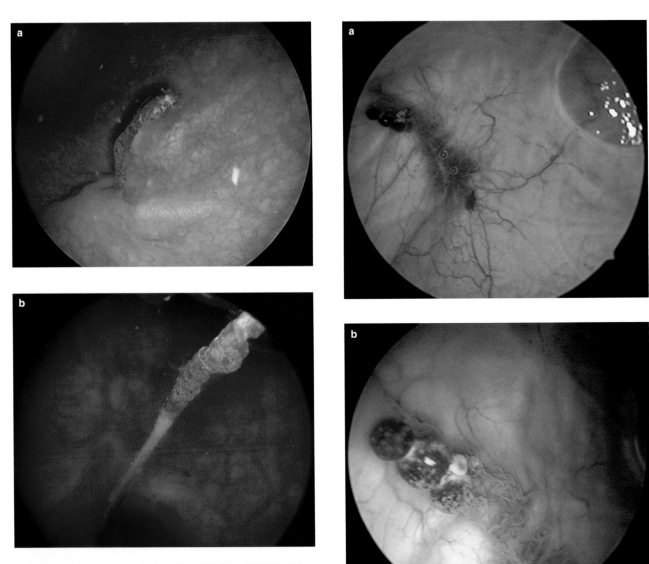

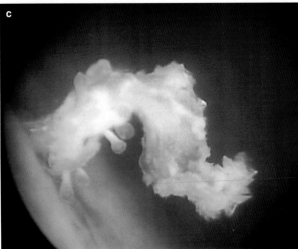

Figure 9.1
(a) Braided nylon Ethibond suture through the base of the bladder following Burch colposuspension. (b) Note early encrustation and calculi formation on suture, which has been partly pulled through bladder mucosa. (c) Another Ethibond suture with encrustation and calculi formation.

Figure 9.2
A tension-free vaginal tape (TVT) midurethral sling penetrated the bladder wall at 11 o'clock through the bladder dome; note the bubble on the bladder dome. (b) A closer view of encrustation on the TVT sling.

time following stress incontinence surgery using nonabsorbable sutures or synthetic slings, should have early cystourethroscopy to exclude the possibility of intravesical perforation or erosion and stone formation.

Diagnosis and management

Cystoscopic examination of the lower urinary tract will usually confirm the presence of any calculi and will allow

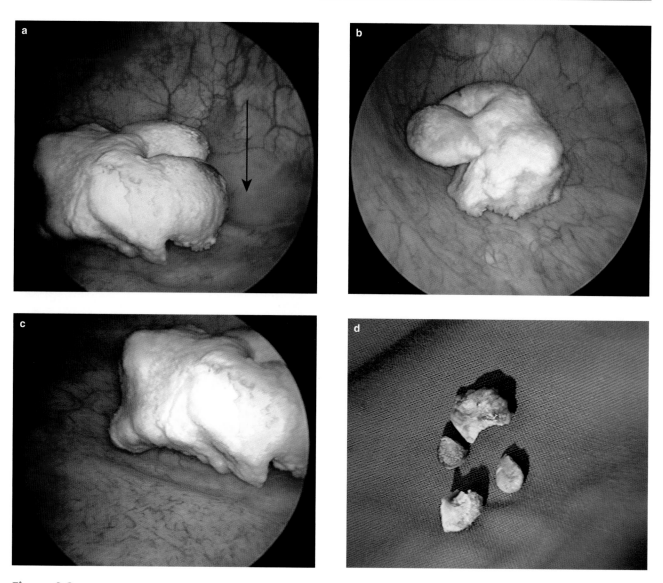

Figure 9.3
(a) Intravesical calculus in a woman who had a previous vesicovaginal fistular repair; note diverticulum (arrow). (b) Calculus. (c) Calculus on bladder base next to right ureteric orifice. (d) Following removal with lithoclast forceps.

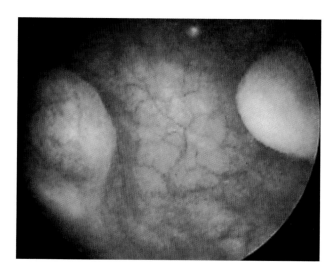

Figure 9.4
Woman with right ureterocele and left-sided bladder calculus.

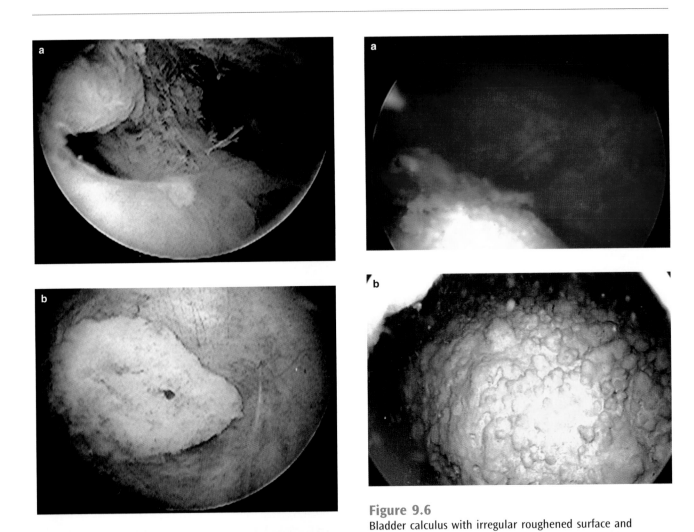

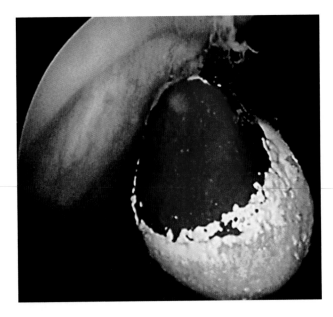

Figure 9.5
(a) Urethral diverticulum with (b) tissue debris and early calcification at diverticulum base. (c) Multiple small calculi seen with a urethroscope in a necrotic urethral diverticulum.

Figure 9.6
Bladder calculus with irregular roughened surface and inflamed mucosa (a), and filling most of bladder (b).

Figure 9.7
Bladder calculus hanging by an Ethibond suture in a woman with a recurrent UTI and previous Burch colposuspension.

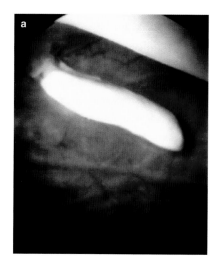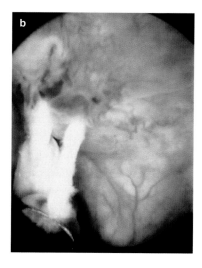

Figure 9.8(a,b)
Calculus on permanent suture post-Burch colposuspension, (b) removed with biopsy forceps.

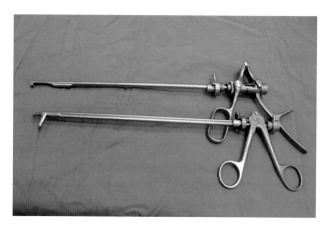

Figure 9.9
Lithoclast forceps.

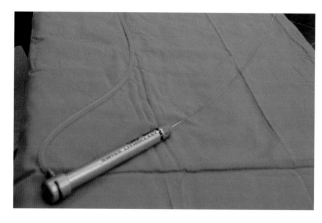

Figure 9.10
A Swiss electrohydraulic lithotripsy probe can be inserted under cystoscopic vision into the bladder through the axillary channel to break up the calculus.

removal of the stone and any associated foreign body. Intravesical sutures occurring as a result of a Burch colposuspension or Marshall–Marchetti–Krantz procedure are usually found above the bladder neck at 1 and 11 o'clock with a 70° cystoscope[6] (Figure 9.7). It is also in this area that perforation of a tension-free vaginal tape (TVT) and other minimally invasive retropubic slings occur (see Figure 9.2a). Transobturator tapes can also inadvertently penetrate the lower urinary tract and are usually found in the urethra or bladder neck area. Calculi adherent to sutures or sling can be removed by grasping forceps (Figure 9.8). If the calculus is large, fragmentation (cystolithola-paxy) usually occurs relatively easily with grasping lithoclast forceps (Figure 9.9). Ultrasonic, electrohydraulic, pneumatic (Figure 9.10), or laser lithotripsy probes can be inserted under cystoscopic vision through the axillary channel into the bladder to break up the calculus, and the fragments removed with grasping or basket forceps. The pneumatic lithoclast was found to be more efficient than ultrasonic or electrohydraulic lithotripsy for large or particularly hard stones.[1] Other surgical options for large stones are percutaneous or open cystolithotomy. Any suture material or synthetic sling should also be removed either by grasping forceps or with scissors cutting the suture material or sling flush with the bladder mucosa. Calculi of different composition may fragment with different degrees of success, calcium oxalate dihydrate, struvite, and uric acid calculi being the easiest to fragment. Women with bladder calculi can also be managed successfully with external shock-wave lithotripsy, which is usually applied in the prone position under ultrasonic guidance or fluoroscopy. This procedure is contraindicated in women during the reproductive years, because the shock-wave energy can damage the ovaries. Moreover, this procedure is relatively contraindicated in patients with huge stones or with bladder outlet obstruction, because retained fragments necessitate multiple endoscopic ancillary procedures to achieve stone-free status.[7]

Plain X-ray films of the kidney, ureter, and bladder will reveal the number, position, and size of radiopaque calculi.

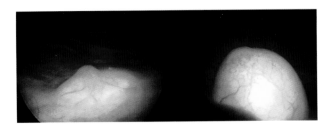

Figure 9.11
Left-sided ureterocele before and after ureteric contraction.

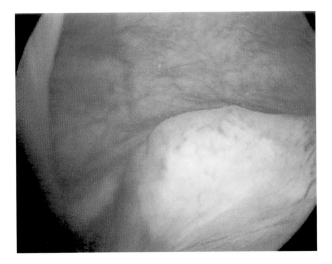

Figure 9.12
Right ureterocele.

Calculi that contain calcium are radiopaque, with calcium phosphate (apartite) stones followed by calcium oxalate calculi, the most radiodense. Magnesium ammonium phosphate (struvite) is less radiopaque and pure uric acid stones are radiolucent. Ultrasonic imaging may reveal radiolucent stones and can detect hydronephrosis and ureteric dilation and confirm the presence of ureteric patency by visualization of ureteric jets. However, the gold-standard diagnostic tool for urolithiasis is non-contrast computed tomography (NCCT), which is more sensitive and specific than any other imaging modality. Other investigations which may be appropriate are urine analysis and culture, and blood chemical profile, including calcium, uric acid, electrolytes, and creatinine and urea levels.

Ureteroceles

A ureterocele is a cystic dilatation of the terminal ureter and a ballooning of the intravesical submucosal ureter (Figures 9.11 and 9.12). Ureteroceles are thought to be developmental abnormalities that lead to stenosis of the ureteric orifice.[8] Not surprisingly, ureteroceles often have associated congenital abnormality, including duplex upper urinary tracts, and frequently present to the pediatric urologist in childhood with obstruction, urinary infection, incontinence, or impaired renal function. Adult women diagnosed with ureterocele usually have a single system upper urinary tract which has some degree of proximal dilatation and is bilateral in 10% of cases (Figure 9.13a). Most simple ureteroceles have obstructing pinpoint orifices, although unobstructed ureteroceles do occur.[8] The commonest presentation to the gynecologist would be as an asymptomatic finding on cystoscopy performed as part of another procedure or less commonly for investigation of urinary incontinence, voiding difficulty, or urinary tract infection. The incidence of bladder calculi is increased in women with ureteroceles (see Figure 9.4). A calculus may form inside the ureterocele, aggravated by stasis and infection inside the 'ballooning' ureterocele, resulting in chronic dilatation and atrophy of the ureteral wall. Ureteroceles vary in size from a small 1 cm swelling to a large balloon-shaped mass that fills the bladder. If large, they may cause urethral obstruction and incontinence. The stenotic ureteroceles have a narrowed orifice on the dome of the intravesical mass which swells rhythmically with each ureteric peristalsis and then deflates as urine dribbles through the stenosed ureteric orifice (Figure 9.13a–d). On intravenous pyelography, the typical cobra head deformity is seen, the radiodense contrast material surrounded by the radiotranslucent ureterocele wall with varying degrees of hydroureter and hydronephrosis (Figure 9.14). On ultrasound imaging, a filling defect will be seen in the bladder.

Once the diagnosis has been made, referral to a urologist would be appropriate. In an asymptomatic adult, treatment of the ureterocele involves little more than regular review. If symptomatic, adult ureteroceles are frequently amenable to endoscopic incision[9] or transvesical excision and ureteric reimplantation.

Endometriosis of the bladder

Vesical endometriosis is rare and accounts for only 1% of all cases of endometriosis. In 12% of patients with bladder endometriosis, there is no evidence of extravesical endometriosis.[10] Clinically, endometriosis of the bladder may present with irritable bladder symptoms, cyclical hematuria, or an anterior vaginal wall mass that enlarges with menstruation, suggestive of a rapidly growing tumor.[11] Endometriosis can also involve the ureters and cause unilateral and bilateral obstruction. The cystoscopic appearance is that of blue, brown, or red-black cysts or a cystic mass (Figure 11.18). Radiographically, bladder endometriosis manifests as submucosal masses with characteristic magnetic resonance imaging (MRI) features consisting of

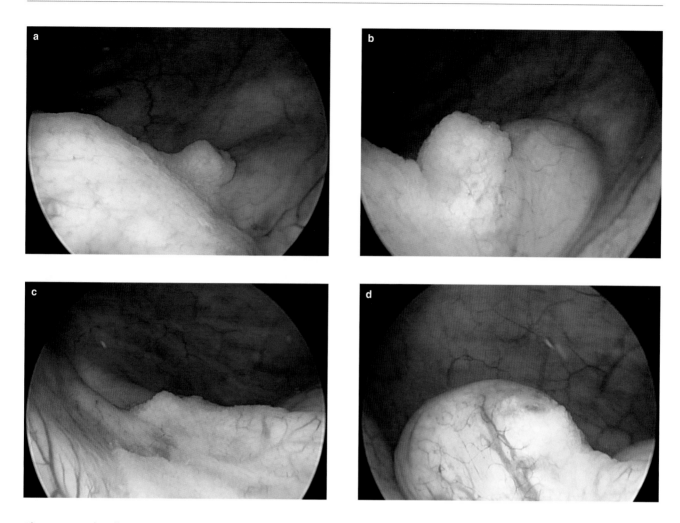

Figure 9.13(a–d)
Bilateral ureteroceles before and with ureteric peristalsis; ureteric jets with indigo carmine in (b) and (d).

hemorrhagic foci and reactive fibrosis.[12] Conservative hormonal treatment can be used but is frequently unsuccessful. Surgical excision of the endometriosis and bladder repair can be performed by cystoscopic excision and fulguration, transvaginal excision, or using the laparoscopic/abdominal approach. The method of choice will depend on the site of the endometriosis and the surgical experience and skill of the surgeon. Excision with histological confirmation of endometriotic tissue is required to confirm the diagnosis and exclude malignancy.

Extravesical pathology

Pelvic masses or inflammatory conditions extrinsic to the bladder can impact on the bladder and cause urinary symptoms. These conditions can also induce inflammatory changes in the bladder wall that mimic other bladder pathology such as UTI, cancer, or interstitial cystitis.

The bladder is a relatively thin-walled viscus when distended, on which external structures, whether normal or pathological, can cause indentations. The symphysis pubis, especially when prominent, causes an indentation in the anterior aspect of the dome (Figure 9.15). The cervix and uterus, especially when enlarged by pregnancy or fibroids, can impact on the bladder base and bladder neck, causing symptoms such as voiding difficulty, urinary retention, frequency, urgency, and incontinence. Pelvic cysts, tumors, abcess (Figure 9.16), and hematomas (Figure 9.17) can also press against the bladder wall and distort the bladder anatomy and function. These indentations normally have healthy bladder mucosa over their surface (Figure 9.17). When the process is one of inflammation and infection, the bladder wall may become secondarily involved. Pelvic infection with or without abscess formation can occur as a result of an infected synthetic graft used for stress incontinence or prolapse (Figure 9.18) or a retained swab. This process is usually confined to one area of the bladder and

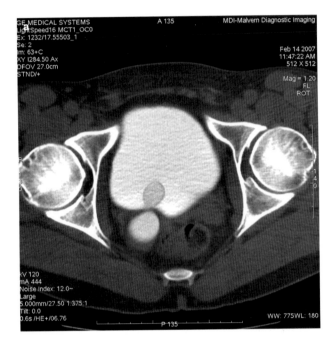

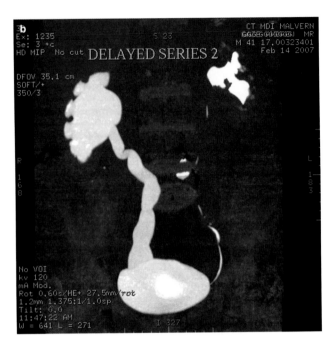

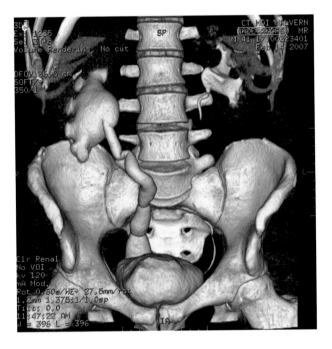

Figure 9.14

(a) Transverse CT scan image following administration of intravenous contrast (delayed excretory phase) demonstrating markedly dilated right-sided ureter, and ureterocoele within bladder, on wide window settings. (b) Delayed excretory phase average intensity projection image from MDCTU (multidetector row computed tomography urogram) demonstrating dilated right collecting system, right megaureter with associated right-sided ureterocoele. (c) 3D volume-rendered image generated from MDCTU of same patient, to demonstrate the dilated right collecting system and ureter, the bladder and normal left collecting system.

does not involve the whole unlike systemic conditions such as interstitial cystitis or drug-induced cystitis. Long-standing vaginal prolapse and bladder evisceration can cause edema of the bladder base (Figure 9.19), producing irritable bladder symptoms. Imaging of the pelvis using ultrasound or CT scanning or MRI will help in establishing the correct diagnosis, although it is essential that the clinician keep an open mind or misdiagnosis may occur and inappropriate surgical treatment be undertaken.

Bladder trabeculation and diverticulum

Trabeculation of the bladder wall has been thought to be caused by hypertrophy of the detrusor musculature, which is frequently associated with functional or obstructed voiding, urinary retention, detrusor overactivity, loss of bladder compliance, and the aging process.

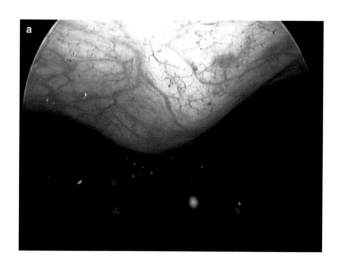

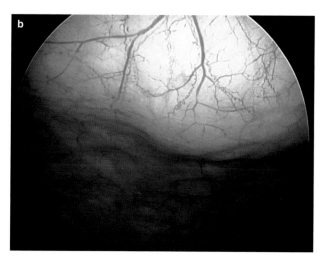

Figure 9.15
Indentation of bladder dome caused by the symphysis pubis.

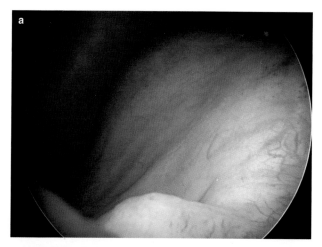

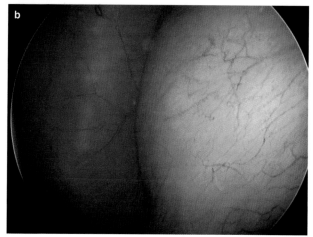

Figure 9.17
Postoperative hematoma 6 days following vaginal hysterectomy and repair pressing on the lateral bladder wall.

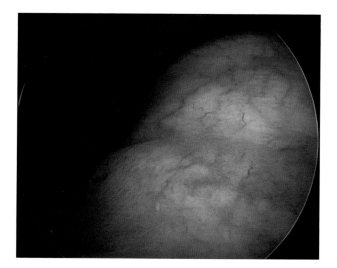

Figure 9.16
Cytoscopic photograph of infected pelvic hematoma indenting the bladder base which was drained 16 days following vaginal hysterectomy.

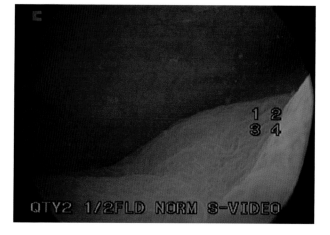

Figure 9.18
Infected intravaginal slingplasty (IVS) sling with left-sided retropubic abscess which was explored and removed through a combined abdominovaginal approach; on cystoscopy preoperatively, the left bladder base was edematous and inflamed and the left ureteric orifice was obscured.

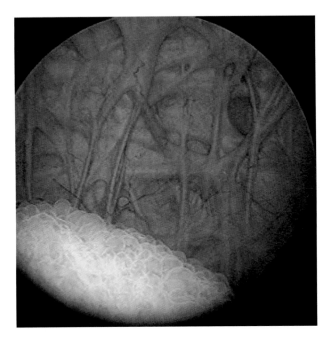

Figure 9.19
An 80-year-old woman with vaginal prolapse, urinary retention, and bladder evisceration through a previous vaginal repair. On cystoscopy, the bladder base was edematous but not inflamed, and there was moderate bladder trabeculation.

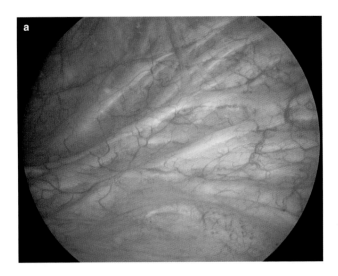

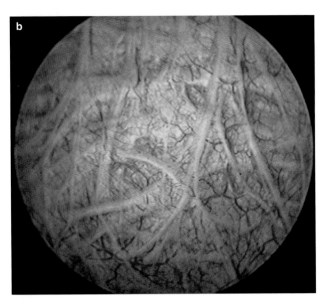

Figure 9.20(a,b)
Mild bladder trabeculation.

However, Gosling and Dixon have demonstrated that severe endoscopic trabeculation is a result of an increase in detrusor collagen,[13] suggesting that incomplete emptying may be the result of increased detrusor collagen rather than impaired muscle function.[14] In experimental animal models, unrelieved obstruction is associated with the development of significant increases in detrusor extracellular matrix (collagen type III).[15] This also appears to be the case in the human, although cause-and-effect relationships have not been established.

Mild trabeculation is present when the normal interlacing detrusor fibers become more accentuated (Figure 9.20). In moderate (Figure 9.21) and severe trabeculation, the bladder wall is thickened, there is marked trellising present with thickened cords of hypertrophied muscle, sacculations, and wide-necked bladder diverticulum, caused by chronically raised intravesical pressure (Figure 9.22). These wide-necked diverticula, can occasionally be the site of calculus formation or a carcinoma. Seven percent of all bladder tumors are sited in diverticulum which may make visualization difficult[16] (Figure 9.23). Women with outlet obstruction, especially in the presence of severe detrusor overactivity with high resting detrusor pressures, are at risk of not only developing multiple bladder diverticulum (Figure 9.24) but also vesicoureteric reflux and renal damage (Figure 9.25).

Women with marked trabeculation should:

- have their overactive bladder (OAB) symptoms treated appropriately – e.g. anticholingeric drugs
- have any significant outlet obstruction treated – e.g. intermittent self-catheterization, urethral dilatation, catheterization
- be monitored to ensure that renal function is preserved.

Single bladder diverticulum can occur and may be congenital or acquired – e.g. post-surgical (see Figure 9.3a). Surgical excision is rarely necessary.

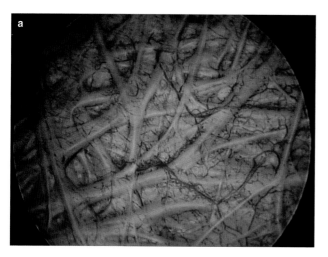

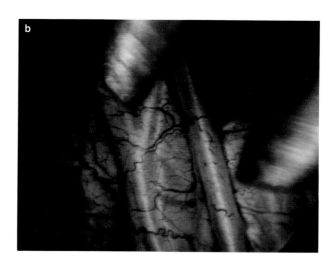

Figure 9.21(a,b)
Moderate bladder trabeculation with biopsy forceps seen in (b).

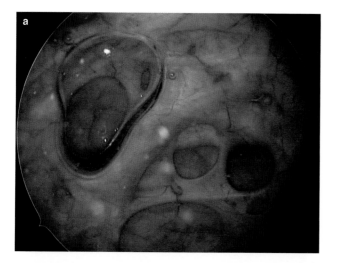

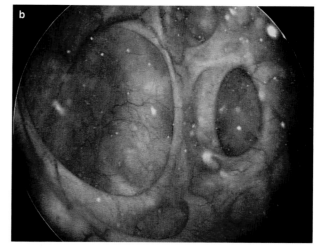

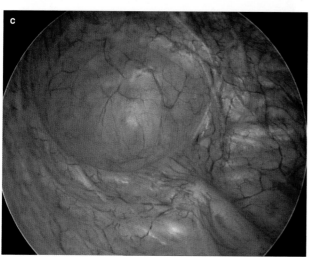

Figure 9.22(a–c)
Severe bladder trabeculation with sacculation and
diverticulum formation.

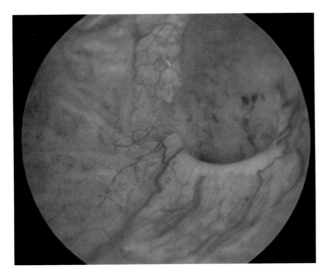

Figure 9.23
TCC diagnosed on cystoscopy in a solitary bladder diverticulum.

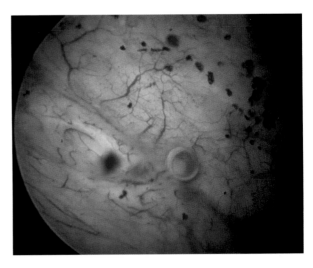

Figure 9.26
Small benign submucosal cyst near right ureteric orifice.

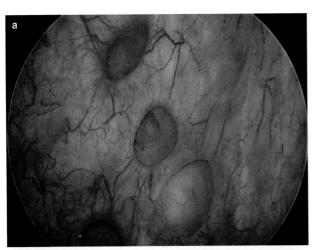

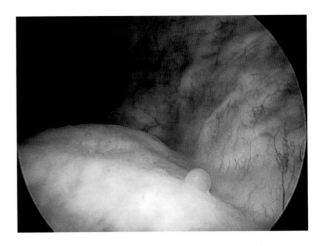

Figure 9.27
Benign solitary inclusion cyst on left side of trigone.

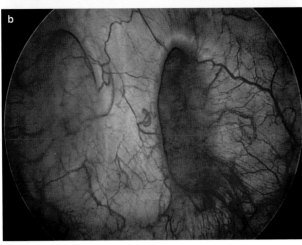

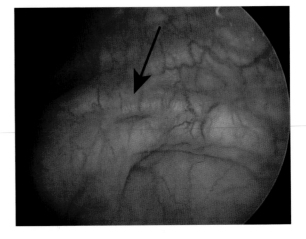

Figure 9.24(a,b)
Multiple bladder diverticulum in women with detrusor overactivity and outlet obstruction.

Figure 9.25
Thickened cord of hypertrophied detrusor musculature with sacculation and diverticulum in women with chronic urinary retention. Right ureteric orifice is highlighted by arrow.

Bladder polyps and mucosa cysts

Benign submucosa inclusion and mucinous cysts are occasionally seen on the bladder trigone and are unexpected findings on cystoscopy (Figures 9.26 and 9.27). They are benign and of no clinical significance. If there are any suspicious signs or clinical doubts, biopsy confirmation is warranted.

References

1. Schwartz BF, Stoller ML. The vesical calculus. Urol Clin North Am 2000; 27(2): 333–46.
2. Gault MH, Chafe L. Relationship of frequency, age, sex, stone weight and composition in 15,624 stones: comparison of results for 1980 to 1983 and 1995 to 1998. J Urol 2000; 164(2): 302–7.
3. Dalela D, Goel A, Shakhwar SN, Singh KM. Vesical calculi with unrepaired vesicovaginal fistula: a clinical appraisal of an uncommon association. J Urol 2003; 170(6 Pt 1): 2206–8.
4. Demirci D, Ekmekcioglu O, Demirtas A, Gulmez I. Big bladder stones around an intravesical migrated intrauterine device. Int Urol Nephrol 2003; 35(4): 495–6.
5. Wai CY, Margulis V, Baugh BR, Schaffer JI. Multiple vesical calculi and complete vaginal vault prolapse. Am J Obstet Gynecol 2003; 189(3): 884–5.
6. Dwyer PL, Carey MP, Rosamilia A. Suture injury to the urinary tract in urethral suspension procedures for stress incontinence. Int Urogynecol J 1999; 10: 15–21.
7. Delakas D, Daskalopoulos G, Cranidis A. Experience with the Dornier Lithotriptor MPL 9000-X for the treatment of vesical lithiasis. Int Urol Nephrol 1998; 30: 703–12.
8. Schlussel RA, Retik AB. Abnormalies of the ureter. In: Walsh PC, Retik AB, Vaughan ED Jr, Wein AJ, eds. ed. Campbell's Urology, 7th edn. Philadelphia: WB Saunders, 1998: 1814–58.
9. Rich MA, Keating MA, Snyder HM 3rd, Duckett JW. Low transurethral incision of single system ureteroceles in children. J Urol 1990; 144: 120–1.
10. Young RH. Pseudoneoplastic lesions of the urinary bladder. Pathol Annu 1988; 23(Pt 1): 67–104.
11. Chertin B, Prat O, Farkas A, Reinus C. Pregnancy-induced vesical decidualized endometriosis simulating a bladder tumour. Int Urogynecol J Pelvic Floor Dysfunct 2007; 18: 111–12.
12. Wong-You-Cheong JJ, Woodward PJ, Manning MA, Davis CJ. From the archives of the AFIP: inflammatory and non-neoplastic bladder masses: radiologic-pathologic correlation. Radiographics 2006; 26(6): 1847–68.
13. Gosling JA, Dixon JS. Structure of trabeculated detrusor smooth muscle in cases of prostatic hypertrophy. Urol Int 1980; 35: 351–5.
14. Barry MJ, Cockett ATK, Holtgrewe HL et al. Relationship of symptoms of prostatism to commonly used physiological and anatomical measures of the severity of benign prostatic hyperplasia. J Urol 1993; 150: 351–8.
15. Levin RM, Monson FC, Haugaard N et al. Genetic and cellular characteristics of bladder outlet obstruction. Urol Clin North Am 1995; 22: 262–83.
16. Cundiff GW, Bent AE. Endoscopic evaluation of the lower urinary tract. In: Walters MD, Karram MM, eds. Urogynecology and Reconstructive Pelvic Surgery, 3rd edn. Philadelphia, PA: Mosby Elsevier, 2007: 114.

10

Malignant conditions of the bladder and urethra

Anita Clarke and Peter L Dwyer

Introduction

Pelvic surgeons may encounter premalignant or malignant disease of the urinary tract in the investigation of hematuria, recurrent urinary tract infection, pelvic pain, or other irritable bladder symptoms. Bladder cancer may be an unexpected finding in women with no related urinary symptoms found during the performance of surgery for coincidental pelvic pathology. Cystourethroscopy is being increasingly performed during gynecological pelvic surgery and stress incontinence and prolapse surgery to detect intraoperative injury to the urinary tract. This offers an opportunity for the early diagnosis of malignant conditions of the lower urinary tract. In one of the authors' gynecological practice (PLD), the diagnosis of bladder cancer during routine endoscopy pelvic surgery is made at least once every year. We also know of a case of a death from bladder cancer in a woman who had a sling procedure performed the previous year. This has had medicolegal consequences, with questions being asked as to why the diagnosis was not made at that time. Therefore, any clinician performing an endoscopy of the lower urinary tract should be able to recognize malignant conditions of the urinary tract, describe and stage the cancer clinically, and perform cytology, and, if appropriate, biopsy for histological diagnosis. Proper tumor description and staging is important for clear communication between clinicians to determine the correct management and to compare results between centers and different modes of treatment.

Malignant bladder conditions
Transitional cell carcinoma of the bladder

Transitional cell carcinoma (TCC) of the bladder is the fifth most common malignancy in women, with an incidence comparable to ovarian cancer.[1] Its pathology varies from small superficial tumors (Figure 10.1) that usually require only endoscopic treatment to muscle invasive disease (Figure 10.2), which is managed with either total cystectomy and urinary diversion or radical radiotherapy.

Although muscle invasive disease is not common, occurring in only 20% of all bladder malignancies, the mortality is very significant, with a 40% 5-year survival rate.[2] Cancer of the bladder is the eighth most common cause of cancer death in women.[3]

In a recent Australian population-based survey by Millar et al[4] of 743 cases of muscle invasive bladder cancer, the male/female mix was 70% to 30%, and the mean age of presentation was 72 years old. Seventy-five percent of cases presented with hematuria and 16% with other bladder symptoms. The 5-year cancer-specific survival rate was 37%, with an overall survival rate of 26%. Curative treatment was more likely to be surgical than by radiation (23% compared with 18%), although 59% received palliative irradiation. One-third of patients received chemotherapy, either palliative or with curative intent.

Etiological factors

Several etiological factors have been identified in patients with bladder cancer.

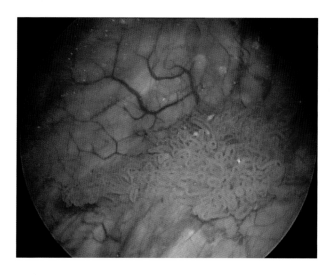

Figure 10.1
Small superficial papillary transitional cell carcinoma with areas of calcification.

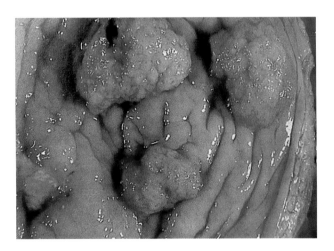

Figure 10.2
Large exophytic bladder tumors from a cystectomy specimen. (Courtesy of R Millard.)

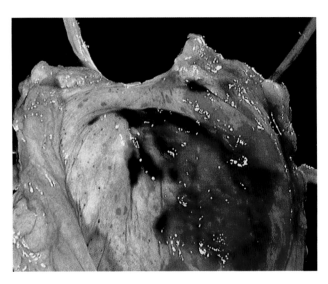

Figure 10.4
Cyclophosphamide cystitis. (Courtesy of R Millard.)

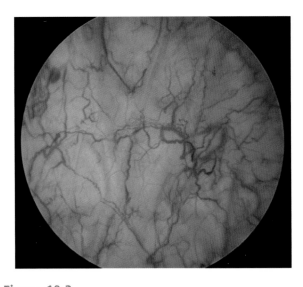

Figure 10.3
Radiation cystitis in a 64-year-old woman with a past history of adenocarcinoma of the cervix treated with surgery and postoperative radiation.

Smoking.   TCC of the bladder is more common in women who smoke cigarettes.[5] The risk increases by two- to fivefold when compared to the general population. With an increase in the number of women who smoke, there is likely to be an increase in the incidence over the next decade or two.

Age.   The incidence of TCC increases with age.[1] Approximately two-thirds of cases of bladder cancer occur

in women over the age of 65 years old. The risk of women developing bladder cancer over the age of 75 years old is 0.5–1%.[3] The life expectancy of women is increasing each year, and as a result we are seeing more transitional cell cancers in the very elderly, particularly in women in their 80s and 90s.

Radiation.   Women treated with high-dose radiotherapy for cervical cancer (Figure 10.3) have a fourfold increase in the risk of developing bladder cancer.[6] These cancers are characteristically of a high grade and are often more locally advanced. As women with radiation symptoms frequently have irritable bladder symptoms and hematuria, cystoscopic surveillance with biopsy of any abnormal area is indicated, particularly if there is a change in symptomatology.

Cyclophosphamide.   The use of cyclophosphamide for both malignant and non-malignant diseases can result in the development of bladder cancer.[7] The risk is dose dependent and is higher in patients who have continuous treatment and receive a total dose of 20 g or more. Acrolein, a metabolite of cyclophosphamide, is believed to be the principal carcinogen. Cyclophosphamide cystitis has a distinct endoscopic appearance (Figure 10.4), and, if seen, a biopsy to confirm the diagnosis should be performed and continuing surveillance of the bladder should be undertaken.

Chronic infection.   Chronic bladder infection has been associated with an increased risk of squamous cell

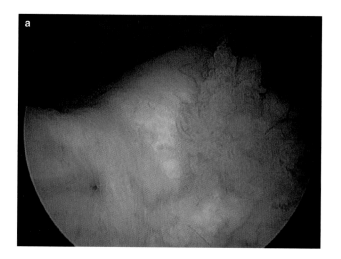
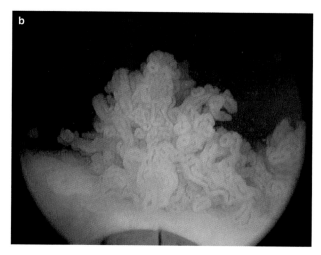
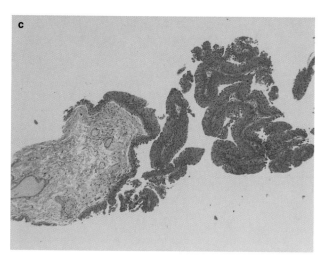
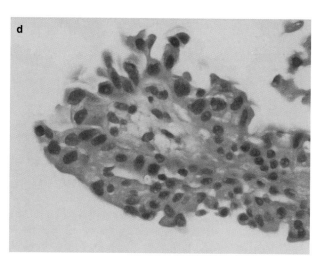

Figure 10.5
A 77-year-old lady with stress incontinence having a tension-free vaginal tape (TVT) sling was found to have this exophytic lesion (a,b) next to the right ureteric orifice. Histology revealed a non-invasive grade 2 papillary transitional cell carcinoma (c,d).

carcinoma (SCC) of the bladder.[8] Patients with long-term indwelling catheters have an increased risk of up to 10%. An increased incidence is also seen in African countries where schistosomiasis is endemic.

Environmental.
A number of occupational exposures have been associated with the development of bladder cancer, including workers in the rubber and dye industries as well as dry cleaners and beauticians.[9]

Histology and staging

Transitional cell carcinomas constitute 90% of all bladder malignancy, with the majority of these being superficial. They are most commonly papillary in appearance (see Figure 10.1), but nodular and sessile forms also exist.

Poorly differentiated muscle invasive tumors appear as a solid mass in the wall of the bladder (see Figure 8.2). The overlying urothelium may have a normal appearance.

Tumor grade.
Transitional cell carcinomas are grouped pathologically according to the degree of cellular atypia and their resemblance to normal bladder urothelium.

They are graded according to their histological features:

- grade 1 – well differentiated (Figure 10.5)
- grade 2 – moderately differentiated
- grade 3 – poorly differentiated/undifferentiated.

Carcinoma in situ.
Carcinoma in situ may be asymptomatic or associated with irritable bladder symptoms of frequency and urgency. The histological

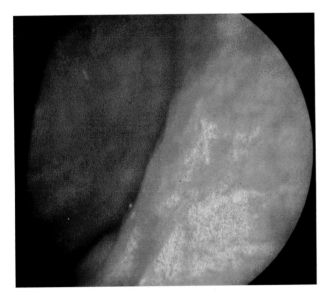

Figure 10.6
Carcinoma in situ of the bladder. Cystoscopy shows velvety patches of erythematous mucosa with a histological picture of poorly differentiated transitional cell carcinoma confined to the urothelium.

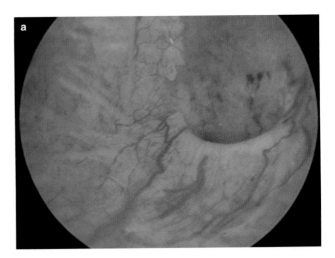

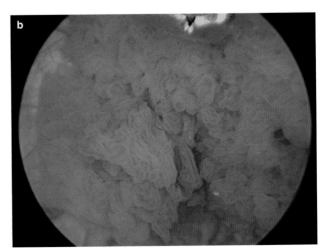

Figure 10.7(a,b)
A 52-year-old woman who is a smoker presented with one episode of hematuria and was found to have microscopic hematuria on urine analysis. On cystoscopy, she has a transitional cell carcinoma in a wide-necked bladder diverticulum situated above the trigone.

appearance of carcinoma in situ is one of flat areas of epithelium composed of cells with anaplastic features without invasion of the basement membrane. It appears at cystoscopy as a red velvety patch or a granular lesion of the bladder wall often in association with papillary or nodular tumor (Figure 10.6). Urine cytology is positive in 80–90% of women with carcinoma in situ.

Tumor stage.   Pathological staging refers to the level of invasion through the bladder wall. The majority of bladder tumors are non-invasive with low malignant potential. However, approximately 20% of TCCs will be muscle invasive with malignant potential. Invasion into adjacent pelvic organs and lymph nodes will also be a predictor of outcome.

Bladder tumors are staged using the TNM system, based on the International Union Against Cancer (UICC 1992), where T denotes tumor size and nodule status and M the presence or absence of distant metastases. A simplified staging system is as follows:

- T0 – non-invasive papillary carcinoma
- Tis – carcinoma in situ
- T1 – tumor invades subepithelial connective tissue
- T2 – tumor invades muscle
- T3 – tumor invades perivesical tissue
- T4 – tumor invades surrounding organs.

Squamous cell carcinoma

Squamous cell carcinoma of the bladder is an invasive tumor demonstrating a nodular growth infiltrative pattern. It constitutes approximately 5% of bladder tumors and is usually associated with chronic infection, stone formation, indwelling catheters, and bladder diverticula. It also occurs in association with chronic schistosomiasis infection, which is seen in migrants from East African countries. It is usually malignant at the time of diagnosis and biopsy will demonstrate ulceration and muscle invasion.

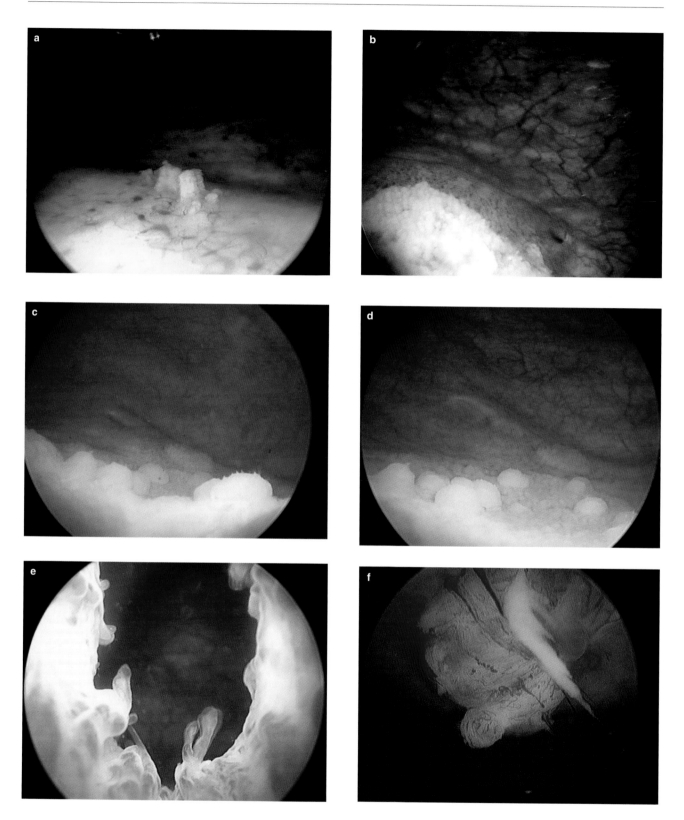

Figure 10.8
Non-maligant bladder conditions which can confuse the endoscopist. (a) Close-up cystoscopic view of small area of squamous metaplasia that was confirmed histologically by biopsy. (b–d) Raised areas squamous metaplasia can be easily mistaken for malignant disease. (e) Benign bladder neck polyps. (f) Close-up cystoscopic view of solitary infected granuloma on the dome of the bladder.

Adenocarcinoma

Primary adenocarcinoma of the bladder is rare and constitutes less than 2% of bladder tumors.

It occurs in three settings:

- in association with bladder exstrophy
- arising from the urachus
- arising in non-urachal epithelium.

Adenocarcinomas are often muscle invasive at the time of presentation. Adenocarcinoma arising from the urachus present with an abdominal mass, umbilical discharge, and hematuria and appears as a polypoid mass at the dome of the bladder.

Presentation

Hematuria

The most common presenting symptom of bladder cancer is painless macroscopic hematuria, which can occur on an intermittent basis and vary in amount. Occasionally, patients with microscopic hematuria are found to have bladder tumors that are small and superficial (Figure 10.7).

Irritative voiding symptoms

Approximately one-third of patients with bladder cancer also have irritative voiding symptoms such as urgency, frequency, and dysuria. These are more commonly seen in patients with muscle invasive disease or carcinoma in situ but may also be seen with tumors at the bladder neck in women.

Incidental finding

We are now seeing a diagnosis of TCC in women undergoing pelvic ultrasound or computed tomography (CT) scan for investigation of non-urological complaints. These 'incidental' tumors are also being seen at the time of cystoscopy performed during a gynecological procedure when checking for injury to the bladder or ureters.

Locally advanced disease

When TCC of the bladder is locally advanced, it may result in obstructive voiding, ureteric obstruction, a pelvic mass, or vaginal bleeding. Occasionally, lower limb edema is also seen, particularly if lymph node metastases have occurred.

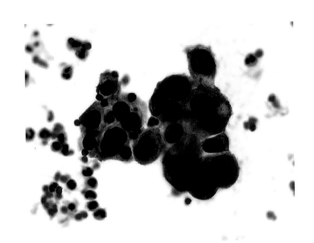

Figure 10.9
High grade TCC in bladder washings - a clump of cohesive transitional cells with marked nuclear enlargement, pleomorphism and hyperchromasia, polymorphs and red blood cells are seen in the background. (Courtsey of J Scurry)

Metastatic disease

TCC generally metastasizes to lymph nodes, liver, bone, and lung.

Diagnosis

In general, TCC of the bladder is diagnosed at the time of cystoscopy, although preoperative imaging and urine cytology are useful adjuncts to the diagnosis. Urine cytology is highly accurate in the diagnosis of high-grade carcinoma (grade 3) and carcinoma in situ but is less helpful in low-grade TCC. Three early morning specimens are taken and the cells are examined for nuclear atypia. Fresh urine samples can be centrifuged and stained by the Papanicolaou technique to detect abnormal cells shed from the surface of bladder cancers (Figure 10.9).

One of the most useful tools available today comprises the images that can be captured using the endoscopic camera. They allow an accurate record to be kept of the patient's tumor as well as facilitating review of the pictures by a urologist if there is doubt about the appearance of the lesion seen. If possible, an overall image of the lesion seen in relation to the rest of the bladder (dome, anterior posterior, or lateral walls as well as ureteric orifices) should be taken as well as a close-up picture. The cystoscopic appearance of the tumor is an important indicator of the nature of the lesion and its histological diagnosis. It is important that any clinician performing cystoscopy be able to differentiate between benign and malignant conditions. This may not always be possible even for experienced cystoscopists, so histological confirmation following biopsy is necessary when there is doubt.

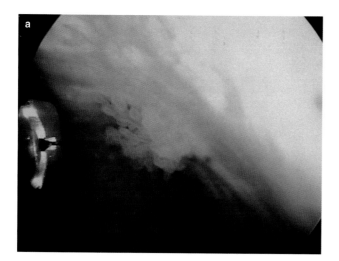

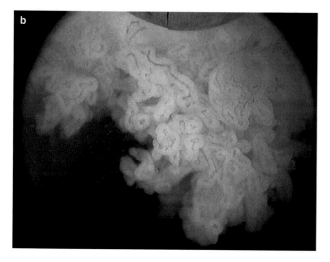

Figure 10.10
(a,b) Biopsy of non-invasive grade 1 papillary transitional cell carcinoma diagnosed on routine cystoscopy in a 67-year-old woman at the time of vaginal repair.

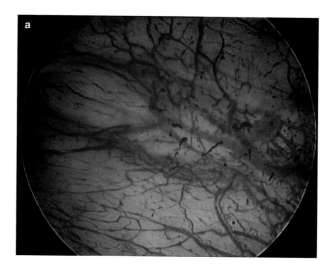

Figure 10.11
The 1–2 mm TCC next to the left ureteric orifice was detected on cystoscopy at the time of vaginal repair and was completely excised by cold-cup biopsy.

Benign conditions such as squamous metaplasia (Figure 10.8), cystitis cystica, or infected cysts or granulomas (Figure 10.9) can be mistaken for malignant disease.

A biopsy is required to confirm the diagnosis, to grade the tumor, and to determine the level of invasion: this should only be performed by operators with some experience. The bladder wall, particularly in the elderly, can be very thin and perforation or significant bleeding can occur at the time of biopsy, especially when using the resectoscope.

Biopsies can be performed in two different ways, depending on the size of the tumor.

Small tumors can be biopsied using the biopsy forceps, which attach to the cystoscope in place of the bridge (Figure 10.10). The tumor is grabbed at its base and removed in a single motion. Small tumors are frequently

completely removed by the biopsy process (Figure 10.11). The biopsy site, if bleeding, is then cauterized using a flexible electrode or a rollerball diathermy; the advantage of this is a more complete biopsy as well as less diathermy artifact, which can make interpretation of the pathology difficult.

Large tumors require resection with a resectoscope (Figure 10.12), which is a similar instrument to the hysteroscope and consists of a cutting/coagulation loop. The cutting loop is used to remove the tumor, often in several pieces, and the coagulation is used to obtain hemostasis. Deep muscle biopsies are sent separately, in order to determine the level of invasion. Resection of large bladder tumors requires significant endoscopic skills. It is not advisable to take a small biopsy from the surface of these tumors as they are often vascular and bleeding may occur. A small biopsy will not give any information with regard to the depth of invasion and therefore is incomplete from a pathological point of view. It is best to either call a urologist at the time of the cystoscopy or to take accurate photographs of the tumor endoscopically and refer the patient appropriately.

Following cystourethroscopy, careful examination under anesthesia should be performed to assess the size of the mass and spread to surrounding organs. Once the histopathology is obtained, further staging as appropriate is then performed. In patients with muscle invasive disease, a computed tomography (CT) scan of the abdomen and pelvis as well as a bone scan are performed prior to planning definitive treatment (Figure 10.13).

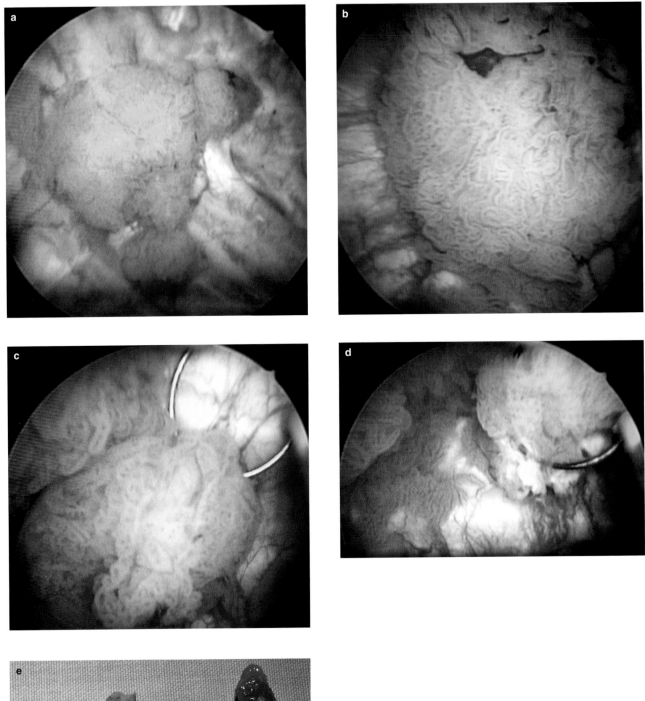

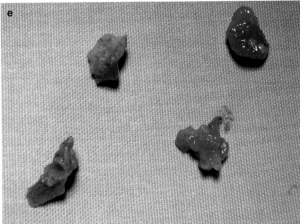

Figure 10.12(a–e)
This combined papillary and solid muscle invasive tumor was excised with a resectoscope; macroscopic chips following resection are seen in (e). (Courtesy of K Stav.)

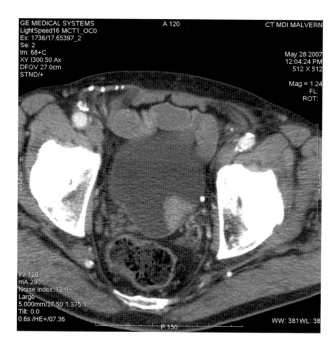 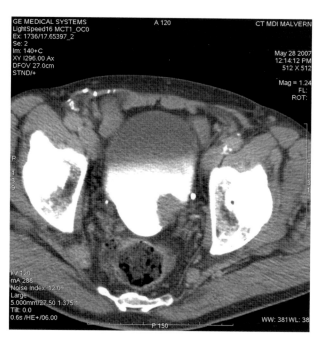

Figure 10.13
CT axiel scan of the peluis during contrast injection (a) and post contrast injection in the delayed excretion phase. The tumor on the right bladder wall can be clearly seen in both scans, but especially when contrast was present in the bladder (b). (Courtesy of A Lavoirpierre.)

Treatment

Further treatment and evaluation depends on the pathological staging of the tumor biopsy.

For low-grade non-invasive tumors, once the tumor has been removed patients are generally allocated to a surveillance program. This usually consists of regular flexible cystoscopies starting at 3 monthly for 1 year and then 6 monthly performed over a 5–10-year period. Approximately, 60% of pTa tumors will locally recur and 20% progress to higher-stage disease.[11]

For patients with lamina propria invasion or carcinoma in situ, there is a much higher probability of progression in the order of 70–80%. These patients are then treated with intravesical therapy, either with bacille Calmette-Guérin (BCG) therapy or with mitomycin C. After this treatment, a further cystoscopy and biopsy is performed and, if clear, the surveillance program is instituted. If carcinoma in situ persists, a second course of intravesical treatment is given. If this is not curative, the patient is treated with radical cystectomy.

In patients with muscle invasive disease, the most common form of treatment is by radical surgery with cystectomy, hysterectomy, removal of anterior one-third of the vagina, urethrectomy, and formation of an ileal conduit. In patients where the primary lesion is at the dome or a good distance from the bladder neck, ileal neobladder formation

and attachment to the urethra may be appropriate. If the patient is not fit for surgery, radiotherapy can be used alternatively as a definitive treatment.

Chemotherapy is generally used for patients with inoperable or metastatic disease. Cisplatinum-based chemotherapy is used either as M-VAC (methotrexate, vinblastine, doxorubicin, and cisplatin) or in combination with gemcitabine. Its use as a neoadjuvant or adjuvant treatment to radical surgery is still being evaluated.

Urethral cancer

Urethral cancer in women occurs mainly in the elderly and is uncommon, accounting, for less than 1% of all female cancers. Although the cause is unknown, chronic irritation, urinary tract infection and proliferate lesions such as caruncles, papillomas, adenomas, and leukoplakia have been associated with subsequent malignancy[12]. Women may present with haematuria, frequency, hesitancy, and slow stream, or as a palpable urethral mass in the anterior vaginal wall (Fig 10.14) or a urethral caruncle. Early biopsy with excision and cystourethroscopy is important for early diagnosis and best outcome.

The tumor may have a papillary or ulcerative appearance with local spread present to the bladder, vagina, or vulva, which can make it difficult to accurately diagnose

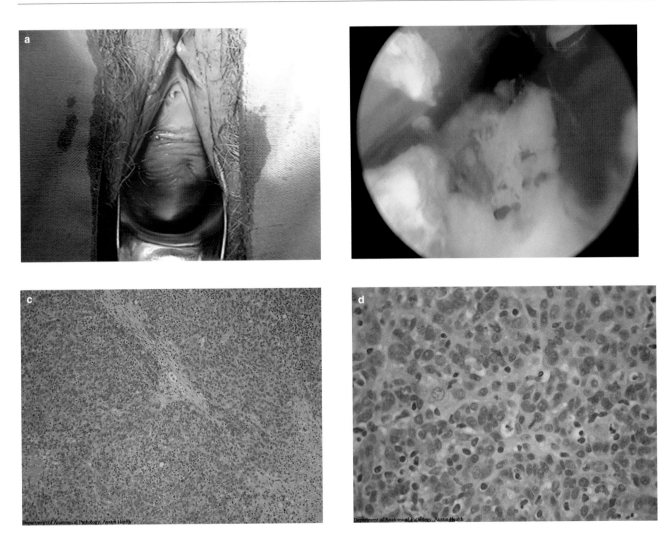

Figure 10.14

A 67-year-old women who was refered with possible vaginal prolapse was found on examination to have an anterior vaginal wall mass (a). On cystourethroscopy there was necrotic tumor extending from the posterior urethra onto the trigone (b). Histological analysis of the urethral biopsy revealed a high grade invasive transitional cell carcinoma, with papillary structures within a desmoplastic and necrotic stroma (c). The tumor cells have large pleomorphic nuclei, with variably prominent nucleoli and mild polygonal amphophilic cytoplasm. Mitosese are numerous, with atypical forms found (d).

the initial source of the cancer. Lymph node spread is to inguinal, external iliac, and obturator lymph nodes. Squamous cell carcinoma is the commonest histological type followed by transitional cell carcinoma and adenocarcinoma. Treatment is by extensive local excision with lymphadenectomy with or without radiation therapy. The 5-year survival rate for early urethral cancers is over 80%.

Conclusion

Cystoscopy remains the most important diagnostic tool in patients with bladder malignancy. It is imperative that

gynecologists who perform cystoscopy can identify the endoscopic features of both superficial and invasive disease in order to ensure prompt and effective treatment of bladder cancer. Hematuria, persistent irritable bladder symptoms, or the presence of an anterior vaginal wall mass are indications for an early cystoscopy.

References

1. Silverman DT, Hartge P, Morrison AS, Devesa SS. Epidemiology of bladder cancer. Hematol Oncol Clin North Am 1992; 6: 1–30.
2. Boring CC, Squires TS, Tong T, Montgomery S. Cancer statistics, 1994. CA Cancer J Clin 1994; 44: 7–26.

3. Kirkali Z, Chan T, Manoharan M et al. Bladder cancer: epidemiology, staging and grading and diagnosis. Urology 2005; 66 (6 Suppl 1): 4–34.

4. Millar JL, Frydenberg M, Toner G et al. Management of muscle-invasive bladder cancer in Victoria, 1990–1995. ANZ J Surg 2006; 76: 1113–19.

5. Augustine A, Hebert JR, Kabat GC, Wynder EL. Bladder cancer in relation to cigarette smoking. Cancer Res 1988; 48: 4405–8.

6. Boice JD Jr, Engholm G, Kleinerman RA et al. Radiation dose and second cancer risk in patients treated for cancer of the cervix. Radiat Res 1988: 116: 3–55.

7. Levine LA, Richie JP. Urological complications of cyclophosphamide. J Urol 1989; 141: 1063–9.

8. Kantor AF, Hartge P, Hoover RN et al. Urinary tract infection and risk of bladder cancer. Am J Epidemiol 1984; 119: 510–15.

9. Cohen SM, Johansson SL. Epidemiology and etiology of bladder cancer. Urol Clin North Am 1992; 19: 421–8.

10. Fitzpatrick JM. The natural history of superficial bladder carcinoma. Semin Urol 1993; 11: 127–36.

11. Heney NM, Ahmed S, Flanagan MJ et al. Superficial bladder cancer: progression and recurrence. J Urol 1983; 130: 1083–6.

12. Herr HW. Campbells urology. Walsh PC, Recik AB, Vaughan EW, Wein AJ (eds). Seventh edition. WB Saunders Company 1997: 3407–8.

11

Laparoscopy in urogynecology

Christopher F Maher and Peter J Maher

Introduction

The key advantages of the laparoscopic approach to surgery include improved exposure and magnification deep in the pelvis. These advantages make the laparoscopic approach ideal for evaluating and treating pathology of the peritoneal surface of the bladder, uterus, bowel, and ureters and the extraperitoneal spaces of the bladder, vagina, and rectum.

While gynecologists led the surgical specialties in understanding the importance and benefits of the laparoscope in diagnosing and treating our patients, the early phase of laparoscopic surgery was hindered by limited optical and instrumental technology. Important milestones in laparoscopic surgery technology include the first tube camera in 1981 and the solid state medical video camera in 1981 by William Chang. The first three-digital-chip camera,

introduced in 1989, significantly improved clarity of vision and digital enhancement and zoom technology, again, improved our capabilities in 1999. Improved instrumentation and better understanding of energy sources have made laparoscopy safer and suitable for a wider range of pelvic surgeries.

Laparoscopic pelvic floor surgery

The loose areolar tissue of the cave of Retzius allows expandability of the bladder and also ensures excellent vision and exposure at laparoscopy (Figure 11.1). Vancaille and Schuessler first reported laparoscopic colposuspension in 1991,[1] as demonstrated in Figure 11.2. Well-conducted randomized controlled trials (RCTs), where similar operating procedures are performed in both arms by suitably

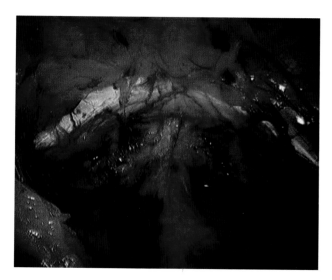

Figure 11.1
Excellent exposure of the cave of Retzius at laparoscopy.

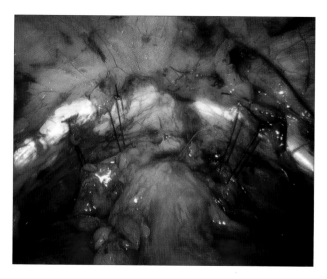

Figure 11.2
The completed laparoscopic colposuspension.

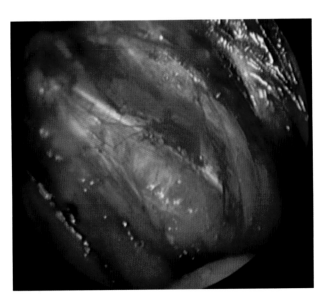

Figure 11.3
Left paravaginal defect with separation of the vagina from the arcus tendineous fascia pelvis.

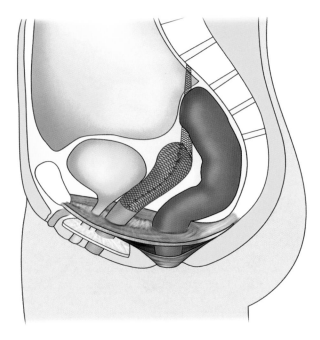

Figure 11.5
Sacral colpopexy. (Published with permission of Maher & Francis.)

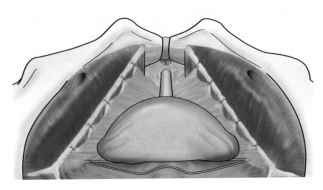

Figure 11.4
Paravaginal repair. (Published with permission of Maher & Francis.)

trained surgeons, have demonstrated that the laparoscopic colposuspension is as effective as the open procedure, with reduced pain, length of admission, and quicker return to daily activities.[2,3] Laparoscopic colposuspension in well-conducted studies has been shown to be affective as the tension-free vaginal tape (TVT) in primary[4] and repeat continence surgery.[5]

The excellent exposure and magnification of the laparoscope in the cave of Retzius also allows the identification and treatment of paravaginal defects, as demonstrated in Figures 11.3 and 11.4. There is a paucity of data on the efficacy of this procedure performed via the laparoscope.

Sacral colpopexy was first described by Lane over 40 years ago. He described the post-hysterectomy upper vagina being suspended from the sacral promontory using permanent mesh, as illustrated in Figure 11.5. Three RCTs compared abdominal sacral colpopexy with vaginal

reconstructive surgery.[6–8] The Cochrane review meta-analysis concluded that abdominal sacral colpopexy was associated with lower recurrent prolapse but longer operating time, length of admission, morbidity, and cost than vaginal sacrospinous colpopexy.[9] In an attempt to reduce hospital stay, postoperative pain, and recovery time, the laparoscopic approach has been championed.[10] In a retrospective case control study, Paraiso et al have demonstrated that the laparoscopic approach was as successful as the open approach with prolonged operating time but significantly reduced hospital stay and blood loss.[11]

The laparoscopic approach is ideal for the sacral colpopexy. The magnification and digital zoom allow the surgeon, assistant, operating nurses, anesthetist, and trainees excellent visualization of the operating field. This has several advantages: it facilitates better exposure of the surgical field and the ability of assistants to predict the next steps of the surgery, improves teaching of trainees and students, is more inclusive of all in the operating team, and increases accountability of the surgeon. The CO_2 used to distend the abdomen also facilitates retroperitoneal dissection planes, as shown in Figure 11.2, which may explain the reduced blood loss associated with the laparoscopic approach.

Figures 11.6–11.11 demonstrate the steps associated with the sacral colpopexy, including opening the peritoneal space from the sacrum to the vaginal vault. The bladder and bowel are mobilized from the vagina. Mesh is secured to the anterior and posterior vaginal wall using absorbable sutures. The mesh is placed retroperitoneally, secured to

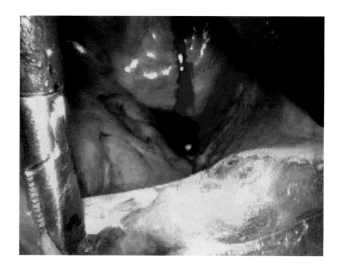

Figure 11.6
Opening peritoneum from sacrum to vaginal vault.

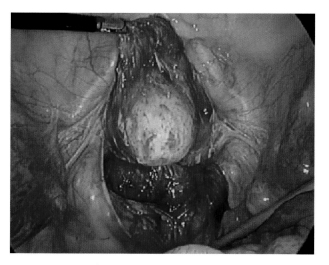

Figure 11.7
Bladder and bowel dissected from vaginal vault.

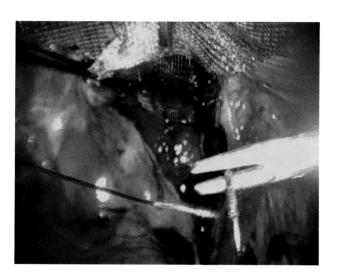

Figure 11.8
Prolene mesh secured to posterior vaginal wall.

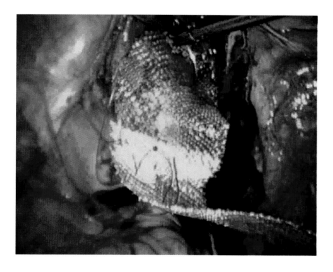

Figure 11.9
Prolene mesh secured to anterior vaginal wall.

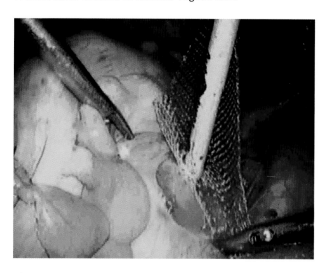

Figure 11.10
Mesh secured to sacral promontory.

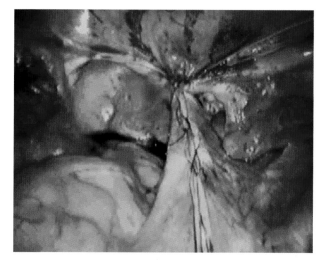

Figure 11.11
Peritoneum closed over mesh.

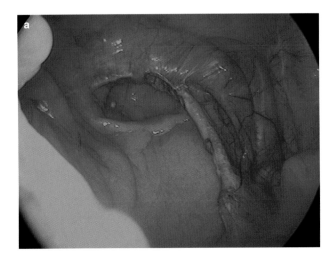 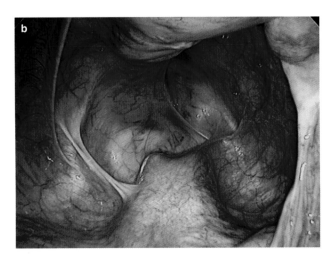

Figure 11.12(a,b)
Laparoscopic appearance of polypropylene mesh following abdominal colposacropexy in the pouch of Douglas many months following surgery.

the sacral promontory using tacks or sutures, and the peritoneum closed, as in the open procedure. The polypropylene mesh used for suspension of the vagina to the sacrum is 20 cm long, which allows vaginal support without tension. Excessive tension can predispose to de-novo stress incontinence and possibly anterior compartment prolapse. The appearance of the mesh viewed at follow-up laparoscopy is shown in Figure 11.12. The efficacy of the laparoscopic approach to pelvic floor surgery requires further ongoing evaluation.

All gynecologists, including those trained in endoscopy, consider ureteric injury to be one of the most serious complications associated with surgery. The reported incidence of ureteral injury related to gynecological surgery varies between 0.4% and 2.5%,[12] whereas the rate of injury to the bladder varies between 1% and 5%.

The majority of injuries to the ureter occur during the operation of hysterectomy. Since the introduction of the laparoscopic approach to remove the uterus in 1989,[13] there has been an increase in ureteric morbidity when compared to the traditional routes of removal by either the abdominal or vaginal route.[14] An estimated 600 000 women undergo hysterectomy in the United States each year, with 37% of the female population having hysterectomy performed by the age of 65 years old.[15] Intraoperative and postoperative complications, including bleeding, infection, and vessel injury, occur in as many as 23% of these cases; 75% of iatrogenic injury to the ureter occurs during gynecological surgery. Many conditions predispose to ureteric injury and include malignancy, previous surgery, and severe peritoneal or infiltrating endometriosis, although it has been reported that at least half of all ureter injuries have no identifiable risk factors.

Many ureteric injuries are not detected intraoperatively, with rates below 15% reported.[16] Lack of diagnosis can

have a profound influence on the patient's postoperative course, with further operative intervention necessary, prolonged hospitalization, and very protracted recovery time.

In a report by Tamussino et al, of 790 consecutive major operative procedures in 711 patients, the reported incidence of urethral injury was 0.38%;[17] all injuries occurred during the operation of laparoscopic hysterectomy – of the 4 injuries reported, 2 were delayed in diagnosis. The site of injury in the delayed cases was in the lower segment of the ureter after laparoscopic bipolar coagulation and division of the entire cardinal ligament. This site has similarly been implicated with the application of staples, caused by the close approximation of the ureters to the anatomical site of the uterine vessels. In contrast to other reports,[18] the authors (CFM and PJM) had no ureteric complications in more than 700 adnexal operations, which is rather surprising considering that the ureter is also considered at risk during division of the infundibulopelvic ligament during adnexectomy. Although not clearly stated in this review, it is strongly recommended to completely identify the ureter and its relationship to the ovarian (gonadal) vessels at the pelvic brim before attempting to secure closure of these vessels with either suture, bipolar diathermy, or staples. Even with clear delineation of the ureter, it is important to ensure that adequate protection is afforded to this structure, particularly when bipolar electrosurgery is used. Thermal damage, with subsequent necrosis and eventual fistula formation, cannot be ruled out, even when 5 mm bipolar instruments are used.

In a further earlier report by Grainger et al,[19] of 13 ureteral injuries, 12 related to the use of cautery. Attempts have been made to avoid these thermal injuries by the use of staples but they too have been implicated. The EndoGIA has a width of 1 cm but the distance between the side of the

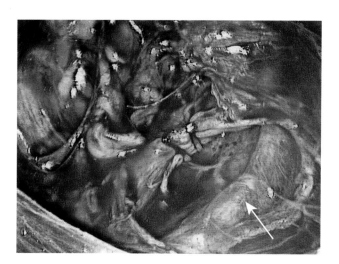

Figure 11.13
Ureteric identification (arrow) followed by individual clipping of the left uterine artery during laparoscopic hysterectomy.

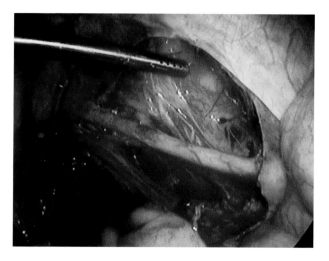

Figure 11.14
Extensive dissection of the pelvic side wall to identify the ureter during side-wall peritonectomy for peritoneal endometriosis.

uterus and the inner edge of the ureter has been reported to be as little as 6 mm.

In an attempt to minimize the risk of ureteric damage during laparoscopic-assisted hysterectomy, this author introduced the routine insertion of ureteric catheters at the commencement of the laparoscopic procedure. The intention was that, at the time of applying the stapling device to the ureteric vessels, the stapling device could be closed but not fired and then the catheters would be moved. Failure to move the catheters alerted the surgeon to the fact that the stapling device had incorporated the ureter together with the vessel to be occluded. The stapling device could then be opened, the ureter freed, and the device reapplied again, checking the position relative to the vessel.

A series of 492 patients undergoing laparoscopic hysterectomy, of whom 92 had ureteric catheters passed prophylactically, was reported by the author (PJM) and his colleagues.[20] The importance of this series was that – although there were no ureteric injuries reported – there was morbidity in 7 of the 92 patients to have ureteric catheterization. Ureteric catheters have been reported to cause trauma to the urothelium and even perforation.[21] The trauma may result from the passage of the catheter, the need to move the catheter upwards and downwards before firing the staple gun, or applying electrocoagulation during the laparoscopic hysterectomy.

In this series, the 7 patients experienced symptoms ranging from oliguria to complete anuria, with resultant anxiety for both the surgeon and the patient. Further investigations, including intravenous pyelography, renal ultrasound, and recatheterization, were required in 5 of the 7 patients who were affected.

Intraoperative cystoscopy may be helpful in confirming ureteric patency as well as detecting any bladder trauma. The absence of ureteric trauma in the 400 patients in the above series who did not have ureteric catheterization convinced the authors that the routine use of this procedure in laparoscopic hysterectomy was most probably not warranted. Primary ureteric dissection before the commencement of the hysterectomy may avoid trauma by displaying the ureters close to where the uterine arteries are divided[22] (Figure 11.13).

Cystoscopy was performed in 292 patients of the series of 400. It is helpful in identifying the passage of urine from the ureters as well as identifying any evidence of bladder trauma that may have occurred during the course of the operation. Cystoscopy will eliminate the possibility of urinary tract trauma during the course of laparoscopic hysterectomy, except in the case of ischemic necrosis. Unfortunately, this complication will only manifest itself in the days subsequent to the day of surgery.

The other main surgical procedure performed by general gynecologists is the laparoscopic removal of moderately severe endometriosis. It is timely to review the surgical treatment of this disease because of the difficulty expressed by gynecologists in removing the endometriosis tissue when there is extensive involvement, particularly on the bladder and ureter. In a review of 198 patients who had been referred to an endometriosis clinic, Wood[23] reported that these patients had on average 5–7 previous surgical interventions. Further surgical therapy that followed initial referral revealed disease mainly over the course of the ureter, bladder, vagina, and rectum. He reported that these findings were suggestive that earlier surgery performed may have avoided these vital structures in order to avoid risk of damage to them.

The ureter is at risk during endometriosis surgery; in particular, its integrity is challenged during peritoneal resection and dissection of the pelvic side wall (Figure 11.14). The mobilization of peritoneum over the pelvic

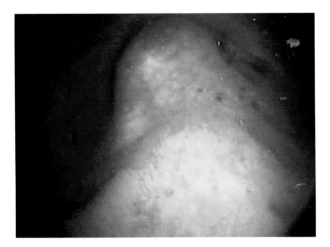

Figure 11.15
Cystoscopic view of infiltrating endometriosis.

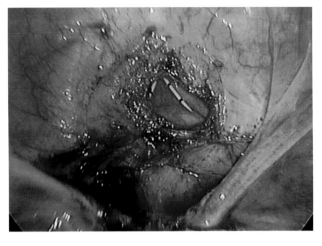

Figure 11.17
Ureteric catheters laparoscopically identified intravesically during full-thickness excision of bladder endometriosis.

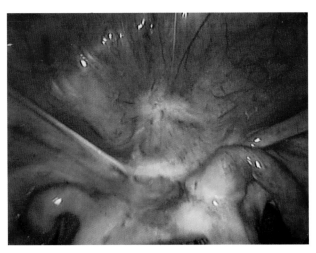

Figure 11.16
Adenomyosis infiltrating from the anterior wall of the uterus into the bladder.

side wall displays the anatomy of the ureter as it traverses from the pelvic brim to the tunnel adjacent to the lateral cervix and also the hypogastric vessels and their branches. When the peritoneum is extremely thick or opaque, passage of a ureteric catheter may be necessary. In this circumstance, the catheter is placed and then not moved (see above) but felt with laparoscopic forceps on the pelvic side wall. Dissection can then occur along the path of the now-identified catheter. This procedure does not generally have the morbidity that has been reported with catheter use during laparoscopic hysterectomy because the catheter is left dormant and not continually moved upwards or downwards as occurs during the application of the stapling device during hysterectomy.

In severe cases of uterosacral endometriosis, it is also imperative to identify and isolate the ureter laterally before attempting to excise the affected ligament.

The other organ relative to this section for the general gynecologist is the bladder. The incidence of bladder endometriosis is relatively rare and represents only 1% of all cases of this disease. Small implants are relatively common on the peritoneal surface of the bladder but it is particularly important to define lesions that have infiltrated into the detrusor muscle. The most common symptom associated with infiltrating bladder endometriosis is pain during micturition, which has been reported in as many as 76% of patients affected.

Cystoscopy is necessary to confirm full-thickness disease and to clarify the relationship of the endometriotic lesion to the trigone and the ureters (Figure 11.15). Bladder endometriosis is often associated with gross distortion of the vesicoureteric fold, with bilateral 'drawing in' of both round ligaments centrally (Figure 11.16). If laparoscopic suturing skills are of a high standard, then electrosurgical incision of the lesion can be undertaken followed by single-layer closure of the defect. The authors would pass ureteric catheters before excision takes place, which would be removed at the end of the procedure (Figure 11.17). At the conclusion of the excision, the musculature of the bladder is closed with 2/0 Monocryl sutures, either with an interrupted or continuous technique (Figures 11.18 and 11.19). A urinary catheter is left in situ for 10 days after the surgery and a cystogram is performed prior to its removal.

It has been suggested that bladder endometriosis results from an adenomyotic extension from the anterior uterine wall[24] or a primary bladder adenomyoma.[25] Although medical therapy may have some role, the primary management, irrespective of the origin of the disease, is surgical excision.

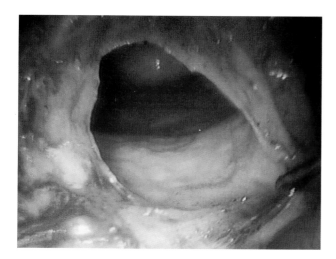

Figure 11.18
Large endometriotic lesion of the bladder fundus excised
laparoscopically.

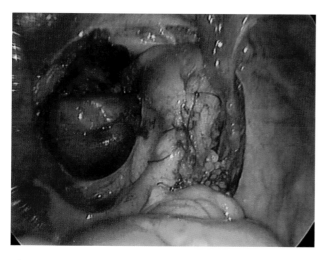

Figure 11.19
Single-layer closure of detrusor muscle following laparoscopic
excision of full-thickness bladder endometriosis.

Improved technology has allowed the benefits of
laparoscopy of reduced pain and postoperative hospitalization in performing abdominal surgery on more patients with
pelvic pathology and pelvic floor disorders who would otherwise have undergone laparotomy. There is considerable
debate within the gynecological specialty on the best
approach to pelvic surgery: whether this should be vaginal,
open abdominal, or laparoscopic surgery. However, patient
benefits are likely to be maximized when clinicians are profi-
cient in all techniques and are able to vary their approach to
meet the needs of the individual patient. Laparoscopic and
cystoscopic endoscopy are complementary skills and are frequently needed together in the diagnosis and surgical treatment of pelvic disorders in the female.

References

1. Vancaille T, Schuessler W. Laparoscopic bladder-neck suspension. J Laparoendosc Surg 1991; 1: 169–73.
2. Cheon W, Mak K, Liu J. Prospective randomised controlled
   trial comparing laproscopic and open colposuspension.
   J Am Assoc Gynecol Laparosc 2001; 8: 99–106.
3. Fatthy H, El Hao M, Samaha I, Abdallah K. Modified Burch
   colposuspension: laparoscopy and open colposuspension.
   Hong Kong Med J 2001; 8: 99–110.
4. Ustun Y, Engin-Usten Y, Gungor M, Texcan S. Tension-free
   vaginal tape compared with Burch urethropexy. J Am Assoc
   Gynecol Laparosc 2003; 10: 386–9.
5. Maher C, Qatawneh A, Baessler K, Cropper M, Schluter
   P. Laparoscopic colposuspension or tension-free vaginal
   tape for recurrent stress urinary incontinence and/or ISD: a
   randomised controlled trial. Neurourol Urodyn 2004; 5:
   Abstract 25.
6. Maher CF, Qatawneh AM, Dwyer PL et al. Abdominal sacral
   colpopexy or vaginal sacrospinous colpopexy for vaginal
   vault prolapse: a prospective randomized study. Am J Obstet
   Gynecol 2004; 190(1): 20–6.
7. Benson JT, Lucente V, McClellan E. Vaginal versus abdominal reconstructive surgery for the treatment of pelvic support defects: a prospective randomized study with long-term
   outcome evaluation. Am J Obstet Gynecol 1996; 175(6):
   1418–21.
8. Lo TS, Wang AC. Abdominal colposacropexy and sacrospinous
   ligament suspension for severe uterovaginal prolapse: a
   comparison. J Gynecol Surg 1998; 14(2): 59–64.
9. Maher CF, Baessler K, Glazener C, Adams E, Hagan S.
   Surgical management of pelvic organ prolapse in women.
   Cochrane Database System Rev 2004; (4): CD004014.
10. Higgs PJ, Chua HL, Smith AR. Long term review of laparo-
    scopic sacrocolpopexy. BJOG 2005; 112(8): 1134–8.
11. Paraiso MFR, Walters MD, Rackley RR, Melek S, Hugney C.
    Laparoscopic and abdominal sacral colpopexies: a compara-
    tive cohort study. Am J Obstet Gynecol 2005; 192(5):
    1752–8.
12. Thompson J. Operative injuries to the ureter: prevention,
    recognition and management. In: Thompson AD, Rock JA,
    eds. TeLinde's Operative Gynecology, 7th edn. 1992; 759–83.
13. Reich H, DeCaprio J, McGlynn F. Laparoscopic hysterec-
    tomy. J Gynaecol Surg 1989; 5(2): 213–15.
14. Garry R, Fountain J, Brown J et al. EVALUATE hysterectomy
    trial: a multicentre randomized trial comparing abdominal,
    vaginal and laparoscopic methods of hysterectomy. Health
    Technol Assess 2004; 8(26): 1–154.
15. Wilcox L, Koonin L, Polvas R et al. Hysterectomy in
    the United States, 1988–1990. Obstet Gynecol 1994; 83:
    549–55.
16. Gilmour DT, Dwyer PL, Carey MP. Lower urinary tract
    injury during gynecologic surgery and its detection by intra-
    operative cystoscopy. Obstet Gynecol 1999; 94: 883–9.
17. Tamussino KF, Lang PE, Brein E. Ureteral complications
    with operative gynecologic laparoscopy. Am J Obstet
    Gynecol 1998; 178(5): 967–70.
18. Saidi MH, Sadler RK, Vancaillie TG et al. Diagnosis and
    management of serious urinary complications after major
    operative laparoscopy. Obstet Gynecol 1996; 87: 272–6.

19. Grainger DA, Soderstrom RM, Schiff JF et al. Ureteral injuries at laparoscopy: insights into diagnosis, management and prevention. Obstet Gynecol 1990; 75: 839–43.

20. Wood EC, Maher PJ, M P. Complications of ureteric catheters at laparoscopic hysterectomy. J Am Assoc Gynecol Laparosc 1996; 3: 393–7.

21. Buchsbaum HJ, PS B. Office and surgical gynecology. Gynecol Obstet Urol 1993: 41.

22. Reich H, McGlynn FM, L L. Total laparoscopic hysterectomy. Gynecol Endosc 1993; 2(2): 59–63.

23. Wood C. Radical laparoscopic surgery for endometriosis. Endometriosis Today – Advances in Research and Practice 1996; 289–96.

24. Fedele L, Piazzola E, Raffaeli R, Bianchi S. Bladder endometriosis: deep infiltrating endometriosis or adenomyosis? Fertil Steril 1998; 69: 972–5.

25. Donnez J, Spada F, Squifflet J, Nisolle M. Bladder endometriosis must be considered as bladder adenomyosis. Fertil Steril 2000; 74: 1175–81.

12

Urogenital fistulae

Lore Schierlitz and Peter L Dwyer

Introduction

In this chapter we review fistulae of the lower urinary tract, their etiology, and the role of endoscopy in their diagnosis and treatment. Urogenital fistula is an uncommon but important cause of urinary incontinence in urogynecological practice in industrialized countries and is in most cases related to trauma during pelvic gynecological surgery. In developing countries, urinary fistula related to neglected labor is commonplace. Endoscopy of the urinary tract plays an important role in prevention, diagnosis, and treatment of urogenital fistulae. Intraoperative endoscopy will detect injury to the urethra, bladder, or ureters and allows early diagnosis and repair, and lessens the risk of postoperative morbidity and medicolegal sequelae. The place of endoscopy in prevention of urinary tract injury is addressed in Chapter 14.

A urogenital fistula is an abnormal communication between the urinary (urethra, bladder, and ureter) and genital tract (vagina, cervix, and uterus). An enterovesical fistula is an abnormal communication between the bladder and the intestinal tract, including small bowel, appendix, and large bowel.

Historically, the first urinary fistula was identified in a 4000-years-old Egyptian mummy, caused by obstructed labor due to cephalopelvic disproportion. In European medical history, vesicovaginal fistula and its surgical repair was first described in 1663 by Van Roonhuyze, a Dutch gynecologist.[1] He clearly described the technique of surgical closure, including fistula exposure with appropriate patient positioning, the use of metal ligatures, silk sutures, and braided sutures, and the need for continuous postoperative drainage of the bladder through the suprapubic or transurethral route. In spite of these efforts, surgery was rarely successful. JM Sims from the United States was the first surgeon to describe a procedure to treat vesicovaginal fistulae in 1852 that showed good success, in no small part, due to meticulous surgical technique and better intraoperative fistular exposure and visualization from

patient positioning.[2] The development of modern endoscopic equipment for cystourethroscopy, and better surgical instrumentation and techniques, have played an important part in improving successful surgical repair of urogenital fistulae, which is now above 90% in most series.

Cystourethroscopy, usually with examination under anesthesia, is important in the diagnosis, assessment, and treatment of urogenital fistulae. Careful vaginal examination will determine the vaginal site and condition of the fistula, the mobility of the tissues, and the ease of access for vaginal repair (Figures 12.1 and 12.2). Direct endoscopic visualization of the lower urinary tract allows accurate diagnosis of site, size, and number of fistulae (Figures 12.3

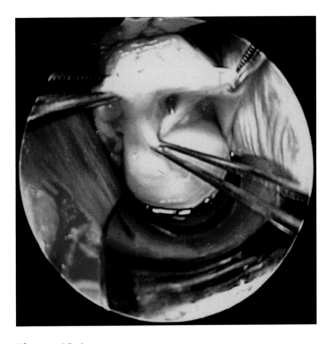

Figure 12.1
Vesicovaginal fistula caused by inappropriate placement of a Shirodkar cervical suture inserted for cervical incompetence during pregnancy.

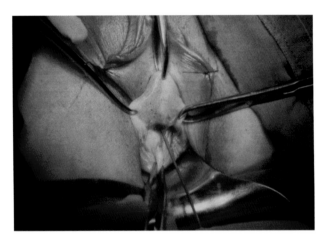

Figure 12.2
Post-hysterectomy vesicovaginal fistula in a woman with
vaginal vault prolapse.

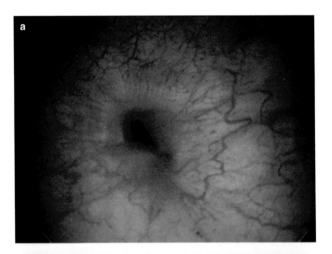

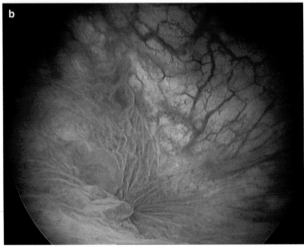

Figure 12.3
(a) Cystoscopic photograph of chronic vesicovaginal fistula ready
for surgical repair; healed fistulous tract with no active
perifistular infection. (b) A more recent vesicovaginal fistula of 5
weeks' duration, with an erythematous fistulous tract but no
active perifistular infection, ready for surgical repair.

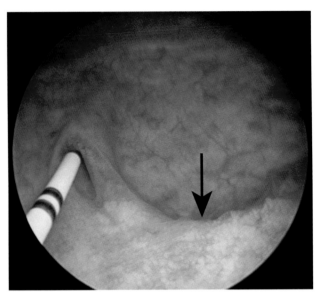

Figure 12.4
Vesicovaginal fistula (arrow) above interureteric ridge and to
left of right ureteric orifice. Ureteric catheter passed to 10 cm
(2 bar marker on catheter) to protect ureter during surgical
repair.

and 12.4). The anatomical relation to urethra, bladder
neck, and ureteral orifices as well as tissue condition, scarring, and adhesions can be assessed. The use of a 0° cystoscope and straight Sasche sheath can improve the
visualization of the urethra in women with a urethrovaginal fistula (Figure 12.5a,b). A 30° and 70° cystoscope
should be used to assess bladder integrity and the patency
and function of the ureters. Indigo carmine, given intravenously, will enable easy visualization of the bilateral
ureteric jets (Figure 12.6); absence may indicate ureteric
obstruction with or without a ureteric fistula. A small
lacrimal probe or urethral probe may be used to pass
through the fistula from the vagina to the bladder, as this
may improve the visualization of a small fistula and its
track (Figure 12.7). When there is postoperative development of urinary leakage from a fistula, the exact site needs
to be established, whether bladder, one or both ureters,
and urethra. Direct visualization will determine the condition of the surrounding bladder wall by detecting the presence of infection, tissue necrosis, and excessive fibrosis,
and help in the planning of the most appropriate timing
and type of repair. The presence of infected, necrotic tissue
and slough would be an indication for delaying surgical
repair. Bladder biopsy of suspicious-looking bladder wall
may be appropriate, particularly in fistulae related to cancer or its treatment with radiation and/or surgery. Calculi
can also be associated with vesical fistula (Figure 12.8),
and may even be important in etiology. Cystourethroscopy
is also useful intraoperatively to confirm watertight closure at the time of the repair and patency of both ureters at
the end of the procedure.

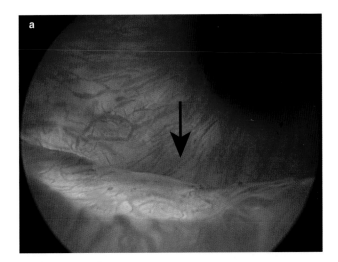

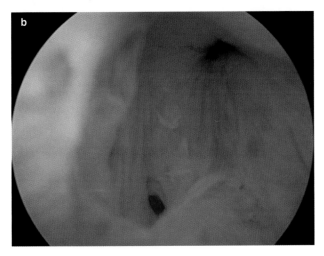

Figure 12.5(a,b)
Urethrovaginal fistula viewed by a 0° cystoscope with Sasche sheath highlighted by arrow in (a), and sited in the right mid-urethral area in (b).

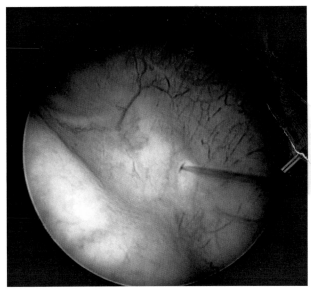

Figure 12.6
Ureteric jet of indigo carmine confirming ureteric patency following surgical repair.

Table 12.1   Etiology of acquired genitourinary fistulae
Obstetrical
Surgical
Malignant
Radiation
Infection
Foreign body
Traumatic
Spontaneous idiopathic

Intravenous indigo carmine, passage of ureteric catheters, and retrograde ureteric urography may also be helpful in the diagnosis of ureteric fistula and in determining the level of obstruction. Intravenous urography, cystography, and hysterosalpingography may be necessary to evaluate complex fistulae. Newer imaging techniques use contrast-enhanced computed tomography (CT) with cystogram (Figure 12.25a,b), magnetic resonance imaging (MRI), and ultrasound.

Etiology

The etiology of urogenital fistulae can be divided into congenital or acquired (Table 12.1). Congenital fistulae are rare. The most common cause of acquired fistulae worldwide is prolonged obstructed labor; however, in developed countries obstetric fistulae secondary to prolonged obstructed labor are very uncommon due to the improvements in modern obstetric care. The majority of fistulae occur as a result of gynecological pelvic surgery. Abdominal hysterectomy, including radical hysterectomy, is the commonest cause of fistulae in industrialized countries, accounting for half of all urogenital fistulae in Hilton's series in the UK,[3] and 81% of all vesicovaginal fistulae in Eilber et al's series in the United States.[4] Vaginal hysterectomy only caused 3 and 8% of fistulae, respectively, in these two series. In a nationwide review of urinary tract injuries after laparoscopic hysterectomy, total abdominal hysterectomy, supracervical abdominal hysterectomy, and vaginal hysterectomy in Finland, Harkki-Siren et al[5] found an incidence of vesicovaginal fistula of 0.8 of 1000 procedures after all hysterectomies: 2.2 of 1000 after laparoscopic, 1.0 of 1000 after total abdominal, 0 of 1000 after supracervical abdominal, and 0.2 of 1000 after vaginal hysterectomy. The incidence of ureteral injury after all hysterectomies was 1.0 of 1000 procedures: 13.9 of 1000 after

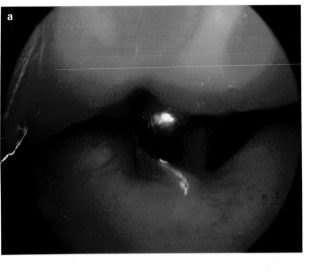

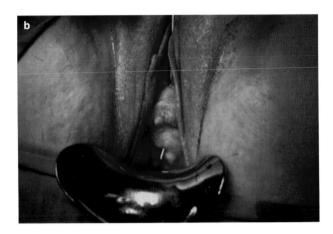

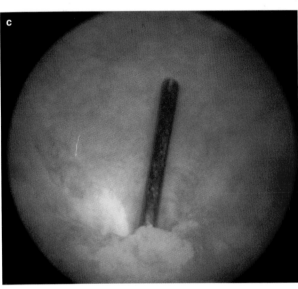

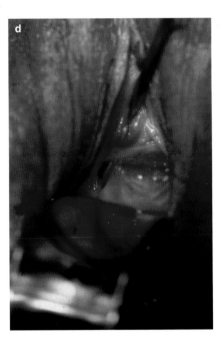

Figure 12.7
Cystoscopic view of vesicovaginal fistula with a sound placed through the fistula transvaginally (a,b). (c,d) Vaginal view.

laparoscopic, 0.4 of 1000 after total abdominal, 0.3 of 1000 after supracervical abdominal, and 0.2 of 1000 after vaginal hysterectomy.

Other pelvic surgery involving the vagina, urethra, uterus, and bladder, such as anterior vaginal repair, urethral diverticulum repair, or surgery for urogenital cancer, is also a significant cause of urinary fistula. Anti-incontinence and prolapse procedures using synthetic meshes and suburethral slings have been associated with the risk of erosion, infection, and development of fistulas.[6]

Classification

At present there is no accepted standardized classification of genitourinary fistulae. Fistula can be described as simple

if only involving two organs, or complex if involving three or more organs (Table 12.2). Another classification is according to etiology (see Table 12.1).

One of the earliest classifications was by Sims (1852), using an anatomical description:

1. Urethrovaginal fistula with defect confined to the urethra.
2. Fistulae involving bladder neck and/or root of the urethra destroying the trigone.
3. Fistulae involving body and floor of the bladder.
4. Uterovesical fistulae communicating with uterine cavity or cervical canal.

Modifications have been made by other authors, and were summarized by Mahfouz in 1930:[7]

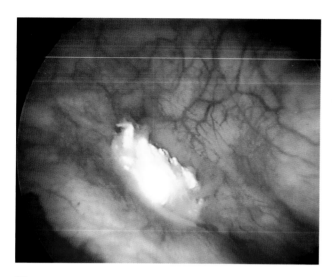

Figure 12.8
Bladder calculi embedded in bladder diverticulum resulting from repair of VVF.

1. Size, form, and variety of the fistula.
2. Scarring of the vagina and mobility of the fistula.
3. Attachment of the fistula to the pelvic side wall.
4. Condition of the urethral sphincter and permeability of the internal orifice of the urethra.
5. Ureteral orifices and their relation to the location of the fistula.
6. Other complicating factors: coexisting rectovaginal fistula; inflammatory lesions in the pelvis, vagina, vulva, or perineum.
7. Number of fistulae.

The development of an accepted classification of urogenital fistulae is important, as this will help in the understanding and comparison of surgical techniques. Cystoscopic and vaginal examination will be an essential element in any classification of urogenital fistulae.

Clinical presentation

The clinical presentation of urinary fistulae depends on the site (ureteral, vesical, urethral), the size of the fistula, and if urethral its relationship to the urethral sphincter. There are variations from slight leakage with a small fistula to severe urinary incontinence with larger fistulae. Women with a ureteric fistula or a moderate to large vesicovaginal fistula usually have continuous urinary leakage day and night and infrequent normal voiding. This can also occur in women with severe intrinsic sphincter dysfunction stress incontinence, so that a high level of suspicion regarding fistula needs to be maintained. Development of skin irritation and malodor is common with larger fistulae.

Table 12.2 Anatomical classification of genitourinary fistulae	
Simple fistulae	*Complex fistulae*
Urethrovaginal	Vesicoureterovaginal
Vesicovaginal	Vesicoureterouterine
Ureterovaginal	Vesicovaginorectal
Vesicouterine	
Ureterouterine	

Urinary leakage may be seen on vaginal examination coming from the upper vagina, and not through the external urethral meatus, as in stress incontinence (Figure 12.9). With small fistulae, the three-tampon test by Moir[8] may be helpful to establish the diagnosis. This involves placement of three tampons in tandem. Methylene blue is instilled in the bladder and the patient is asked to walk for 15 minutes. Then the tampons are removed and examined. Staining of the lowest tampon will indicate urethral leakage or a urethrovaginal fistula, whereas staining of the upper tampons make a vesicovaginal fistula likely. If the upper tampons are wet but not stained blue, a ureterovaginal fistula should be suspected.

Urinary leakage in women with urethrovaginal fistula (UVF) will vary with the site of the fistula in relationship to the urethral sphincter, and the competency of the bladder neck. Where the UVF is in the distal urethra the woman may be continent, but may have post-micturition dribbling or vaginal leakage. UVF in the mid to proximal urethra may still be dry if the bladder neck is competent. If the bladder neck becomes incompetent in pregnancy or with aging, then incontinence can occur.

Ureteric fistulae have a similar presentation and etiology to other urinary fistulae. Postoperative symptoms following hysterectomy such as abdominal or loin pain, distention, paralytic ileus, hematuria, pyrexia, and severe bladder irritability are suggestive of a possible bladder or ureteric injury.[9] Ureteric fistula may present with urinary leakage with minimal other symptoms, so that a high level of suspicion is necessary with early investigation, recognition, and treatment.

Congenital urinary fistula

Congenital urogenital fistulae are uncommon but can be easily overlooked if not considered. Congenital urethrovaginal, vesicovaginal fistula, and ectopic ureters associated with other anomalies of the urinary tract frequently present in adolescent or adult women as urinary incontinence[10,11] (Figure 12.10). A high level of suspicion should be maintained, especially in women with other congenital urogenital anomalies, including uterus didelphys, a solitary

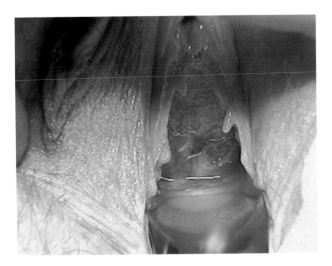

Figure 12.9
Vaginal view of vesicovaginal fistula leaking urine high on anterior vaginal wall with Sims speculum retracting the posterior vaginal wall.

hypoplastic or absent kidney, or unusual urethral diverticulum or Gartner's duct anomalies.[10] The author (PLD) knows of two cases of ectopic ureters that presented after unsuccessful stress incontinence surgery before the correct diagnosis was made. Congenital anomalies and their embryogenesis are discussed in Chapter 5.

Obstetric urinary fistulae

In the developing world, obstetric fistulae caused by obstructed labor are common, occurring as frequently as 1 in 300 deliveries.[12] The incidence of urogenital fistulae secondary to obstructed labor is highest in areas of poor obstetric care where the maternal mortality is high. In labor, the base of the bladder and urethra is compressed between the fetal head and the symphysis, which even in straightforward normal labor results in bruising and swelling of the bladder base (Figure 12.11). In obstructed labor the uterus becomes hypertonic and persistent compression of the soft tissues of the partly dilated cervix, vagina, and base of bladder result in ischemic necrosis of these tissues and fistula formation 5–10 days later (Figure 12.12). Similarly, pressure necrosis can also result from compression of the rectovaginal septum between the fetal head and sacral promontory. Vesicovaginal fistula (VVF) resulting from obstructed labor has coexisting rectovaginal fistula in 6–24% of cases.[13]

The size of these obstetric fistulae makes bladder filling and visualization during cystourethroscopy difficult (Figures 12.13 and 12.14). However, even in a large fistula,

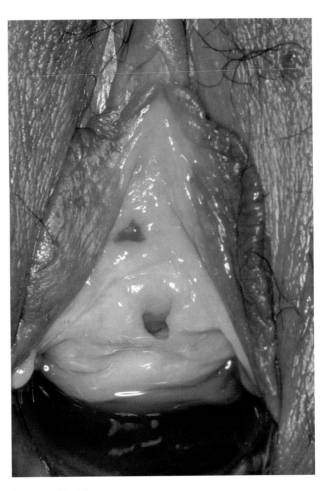

Figure 12.10
Congenital urethrovaginal fistula leaking urine in a woman with renal hypoplasia and left ectopic ureter.

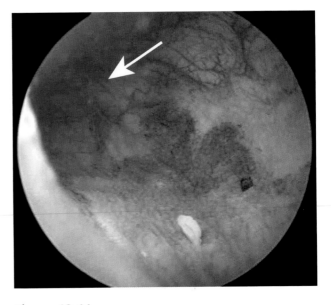

Figure 12.11
Bruising of the trigone and bladder base following a normal vaginal delivery. Arrow shows right ureteric orifice.

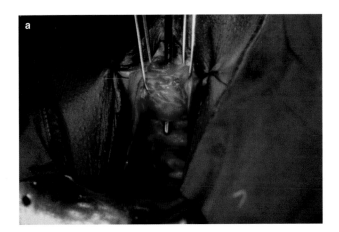

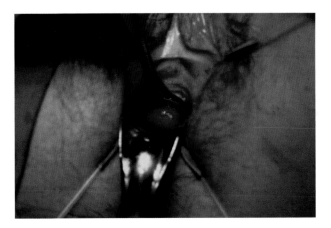

Figure 12.13
Large obstetric vesicovaginal fistula with bladder mucosa and base seen transvaginally on retraction with a Sims speculum. (Ethiopia. Courtesy of C Murray.)

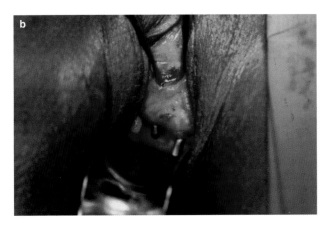

Figure 12.12
Obstetric fistulae with (a) one and (b) two tracts. (Ethiopia. Courtesy of C Murray.)

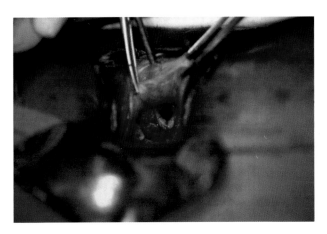

Figure 12.14
Obstetric vesicovaginal fistula. (Ethiopia. Courtesy of C Murray.)

cystourethroscopy and examination under anesthesia can provide useful information on the size and site of the fistula and condition of the surrounding tissue.

In industrialized countries, obstetric fistulae are caused by injury to the urinary tract during forceps delivery, cesarean section, uterine rupture, or cesarean hysterectomy. In Hilton's UK study,[3] obstetric fistulae accounted for 12% of all urogenital fistulae.

Iatrogenic surgically induced fistula

Injury to the urinary tract during surgery is the commonest cause of urogenital fistulae in industrialized countries. In most series of urinary fistulae in industrialized countries abdominal hysterectomy is the commonest cause followed by radical hysterectomy, vaginal hysterectomy, urethral diverticulum, and pelvic floor surgery. Urinary fistulae usually present as urinary leakage postoperatively; early leakage suggests direct injury to the urinary tract with inadvertent

opening of the urinary tract and/or inadequate repair. Later presentation, occurring 7–10 days following surgery, would indicate that ischemic necrosis, hematoma formation, and infection may also play a more important role in causation. The site of the fistula will vary with the procedure performed and the causation. Following abdominal hysterectomy, the location of the fistula is invariably just above the interureteric ridge (Figure 12.15). There may be more than one site of fistula formation (Figure 12.16), so careful endoscopic and urographic evaluation is necessary prior to surgical closure. The fistula may also be in close approximation to the ureteric orifices, necessitating the placement of ureteric catheters. Cystoscopy should also be performed immediately following surgical closure to ensure a watertight closure and that there are no other VVF present.

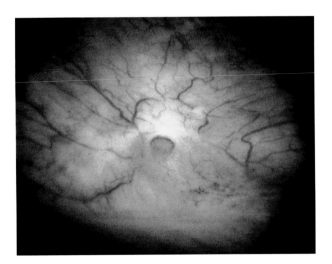

Figure 12.15
Cystoscopic view of vesicovaginal fistula occurring following a total abdominal hysterectomy. These fistulae are typically sited as in the case above just above the interureteric bar at the bottom of the figure.

Injury to the bladder can occur at the time of retropubic surgery for stress incontinence (e.g. Burch colposuspension or sling (Figure 12.17)) and result in fistular communication with the anterior bladder wall or bladder dome. This is the same site where intravesical sutures are sometimes mistakenly placed during Burch cdposuspension or long needle urethral suspension (e.g. Stamey). The placement of intravesical sutures however is an uncommon cause of a urinary fistula. Meeks et al[14] in an eloquent animal study on rabbits found that suture placement through the bladder during closure of the vaginal cuff after transabdominal hysterectomy, as an isolated event, does not appear to be associated with formation of postoperative VVF.

In Hilton's series[3] from the North-East of England, urethral diverticulectomy accounted for 10% of the surgical-induced urogenital fistulae. UVF has been reported to occur in 0.9–8.3% of cases following urethral diverticulectomy.[15–17] This high prevalence emphasizes the surgical care that needs to be taken in diverticular repair. Excision of the urethral diverticulum, meticulous urethral closure using a 4/0 absorbable suture in layers without tension, and postoperative bladder drainage are important in the prevention of this postoperative complication. Infection in the diverticulum can also be a contributing factor to repair breakdown, so that antibiotic cover is frequently necessary. Partial breakdown can lead to the recurrence of a wide-necked diverticulum (Figure 12.18), which may be asymptomatic or be associated with stress incontinence or calculus formation.

A permanent vesicocutaneous fistula may be created intentionally to allow long-term suprapubic catheterization

in women with chronic urinary retention or incontinence (Figure 12.19).

Non-surgical traumatic fistula

Non-surgical injury to the urethra and bladder can occur as a result of accidental trauma to the urinary tract or as a result of sexual misadventure. Trauma to the urinary tract can be self-induced during masturbation alone or during sexual activity with other people.

These are case reports on urogenital fistulae caused by foreign bodies such as aerosol caps,[18] neglected vaginal pessaries,[19] or a raw banana[20] inserted into the vagina. The foreign body may have been used for contraception, conservative treatment for prolapse, sexual gratification, or as part of a complex psychiatric illness such as Munchausen's syndrome.[21,22] Injury can be to either the urethra or bladder by direct trauma, pressure necrosis, or infection from a foreign body resulting in a urethrovaginal (Cases 1 and 2) or vesicovaginal fistula (Case 3).

Case 1

A 17-year-old woman presented to the urogynecological clinic with a history of urinary urgency, urge incontinence, intermittent hematuria, and offensive vaginal discharge. In the past she was investigated for dystonia of the right foot at 13 years of age and she developed unexplained bruising at the age of 16. She was extensively investigated without establishment of a diagnosis, and a psychiatric assessment that was also performed at that time was normal.

On examination, her body mass index (BMI) was 27.5 and the abdominal examination was normal. Gynecological examination was limited to inspection of the genitalia, as she was not sexually active as yet. Vaginal swabs showed heavy growth of enteric flora and mid-stream urine (MSU) repeatedly diagnosed a urinary tract infection: both were treated with repeated courses of oral antibiotics. She was commenced on oxybutynin, 2.5 mg twice daily, and a bladder diary was completed.

As symptoms did not improve, an examination under anesthesia and cystoscopy was performed. A 1 cm VVF was detected above the trigone and communicating with the anterior vaginal wall approximately 3–4 cm from the hymen (Figure 12.20a,b). An indwelling catheter was inserted and remained in situ for 4 weeks. Findings were discussed with the patient and the cause of the fistula could not be established. As trauma due to sexual activity or sexual abuse was considered, the patient was referred for psychiatric evaluation. Further evaluation of the renal tract with intravenous pyelography (IVP) was arranged. The IVP demonstrated a normal renal system, but on the premicturition film, a 5 cm long screw was seen within the vagina (Figure 12.20c,d).

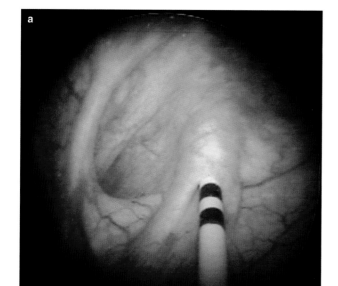

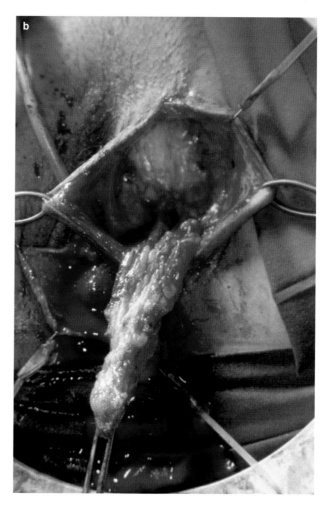

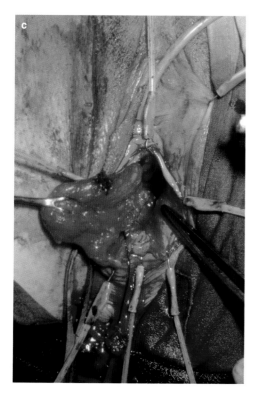

Figure 12.16
Cystoscopic photographs of a woman with bilateral vesicovaginal fistulae sited medially to the left (a) and right ureteric orifice, taken 3 months following a difficult abdominal hysterectomy. The bladder was inadvertently opened during the hysterectomy and then repaired. Vaginal leakage was noticed 7 days following surgery. One fistula was sited next to the right (a) Repair was performed transvaginally and both fistulae were closed in multiple layers. This repair was reinforced with a Martius labial fat graft; an incision was made on the left labia major; the fat pad was fashioned (b), tunneled between the inferior border of the pubic ramus and vulval skin, and laid over the repaired fistula (c).

Further psychiatric assessment over a period of 3 months established the diagnosis of Munchausen's syndrome.

After discussion with the psychiatrist, a layered fistula repair was performed and closure was achieved with a Martius graft from the left labia majora. Psychiatric treatment was continued throughout. The fistula site did heal well, but the graft site at the labia broke down due to patient manipulation, but subsequently healed by secondary intention. One year following the surgery, the fistula remained healed and no other urogynecological problems were detected.

Case 2

A 30-year-old primigravid woman did have normal vaginal delivery at term. The infant weighed 3.5 kg. Post-delivery a catheter was inserted through the external urethral meatus into the vagina, indicating a urethro- or

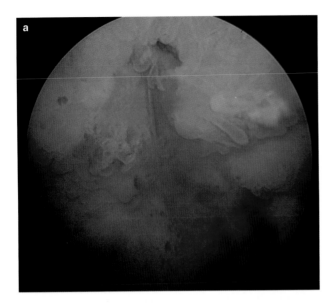

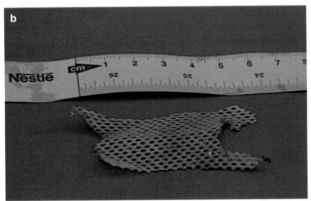

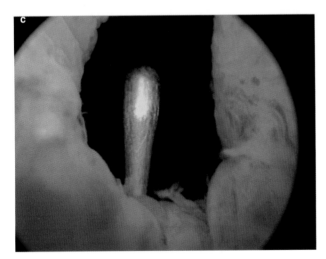

Figure 12.17
(a) Vesicovaginal fistula (VVF) present at bladder dome following insertion of silicone-coated sling; note edematous bladder mucosa around fistula and purulent discharge. However, she continued to be incontinent postoperatively and 6 months later was found to have posterior vesicovaginal fistula just above the bladder neck (probe). This was repaired vaginally with layered closure and Martius graft. (b) Intac sling was removed transvaginally and the VVF healed spontaneously following 2 weeks of continuous bladder drainage. (c) Probe.

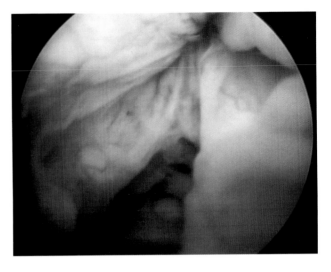

Figure 12.18
This woman developed a urethrovaginal fistula following excision of a urethral diverticulum. The UVF was successfully closed but she had persistent stress incontinence and on urethroscopy had a wide necked urethral diverticulum.

vesicovaginal fistula. On examination under anesthesia, a long-standing urethrovaginal fistula (Figure 12.21a,b) was found which was not caused by childbirth trauma as was suspected. On cystourethroscopy, there was bruising of the trigone and bladder base, presumably a consequence of the normal vaginal delivery. A layered repair of the fistula was performed (Figure 12.21c,d). Afterwards, the patient reported that at the age of 1 year she suffered a vaginal injury due to the insertion of a pen top by a 5-year-old sibling. A repair by a gynecologist was performed at the time. She did have urinary leakage 2–3 times per week during her childhood and prior to the pregnancy, but thought this to be normal. During pregnancy, urinary leakage worsened, presumably as the bladder neck became less competent.

Eight weeks post repair the fistula did heal well and incontinence episodes had reduced to minimal leakage, occasionally with lifting.

Case 3

A 72-year-old woman presented with a large ulcerated post-hysterectomy vaginal vault prolapse and urinary incontinence. The incontinence was caused by a large chronic urethrovaginal fistula (Figure 12.22a,b). The cause of the urethrovaginal fistula was not clear but it may have been caused by forceful urethral catheterization in a woman with marked urethral distortion secondary to prolapse. The inappropriate use of a vaginal pessary causing ulceration and ischemic necrosis may also have been a contributing factor in this patient. The prolapse was treated

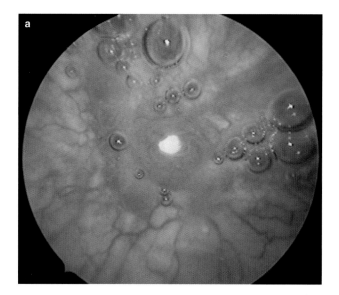 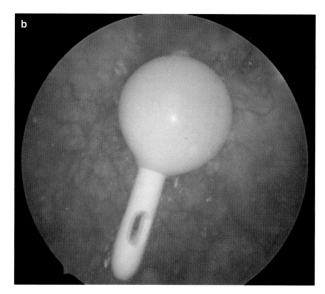

Figure 12.19
(a) Cystoscopic view of vesicocutaneous fistula intentionally made for long-term suprapubic bladder drainage in a woman with urinary retention. (b) With Foley catheter in situ.

surgically with a transvaginal extraperitoneal uterosacral vault suspension, and the fistula with a layered transvaginal urethral repair (Figure 12.22c).

Radiation-induced and cancer-related fistulae

Cancer is an important cause of urinary fistulae, occurring either secondary to tumor invasion and necrosis or as a secondary result of treatment using radiation or surgery or both. Ionizing radiation can cause major damage to the urinary tract and is a significant cause of vesicovaginal fistula, being the primary etiological factor in 12% of urogenital fistulae reported by Hilton[3] in the UK and 4% of all vesicovaginal fistulae in a series by Eilber et al[4] in the United States. Vesicovaginal fistulae have been reported to occur in between 0.6 and 2.4% of women having radiation for treatment of cervical cancer.[23,24] The incidence of radiation fistulae varies with the dosage of irradiation given, stage of the cervical cancer, and whether cancer surgery is also performed. Perez et al,[23] in their series, found that the incidence of vesicovaginal fistula with irradiation alone was 0.9% compared with 1.6% with irradiation + surgery.

Radiation fistulae usually occur within 12 months of the completion of treatment; however, they can occur many years following radiation therapy because of the ongoing ischemic effects caused by obliterative arteritis (Case 4).

In the acute phase (<6 months), radiation cystitis may present with intermittent hematuria, dysuria, and irritable bladder symptoms. The cystoscopic appearance in acute cases is diffuse mucosal hyperemia with partial desquamation and superficial ulceration. When tissue necrosis is severe, severe ulceration can occur with fistula formation. Chronic radiation cystitis may present with urinary incontinence, urinary frequency, and urgency or voiding difficulty. Radiation injury may result in bladder wall fibrosis and loss of bladder compliance, damage to the urethral sphincter mechanism, or the development of a fistula. In chronic cases, the bladder mucosa is pale and atrophic with tortuous dilated blood vessels, telangiectasia, and occasionally ulceration (Figure 12.23).

Cystourethroscopy is important in the diagnosis and evaluation of radiation fistulae but can be difficult because of the inability to fill the bladder completely, especially if the fistula is large. However, cystoscopy can provide much useful information. First, cystoscopy should confirm the diagnosis of vesicovaginal fistulae secondary to radiation and exclude the possibility of recurrent cancer. If the surrounding bladder mucosa appears suspicious, a biopsy should be taken. The site and location of the fistula should be described and the degree of surrounding inflammation and bladder fibrosis should also be assessed.

Case 4

An 80-year-old woman had an endometrial adenocarcinoma treated with abdominal hysterectomy, bilateral salpingo-

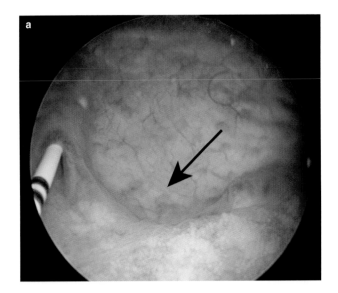

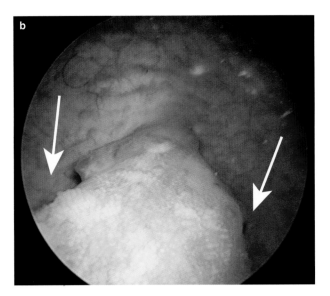

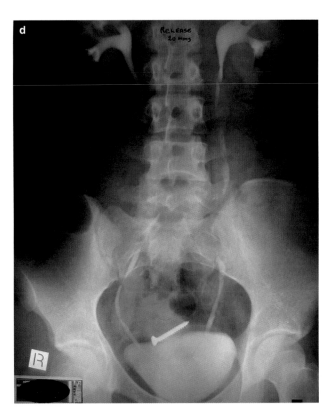

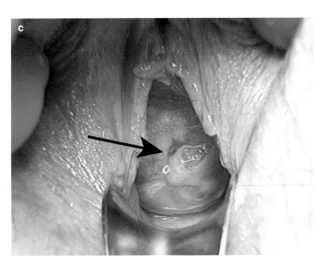

Figure 12.20

(Case 1) (a) Vesicovaginal fistula (VVF) caused by a screw placed intentionally into the vagina by a 17-year-old girl with Munchausen's disease. (b) Cystoscopic view of the VVF and left ureteric orifice. (c) Vaginal view of the VVF. (d) Unexpected finding of a 5 cm screw in the vagina at the time of IVP.

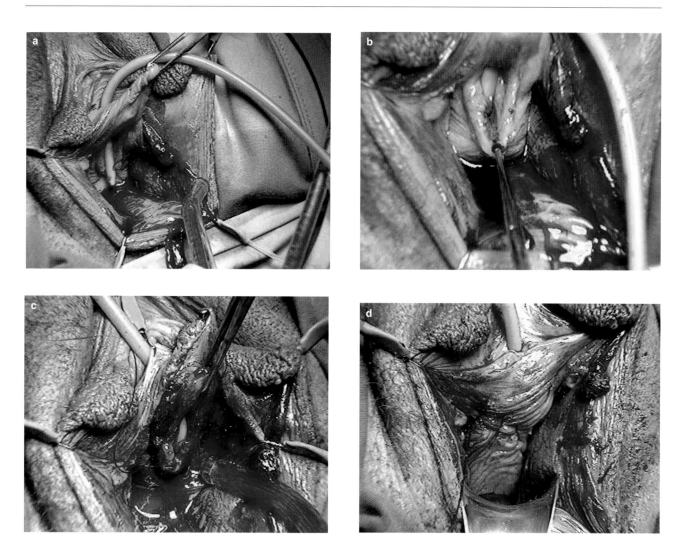

Figure 12.21(a–d)
(Case 2) Urethrovaginal fistula discovered in a 30-year-old primigravida at time of normal vaginal delivery which was subsequently found to be caused by a childhood accident. (c,d). The UVF was repaired in a layered closure using 3/0 Vicryl.

oophorectomy, and lymphadenectomy followed by pelvic irradiation in 1995. She developed severe radiation proctitis in 1998. She presented with severe sudden-onset continuous urinary leakage of 8 months' duration in 2004. She was very difficult to examine, as she had a small stenosed vagina. Examination under anesthesia and cystourethroscopy revealed a 1 cm vesicovaginal fistula present between the posterior bladder wall and the vault of a stenosed vagina (see Figure 12.23). The bladder mucosa was pale and edematous, typical of a post-irradiation bladder. There was no evidence of malignancy in the bladder, vagina, or pelvis. A bladder biopsy was taken and showed active chronic cystitis with dilated thickened blood vessels typical of radiation effect.

Following discussion of her options, she requested no further surgical treatment. Surgical repair of radiation-induced vesicovaginal fistulae is particularly difficult because of the size of the fistula and poor healing secondary to poor blood supply and vasculitis of the radiation- damaged surrounding tissue. Moreover, mobilization of the tissues and closure without tension is difficult because of radiation-induced fibrosis. Therefore, whether surgical repair is performed abdominally or vaginally, healthy non-radiated well-vascularized tissue needs to be interposed between the affective organs to improve closure and healing. This is usually performed abdominally using omental grafts or vaginally with a Martius labial fat pad graft (Figure 12.16 b,c).

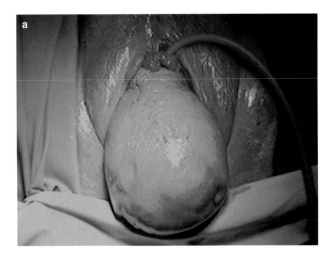

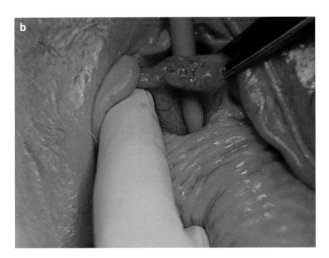

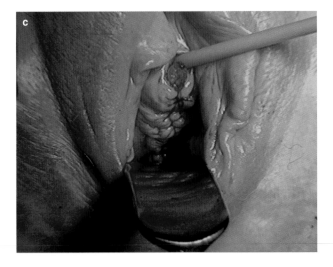

Figure 12.22(a–c)
(Case 3) (a,b) Large ulcerated post-hysterectomy vault prolapse and urethrovaginal fistula. (c) Following transvaginal repair of the UVF and prolapse with extraperitoneal bilateral uterosacral suspension.

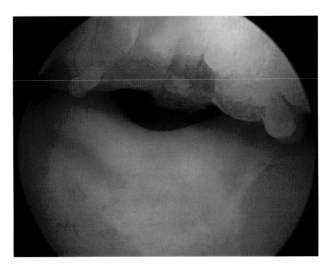

Figure 12.23
(Case 4) Large vesicovaginal fistula in an 80-year-old woman who became incontinent 8 years following hysterectomy and radiation treatment for adenocarcinoma of the uterus. Note pale atrophic mucosa on posterior bladder wall and edematous mucosa on the anterior wall.

Treatment

Conservative treatment

Prolonged bladder drainage can achieve spontaneous closure in small vesicovaginal fistulae with reported success rates between 3%[25] and 7%.[26] It is important that any urinary tract or vaginal infection be treated before any attempt to surgical closure of the fistula. Untreated and ongoing infection will jeopardize healing after the repair. Estrogen replacement (where appropriate) may help to improve the vaginal epithelium and vascularity prior to surgery.

Surgical treatment

General principles that apply in the planning of a urogenital fistula repair are:

- The first attempt is the best chance of success.
- The choice of procedure will depend on the etiology of the fistula, the size and position of the fistula, vaginal access, the quality of the tissue available for repair, and the experience and training of the surgeon.
- Follow basic surgical principles such as tension-free closure, uninfected tissues, and good hemostasis and, if the repair is tenuous, use of well-vascularized tissue grafts should be considered.

Prior to surgical fistula closure, cystoscopy may be required to identify the ureters' orifices and, if the fistula is in close

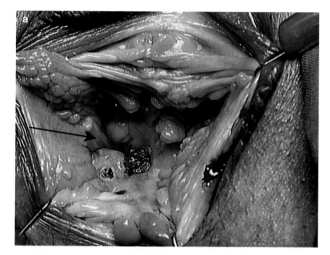

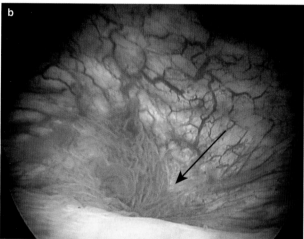

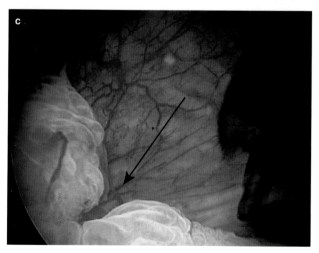

Figure 12.24
A 40 year old woman with vaginal stenosis from repeated prolapse surgery developed a VVF 8 months following a transvaginal procedure with graft to enlarge the vaginal lengh and width. The fistula was thought to be caused by the repeated use of vaginal dilators. The VVF (arrow) can be seen at the vaginal apex (a), and by cystoscopy before (b) and after a Latzko repair and injection of indigo carmen (c).

proximity, pass ureteric catheters. This will allow easy identification of the ureters throughout the surgery and help to prevent intraoperative damage due to unrecognized ligation.

In developed countries vesicovaginal fistulae are the commonest urogenital fistula, usually occurring following gynecological surgery for benign conditions. Post-hysterectomy fistulae are usually located at or just above the interureteric ridge and open into the vagina anterior to the vault. Fistula repair is normally delayed until the tissue conditions are good when local infection and inflammation has settled. The vaginal approach is preferable to the abdominal one, as there is less postoperative morbidity and pain, and a quicker recovery, and therefore less risk of medicolegal sequelae. In the Latzko procedure, the vaginal wall around the fistulous tract is excised in 2 cm radius. The bladder opening is identified and closed with 4/0 Monocryl without excision of the fistula. The fascia and vaginal epithelium is closed in layers with 2/0 Vicryl without tension. The failure rate for primary fistula repair using the Latzko procedure is low and has been reported as 7%.[27,28]

Urethrovaginal fistulae or vesicovaginal fistulae of the bladder base present on the anterior vaginal wall and can be repaired with a layered transvaginal closure. Following wide mobilization of the surrounding tissue, the bladder or urethra are closed with interrupted sutures of 4/0 Monocryl, inverting the bladder or urethral mucosa. This is followed by a layered closure of the bladder/urethral muscularis and fibromuscular wall of the vagina. Watertightness of the repair can be tested by careful bladder distention either by a catheter or by cystourethroscopy (Figure 12.24 a–c). Any additional sutures may be placed at any site of leakage and then the vaginal epithelium is closed in layers.

Flap closures with bulbocavernosus fat pad graft (the Martius graft procedure) or a gracilis/rectus muscle graft will give additional support and introduce healthy, well-vascularized tissue in more complex fistulae or previous unsuccessful closure. The success rate using tissue interposition has been reported as 96–97%.[4] Most vesicovaginal fistulae can be repaired vaginally, even in nulliparous women where the access is limited.

The abdominal or abdominovaginal route is the best choice in cases of complex fistulae such as vesicoureterovaginal, vesicoureterouterine, vesicovaginorectal. Fistulae associated with malignancy and radiation therapy (where the amount of fibrotic-indurated damaged tissue around the fistula is difficult to mobilize) or in women with multiple previous unsuccessful attempts of closure may require an abdominal approach. In these complex cases more complete assessment and imaging using contrast-enhanced three-dimensional CT scans with cystogram[29] (Figure 12.25a and b) or MRI is appropriate to visualize the site of the fistula and its relationship to surrounding organs. The fistula can be accessed through an abdominal incision and sagittal cystotomy. After mobilization of the fistulous

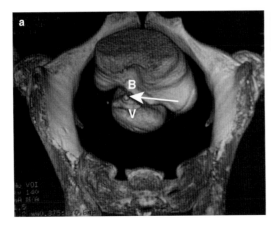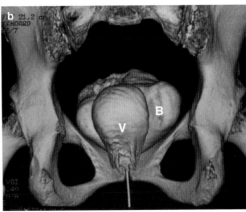

Figure 12.25(a,b)
Volume rendered 3 dimensional reconstruction computer tomograms of 39 year old woman who devevloped a vesicovaginal fistula (arrow) following radical hysterectomy and adjuvant radiation for adenocarcinoma of the uterus. Abdominal repair of the VVF was unsuccessful. The pelvic inlet is viewed from the superior (a) and posterior perspective (b), demonstrating contrast within the bladder (B) and vagina (V), the catheter can be seen entering the bladder in the posterior (b) view.

tract, closure of the bladder and the vagina in separate layers with absorbable, interrupted sutures is recommended. The use of peritoneum or omentum introduces healthy, well-vascularized tissue to separate bladder and vagina. Transperitoneal–transvesical vesicovaginal fistula repair has a reported success rate of 85%.[30] Occasionally, a combined abdominal–vaginal procedure may be necessary.

Early postoperative complications after fistula repair may be fistula recurrence, bleeding, wound infection, and/or dehiscence. Late complications such as urinary stress incontinence, reduced bladder capacity, dyspareunia, and vaginal stenosis can occur.

References

1. Roonhuyse Hv. Operative Gynaecology, 1663.
2. Sims J. On the treatment of vesico-vaginal fistula, 1852. Int Urogynecol J Pelvic Floor Dysfunct 1998; 9(4): 236–48.
3. Hilton P. Fistulae. In: Shaw R, Soutter WP, Stanton SL, eds. Gynaecology, 3rd edn. London: Churchill Livingstone, 2003: 835–56.
4. Eilber KS, Kavaler E, Rodriguez LV, Rosenblum N, Raz S. Ten-year experience with transvaginal vesicovaginal fistula repair using tissue interposition. J Urol 2003; 169: 1033–6.
5. Harkki-Siren P, Sjoberg J, Tiitinen A. Urinary tract injuries after hysterectomy. Obstet Gynecol 1998; 92: 113–18.
6. Kobashi KC, Dmochowski R, Mee SL et al. Erosion of woven polyester pubovaginal sling. J Urol 1999; 162: 2070–2.
7. Mahfouz B. Urinary fistulae in women. J Obstet Gynaecol Br Emp 1930: 566–78.
8. Moir JC. Vesico-vaginal fistulae as seen in Britain. J Obstet Gynaecol Br Commonw 1973; 80: 598–602.
9. Kursh ED, Morse RM, Resnick MI, Persky L. Prevention of the development of a vesicovaginal fistula. Surg Gynecol Obstet 1988; 166: 409–12.
10. Dwyer PL, Rosamilia A. Congenital urogenital anomalies that are associated with the persistence of Gartner's duct: a review. Am J Obstet Gynecol 2006; 195(2): 354–9.
11. Dolan LM, Easwaran SP, Hilton P. Congenital vesicovaginal fistula in association with hypoplastic kidney and uterus didelphys. Urology 2004; 63: 175–7.
12. Harrison KA. Child-bearing, health and social priorities: a survey of 22774 consecutive hospital births in Zaria, Northern Nigeria. Br J Obstet Gynaecol 1985; 92: 1–119.
13. Wall LL, Karshima JA, Kirschner C, Arrowsmith SD. The obstetric vesicovaginal fistula: characteristics of 899 patients from Jos, Nigeria. Am J Obstet Gynecol 2004; 190: 1011–19.
14. Meeks GR, Sams JO 4th, Field KW, Fulp KS, Margolis MT. Formation of vesicovaginal fistula: the role of suture placement into the bladder during closure of the vaginal cuff after transabdominal hysterectomy. Am J Ostet Gynecol 1997; 177(6): 1298–303, discussion 1303–4.
15. Ganabathi K, Leach GE, Zimmern PE, Dmochowski R. Experience with the management of urethral diverticulum in 63 women. J Urol 1994; 152: 1445–52.
16. Mackinnon M, Pratt JH, Pool TL. Diverticulum of the female urethra. Surg Clin North Am 1959; 39: 953–62.
17. Lee RA. Diverticulum of the female urethra: postoperative complications and results. Obstet Gynecol 1983; 61: 52–8.
18. Binstock MA, Semrad N, Dubow L, Watring W. Combined vesicovaginal-ureterovaginal fistulas associated with a vaginal foreign body. Obstet Gynecol 1990; 76: 918–21.
19. Grody MH, Nyirjesy P, Chatwani A. Intravesical foreign body and vesicovaginal fistula: a rare complication of a neglected pessary. Int Urogynecol J Pelvic Floor Dysfunct 1999; 10: 407–8.
20. Ramaiah KS, Kumar S. Vesicovaginal fistula following masturbation managed conservatively. Aust N Z J Obstet Gynaecol 1998; 38: 475–6.
21. Fliegner JR. Munchausen's syndrome and self-induced illness in gynaecology. Med J Aust 1983; 2: 666–7.

22. Edi-Osagie EC, Hopkins RE, Edi-Osagie NE. Munchausen's syndrome in obstetrics and gynecology: a review. Obstet Gynecol Surv 1998; 53: 45–9.

23. Perez CA, Grigsby PW, Lockett MA, Chao KS, Williamson J. Radiation therapy morbidity in carcinoma of the uterine cervix: dosimetric and clinical correlation. Int J Radiat Oncol Biol Phys 1999; 44: 855–66.

24. Mitsuhashi N, Takahashi M, Yamakawa M et al. Results of postoperative radiation therapy for patients with carcinoma of the uterine cervix: evaluation of intravaginal cone boost with an electron beam. Gynecol Oncol 1995; 57: 321–6.

25. Tancer ML. Observations on prevention and management of vesicovaginal fistula after total hysterectomy. Surg Gynecol Obstet 1992; 175: 501–6.

26. Hilton P. Vesico-vaginal fistula: new perspectives. Curr Opin Obstet Gynecol 2001; 13: 513–20.

27. Tancer ML. The post-total hysterectomy (vault) vesicovaginal fistula. J Urol 1980; 123: 839–40.

28. Methfessel HD, Retzke U, Schwarz R, Methfessel G. Occlusion of a vesicovaginal fistula with Latzko-repair. Geburtshilfe Frauenheilkd 1992; 52: 606–10.

29. Lawrentschuk N, Koulouris G, Bolton DM. Delineating the anatomy of oncologic post-radiation vesicovaginal fistula with reconstructed computed tomography. Int J Urogyn 2007 in press.

30. Mondet F, Chartier-Kastler EJ, Conort P et al. Anatomic and functional results of transperitoneal–transvesical vesico-vaginal fistula repair. Urology 2001; 58: 882–6.

13

Role of cystourethroscopy in urogynecological surgery

Brigitte Fatton and Peter L Dwyer

Introduction

Cystourethroscopy to check the integrity of the lower urinary tract has become an essential part of many urogynecological operations if these procedures are to be performed safely, and this has led many gynecologists to see the need to improve their endoscopic skills and knowledge.

Cystourethroscopy may be necessary during surgery:

1. To exclude injury to the bladder or urethra during the procedure, especially during the learning phase.
2. To verify accurate placement of suspension sutures or slings or to safely place suprapubic catheters.
3. To deliver material endoscopically into the wall of the urethra or the bladder to treat urinary conditions: e.g. transurethral collagen or silicone for stress incontinence, transvesical Botox (botulinum A toxin) injections for overactive bladder.
4. To confirm ureteric patency and enable placement of ureteric catheters when needed.

In this chapter we review these urogynecological procedures with an emphasis on the endoscopic aspect of the operation, either in the performance of the procedure or in the treatment of postoperative complications.

Retropubic bladder neck suspension procedures

Retropubic urethropexy operations for stress incontinence were first described by Marshall, Marchetti, and Krantz in 1949[1] and later by Burch in 1961.[2] The aim of both procedures was to stabilize the urethra by suspension sutures and to approximate the periurethral and vaginal tissue to the back of the symphysis pubis or iliopectineal ligaments. The suspension sutures originally used were absorbable, although more recently non-absorbable

sutures have been used to improve long-term outcome. There are numerous technical modifications and refinements, including performing the procedure laparoscopically first performed in the early 1990s.[3] Intraoperative cystoscopy has not been a standard part of the original operations, although urinary tract injury has been a significant complication of these operations, with Burch[2] describing a case of vesicovaginal fistula in a woman who had a Burch colposuspension and abdominal hysterectomy. In recent years many surgeons have performed cystourethroscopy postoperatively to ensure that the bladder or the ureters have not been injured intraoperatively or that suspension sutures have been placed in the correct positions, not distorting or overelevating the bladder neck (Figure 13.1), or not inadvertently being placed through the wall of the bladder (Figure 13.2).

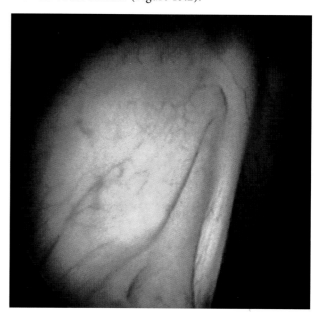

Figure 13.1
Cystoscopic photograph of left ureteric orifice suspended by a misplaced suture from a previous Burch colposuspension.

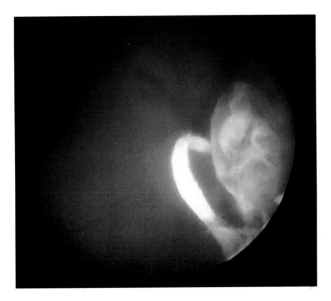

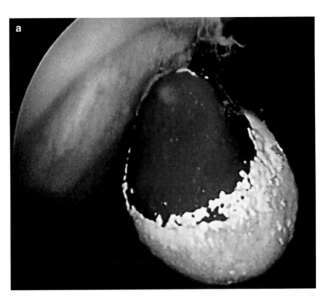

Figure 13.2
Non-absorbable Ethibond multifilament nylon suture of a Burch colposuspension is surrounded by inflamed edematous mucosa penetrating the dome of the bladder. The presenting symptoms were pelvic pain, urinary frequency, and recurrent urinary tract infection.

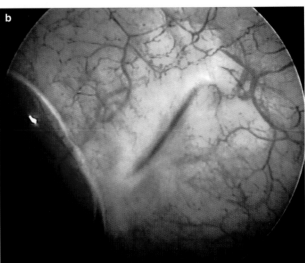

Burch colposuspension

The risk of urinary tract injury with an abdominal open Burch and laparoscopic Burch colposuspension reported in our department was 3/972 (0.03%) and 6/178 (3.0%), respectively.[4] The open Burch colposuspension injuries were 3 intravesical sutures: 1 was detected intraoperatively and 2 postoperatively over a 12-year follow-up. With the laparoscopic Burch colposuspension, there were 3 patients with intravesical sutures diagnosed intraoperatively and 3 ureteric injuries (2 diagnosed intraoperatively and 1 postoperatively). The risk of injury during laparoscopic Burch colposuspension was also higher in other comparative studies,[5,6] but this may have been in part due to the learning phase. The risk of urinary tract injury during Burch colposuspension in other studies has been 1.8%[6] up to 10% in Harris et al.[7] Ureteral injuries are uncommon and may also be attributable to a concomitant procedure such as a paravaginal repair.[8] Nevertheless, ureteral ligations have been described during the Burch colposuspension and are most often managed by releasing the obstructing suture and replacing it appropriately but only if detected intraoperatively.[7]

Cystourethroscopy performed following completion of the Burch colposuspension will require a 70° scope to see the ureteric orifices as the bladder neck is suspended. The commonest site of suture penetration is at 11 and 1 o'clock above the bladder neck (Figure 13.3) on the dome or lateral

Figure 13.3
(a) Large bladder calculus suspended from the right bladder wall at 11 o' clock above the bladder neck by an Ethibond suture of a Burch colposuspension. (b) Prolene suture of a Burch colposuspension passed through the dome which subsequently re-epithelialized.

walls of the bladder. Cystourethroscopy following urethral suspension procedures can also ensure the correct placement of sutures, avoiding inappropriate placement around the bladder base and ureters (see Figure 13.1). Overelevation of the bladder neck (Figure 13.4a) may result in voiding difficulty or de-novo urge symptoms and incontinence. If this is detected intraoperatively, removal of suspending sutures or mesh and replacement would be appropriate. Women with significant persistent voiding

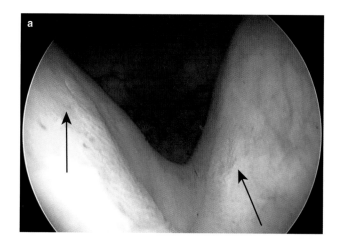

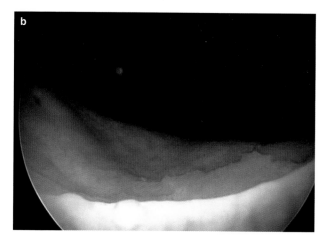

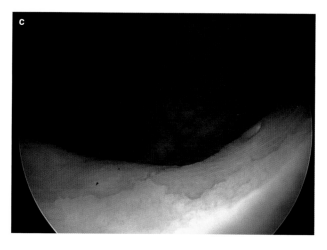

Figure 13.4

(a) View of the bladder neck in a 56-year-old woman who presented with recurrent stress incontinence and voiding difficulty following a mesh abdominal colposuspension 3 years earlier. The bladder base is overelevated and distorted with the left and right ureteric orifices (arrows) pulled forward. (b,c) Bladder base is now in its normal position following a transvaginal urethrolysis, and placement of a mid-urethral sling.

difficulty or urinary retention following urethral suspension or sling procedures may require further surgery performed retropubically or transvaginally to remove the offending suspension sutures or sling and resupport the urethra at a lower level (Figure 13.4a–c). Vaginal or retropubic urethrolysis or takedown is usually effective in improving obstructive symptoms and urinary retention but less effective in improving irritative bladder symptoms. If no resuspension is performed at the time of urethrolysis, over half of women will develop recurrence of their stress incontinence.

Marshall–Marchetti–Krantz procedure

This procedure has been very popular between 1965 and 1985, with many series reported.[9,10] Complications, including urinary tract injury, are similar to those described with the Burch procedure;[11,12] nevertheless, some additional complications can occur, including osteitis pubis,[13] which was an important reason for its decreasing popularity.

Long needle urethropexy

The long needle urethral suspensions of Pereyra, Stamey, Raz, Gittes, and others are closed procedures, performed through small suprapubic and paraurethral incision with intraoperative cystoscopic visualization of the bladder and urethra to avoid urinary tract injury and to allow correct placement of the suspension sutures. Intraoperative cystourethroscopy was seen as an essential part of the procedure. Stamey[14] described the use of an angled long needle passed downwards as close as possible to the posterior aspect of the symphysis pubis onto the surgeon's finger, which was situated lateral to the bladder neck while the bladder neck was visualized with a 70° lens cystoscope. Dacron tubular grafts were placed around the suture to buttress the vaginal loop and prevent pull-through. Originally it was advised that the sutures were tied with considerable tension, although subsequent authors advised minimal or no tension to avoid oversuspension and voiding difficulty. Intraoperative placement could be easily identified and the needle with suture replaced if bladder perforation had occurred.[14, 15]

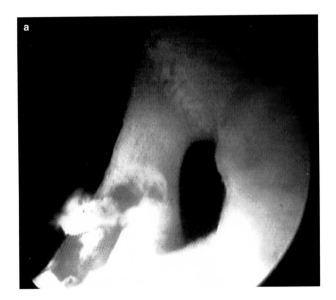

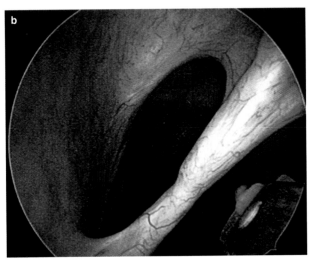

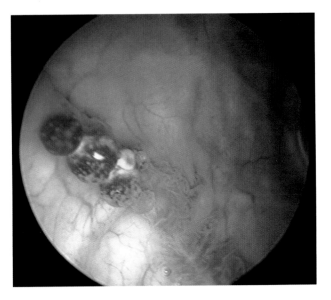

Figure 13.6
Calculus adherent to exposed tension-free vaginal tape (TVT) polypropylene tape penetrating the bladder wall to the right of the dome.

Figure 13.5(a,b)
Cystoscopic photograph showing epithelialization of a nylon suture passed through the bladder neck at the time of the previous Stamey suspension.

Although the initial reports of these procedures have been good, the long-term effectiveness has been disappointing, with cure rates of about 30% at 1–10 years. Complications reported following these procedures are voiding difficulty, suture abscess, and suprapubic pain. The non-absorbable suture material may also be found within the lumen of the lower urinary tract at a later time. This complication may occur due to inadvertent bladder perforation at the time of surgery, or secondary to erosion or migration into the lower urinary tract over time. In any single case, postoperatively, it is frequently difficult to say with certainty what the initial cause was. If there is suture or other foreign body penetration into the urinary tract, the mucosa may re-reepithelialize over the suture (Figure 13.5) or graft material, and the

patient may remain asymptomatic, or the suture or graft material may act as nidus for chronic infection and calculus formation (Figure 13.6), resulting in chronic pelvic pain, frequency, and urgency, and recurrent urinary tract infection (UTI).

Suburethral slings

Retropubic minimally invasive slings (TVT, SPARC)

The new minimally invasive slings of monofilament polypropylene tape which are passed through small suburethral and 2 suprapubic stab incisions can be either passed transvaginally through the retropubic space to the suprapubic incisions (tension-free vaginal tape [TVT] Figure 13.7) or from above down (SPARC procedure, American Medical Systems). Cystourethroscopy is required during the procedure to exclude the possibility of urethral or bladder injury. The area of penetration of the bladder with the passage of a TVT sling through the retropubic space is at 11 and 1 o'clock at the bladder dome usually just anterior to the dome bubble. In this area the needle of the TVT that is introduced can usually be easily seen under the bladder wall (Figure 13.8), especially if the trocar is moved. Bladder perforation rates vary among studies, with up to 10% incidence reported[16–18] (Figure 13.9). However, high perforation rates are no doubt

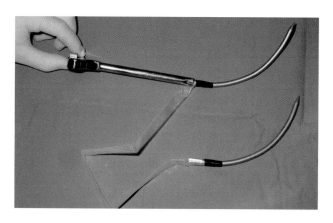

Figure 13.7
TVT sling with introducer, trocar needles, polypropylene mesh tape, and plastic sheath.

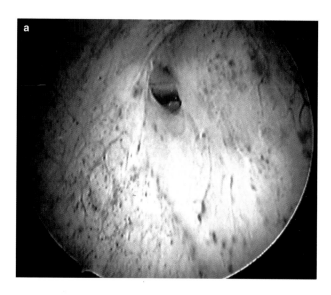

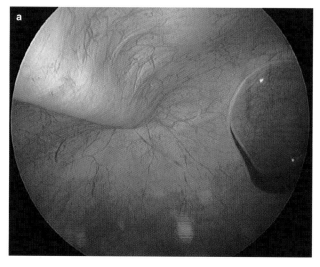

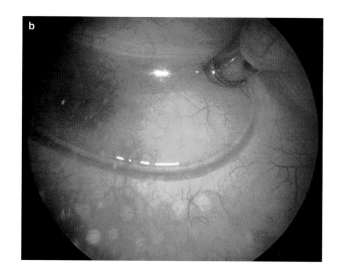

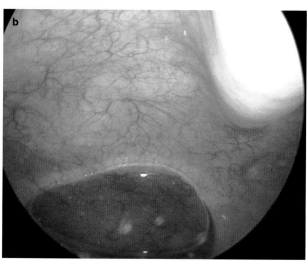

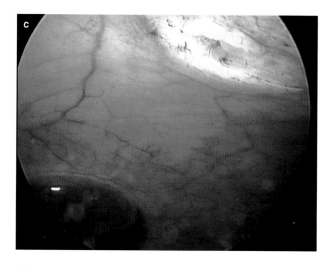

Figure 13.8
Bladder dome with normally positioned trocar needle under the bladder wall to the right (a) and left (b) of bubble.

Figure 13.9
(a,b) Trocar perforations of the bladder dome as the needle was passed through the retropubic space. (c) Small perforation after removal of trocar.

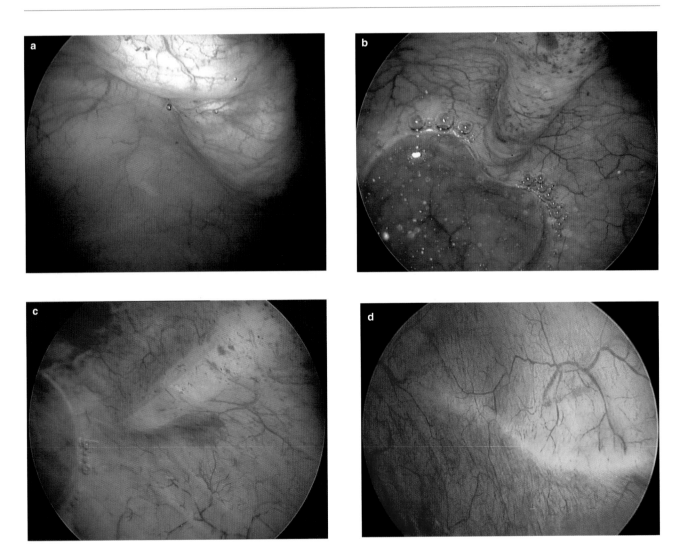

Figure 13.10
(a) The blue cover of the trocar of the Advantage sling (Boston Scientific) can be seen through a defect in the bladder dome caused possibly by a previous bladder injury or biopsy. (b) The full length of the blue cover is seen through the bladder wall, thinned by repeated previous retropubic surgery in a woman who had a previous Burch colposuspension and pubovaginal fascial sling.
(c) Following removal of the trocar and placement of the polypropylene sling. (d) 'Another near miss' intravaginal slingoplasty (IVS) sling visible under the bladder mucosa.

related to the experience of surgeons, with a perforation rate considerably higher during the learning phase. If the wall is thinned by previous surgery (Figure 13.10) or injury, there is an increased risk of sling erosion. When a bladder perforation is identified intraoperatively, the trocar is withdrawn and then replaced. The perforation of the bladder is usually small, and overnight bladder drainage is all that is required. The management of women with sling erosion in the bladder following surgery (Figure 13.11) is discussed below. These bladder intrusions are found in a similar area at the dome and are usually a result of an undiagnosed perforation rather than erosion of the mesh into the bladder. There have been few comparative studies performed with the other minimally invasive retropubic

slings such as the SPARC or Advantage slings (Boston Scientific). The incidence of bladder and urethral perforation would appear to be similar[19] for the above below approach of the SPARC procedure to the below above approach of the TVT.

The rate of urethral injury during the TVT procedure has been shown to range between 0% and 1%, with a 0.7% incidence reported by Kuuva[17] in a nationwide analysis of 1455 procedures. Mistakenly entering the wall of the urethra at the time of suburethral incision or periurethral dissection is particularly a risk in patients with previous stress urinary incontinence (SUI) surgery or urethral scarring such as urethral diverticulum (Figure 13.12), or previous radiotherapy. Secondary transurethral

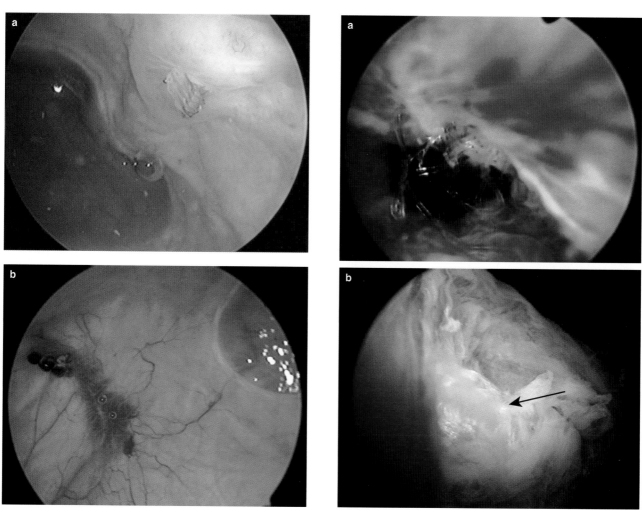

Figure 13.11
Perforation of the bladder dome by an (intravaginal slingoplasty) IVS sling (a) and tension-free vaginal tape (TVT) sling (b).

Figure 13.12
Urethral erosions of the tension-free vaginal tape (TVT) (a) and intravaginal slingoplasty (IVS) (b) slings caused by inappropriate operative placement and diagnosed many months postoperatively. The IVS sling appears as a whitish fibrous cord (arrow) below the bladder neck.

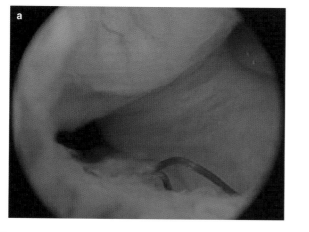

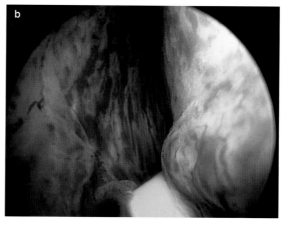

Figure 13.13
(a) Urethroscopic view of an eroded blue tension-free vaginal tape (TVT) sling. (b) The Advantage trocar needle (Boston Scientific) with its blue cover has been inadvertently passed through the proximal urethra and diagnosed on postoperative cystourethroscopy. The trocar needle was removed and replaced, and the urethral defect repaired with 3/0 Vicryl suture.

a
b
1 2
3 4
QTY2 1/2FLD NORM S-VIDEO

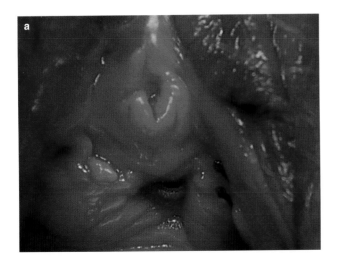

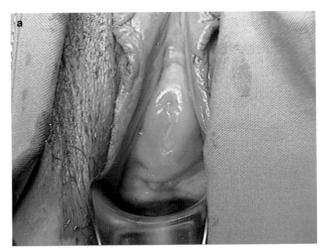

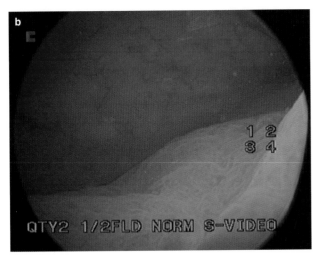

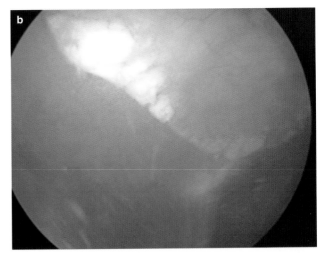

Figure 13.14
(a) Vaginal erosion of infected intravaginal slingoplasty (IVS) sling. (b) A 65-year-old woman with recurrent retropubic infection secondary to an infected IVS sling presenting with severe incontinence, frequency, and urgency. Cystoscopy showed an inflamed edematous bladder base.

penetration of the sling is rare when using polypropylene monofilament tape and when avoiding excessive tension of the tape. A few case reports of urethral erosion have been published[20–22] with the patient complaining of vaginal or urethral pain, vaginal discharge and/or bleeding, irritative bladder symptoms, voiding dysfunction, recurrent urinary tract infection, and hematuria. Usually, symptoms resolve after removal of the eroded sling component,[20–22] but recurrence of SUI may occur. Gynecare (Women's Health & Urology, a division of Ethicon, Inc., Johnson & Johnson) have recently changed the TVT tape (Figure 13.13) from a white to a blue color to enable easier detection either intravesically or during tissue

a
b
c

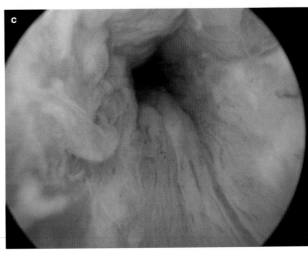

Figure 13.15
A 55-year-old woman presents with frequency, urgency, bladder, and urethral pain, and incontinence. She had a SPARC retropubic sling 2 years earlier. On examination, the external urethral meatus and urethra was inflamed and indurated (a); on cystourethroscopy, the urethra and bladder mucosa were inflamed and edematous, and the sling was visible in the bladder wall of the dome (b).

dissection, e.g. tape removal or division for obstructed voiding. Infection can occur in synthetic slings and cause vaginal erosion of the tape (Figure 13.14a), abscess formation, and bladder inflammation (Figure 13.14b); it is more common in multifilament than monofilament synthetic slings (Figure 13.15). These sling infections, even without penetration of the urinary tract, can cause severe inflammation of the lower urinary tract. Type I monofilament macroporous mesh has been reported to have a lower incidence of infection and vaginal erosion (less than 1%) compared to the multifilament (up to 9%).[23,24] The larger pore size and monofilament nature of the mesh is thought to lessen the risk of infection by allowing easier penetration of inflammatory cells such leukocytes (9–15 µm) and macrophages (16–20 µm) into the graft to phagocytose bacteria (<1 µm) (Figure 13.16).

Early cystourethroscopy should be performed in any woman who has recurrent UTI or persistent irritable bladder following stress incontinence surgery with prosthetic non-absorbable slings or sutures to exclude lower urinary tract penetration.

Transobturator tapes

The transobturator tension-free vaginal tape has been described in 2001 by Delorme[25] with an outside-in approach in which the tape is placed beneath the middle of the urethra in a horizontal plane between the two obturator foramen. This approach has the advantage of avoiding the blind entry of trocar needles into the retropubic space, which is expected to decrease the risk of bladder, bowel, and vascular injury. Delorme et al published a series of 150 patients[26] who underwent a transobturator tape (TOT) procedure for SUI and reported no case of lower urinary tract (LUT) injury. They concluded that routine check cystoscopy is not required with this approach. Since the first description of the technique, variations have been described, including the modification of the synthetic material (monofilament polypropylene mesh is now recommended and the most commonly used) and the use of different introducers (i.e. helical) (Figure 13.17). de Leval[27] described the inside out technique and reported a series of 107 patients operated on without any LUT injury. He also believed there was no need for routine cystoscopy during the procedure (Figure 13.18). All the studies comparing the transobturator approach with the retropubic approach have proven the safety of the procedure, with a significantly lower rate of LUT injury with the transobturator approach.[28–31]

Nevertheless, a few cases of bladder injury have been reported with the transobturator approach.[32–35] This has also been our experience with the out-in approach (e.g. Monarc), which is more likely to injure the lower urinary tract than the inside-out (e.g. TVT-O) (Figures 13.19 and

13.20). Minaglia et al[32] reported 3 cases of bladder perforation, 2 of whom had unsuspected injuries during surgery. In a large retrospective cohort study of 389 women[35] (241 outside-in and 148 inside-out procedures), the rate of LUT injury was 1% (4 patients), including a 0.5% rate of urethral injury and a 0.5% rate of bladder injury. In this study, bladder injuries occurred in women who underwent concurrent prolapse surgery and urethral injuries in women with previous incontinence surgery. Whereas bladder injuries more often occur at the time of tape insertion, urethral injuries usually occur at the time of suburethral incision or paraurethral dissection. The site of urinary tract penetration is different from the retropubic slings, and is usually just above or below the bladder neck (see Figures 13.19 and 13.20). In patients with previous anti-incontinence surgery (e.g. Burch colposuspension) or paravaginal repair, the upward position of the vaginal sulci makes the trocar insertion difficult and may result in urethral or bladder damage and make vaginal penetration and erosion more likely. The risk of LUT injury is greater at the beginning of the surgeon's learning curve.[35]

Despite the fact that LUT is an uncommon complication during TOT sling procedure, intraoperative cystoscopy should be considered, especially in women presenting risk factors such as previous pelvic surgery, concomitant procedures, severe vaginal atrophy, or obesity.

The question of long-term effectiveness of the retropubic vs the transobturator sling remains unanswered, although short term studies to date suggest equal effectiveness.[31] However, women with intrinsic sphincter dysfunction (ISD) stress incontinence (defined as low urethral closure pressure) in one retrospective study[29] were found to have a higher failure rate with the transobturator sling (Monarc) than with the TVT retropubic sling. In a prospective, randomized controlled trial in Melbourne of 162 women with urodynamic stress incontinence (USI) and intrinsic sphincter deficiency (ISD), defined as MUCP (maximum urethral closure pressure) $< 20\,cmH_2O$ and/or ΔALLP (abdominal leak point pressure) $< 60\,cmH_2O$, we found that TVT is objectively superior to Monarc sling, with 8 women requiring repeat sling surgery in the Monarc group compared with none in the TVT group over the first year postoperatively.[36]

Endoscopic injections for urinary incontinence

Injection of material into the LUT through an operating cystourethroscope has had a number of useful applications over recent years. Injections have been used as bulking agents in the urethra for stress incontinence in both sexes and around the ureteric orifices for the treatment of

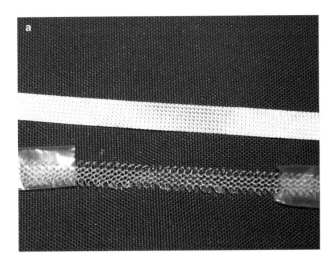

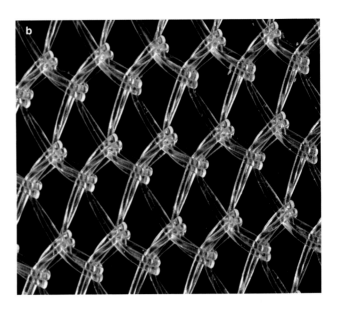

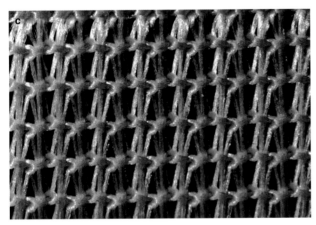

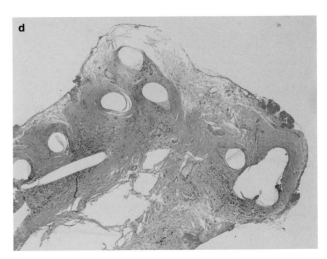

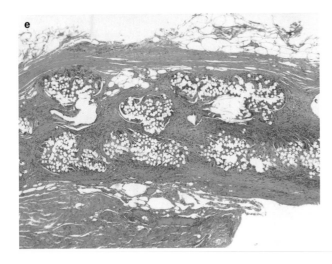

Figure 13.16
TVT monofilament (a lower and b) and intravaginal slingoplasty (IVS) multifilament (a upper and c) polypropylene slings. (d,e) Histology of explant of tension-free vaginal tape (TVT) sling removed for voiding difficulty (d) and IVS sling removed for vaginal erosion (e).

ureteric reflux. Phenol and alcohol has been injected through the trigone to denervate the bladder in women with neurogenic and non-neurogenic overactive bladder. This destroys the vesical plexus of pre- and postganglionic autonomic fibers and cholinergic nerve cell bodies passing under the bladder base before they ramify in the detrusor muscle wall. Case reports of vesicovaginal fistula following

phenol injection have prevented its wider usage.[37] Contraction of the detrusor muscle wall is mediated through muscarinic receptor stimulated by released acetylcholine. The autonomic nerve fibers supplying the bladder form a dense complexus among the detrusor muscle cells, with the majority of the nerves containing acetylcholinesterase. More recently botulinum A toxin, an

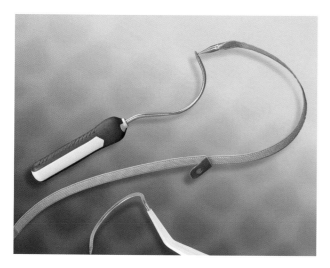

Figure 13.17
The Obtryx transobturator tape by Boston Scientific.

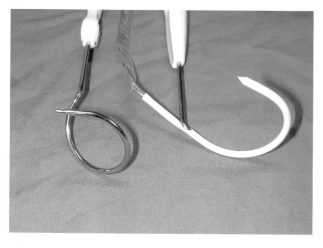

Figure 13.18
The transobturator tapes and introducer needles of the TVT-O (Johnson & Johnson) and Monarc (American Medical Systems).

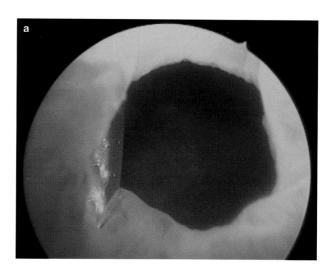

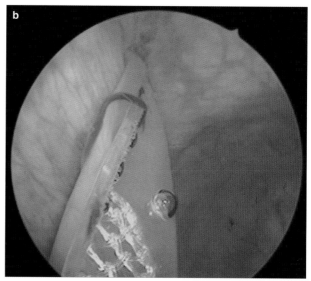

Figure 13.19(a,b)
Perforation of the bladder neck during the performance of a Monarc (American Medical Systems) transobturator sling.

acetylcholine blocker, has been injected into the bladder to treat motor and sensory disorders of the LUT and into the urethral sphincter for obstructed voiding secondary to detrusor sphincter dyssynergia.

Urethral bulking agents

The injection of material into the urethra is not new. Over the last 70 years different materials such as wax, sclerosing agents, and polytetrafluoroethylene (PTFE or Teflon) paste have been used. Shortliffe et al in 1989 were the first to report on periurethral injection of glutaraldehyde cross-linked collagen for urinary incontinence.[38] More recently,

injection of silicone microparticles and microballoons, has been reported.[39] Suitable patients for this therapy are women with stress incontinence and poor urethral function – low maximum urethral closure pressure (MUCP) ($< 20\,cmH_2O$) or low abdominal leak point pressure (ALLP) ($< 60\,cmH_2O$) – with good urethral support and normal detrusor function.

The most commonly used methods of injection into the proximal urethral wall are either transurethral or periurethral. Both routes are performed under urethroscopic vision. Collagen can also be directly injected without cystourethroscopic guidance through a specially designed urethral introducer.[40] Collagen (Bard Inc.) is injected transurethrally through a long 20 Fr gauge needle through the operating channel of the 0° or 30° cystoscope or urethroscope (Figure 13.21) and the highly viscous silicone microparticles (Macroplastique; Uroplasty Inc.,

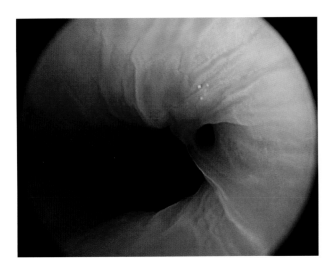

Figure 13.20
Scarred urethra from the previous intraurethral placement of a TVT-O sling (Johnson & Johnson).

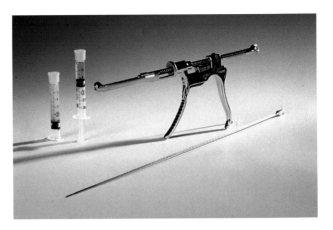

Figure 13.22
The highly viscous silicone microparticles (Macroplastique; Uroplasty Inc., Minneapolis, MN, USA) and gel are passed through a 16 Fr gauge needle with an injection gun.

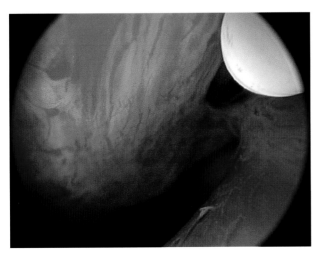

Figure 13.21
The transurethral injection of collagen (Bard Inc.) into the anterior mid-urethral wall using a long needle.

Minneapolis, MN, USA) through a 16 Fr gauge needle with an injection gun (Figure 13.22). Injections can be placed transurethrally, beginning in the mid-urethral area in equal aliquots up to 6 ml at 2, 10, and 6 o'clock until the proximal urethra is closed (Figure 13.23a,b). The material is placed submucosally deep enough so that an intact mucosa is present over the material but superficial enough so that the ballooning effect into the lumen is seen during insertion (Figure 13.23c,d). This can be performed under local anesthesia and antibiotic cover. The patient is then asked to cough and strain to ensure that a watertight closure has occurred or further bulking agent can be given. The bladder is then drained with a small-diameter 8 Fr catheter to avoid any disruption of the injected material. The procedure is safe and has a low morbidity, which makes it suitable for the frail and elderly. Complications are uncommon (~5%),

and include UTI, postoperative voiding difficulty, and, rarely, urethral masses or abscesses,[41,42] and particle migration.[43] The collagen is cross-linked with glutaraldehyde to prevent absorption; however, studies have shown that the implant is at least in part replaced by host collagen over time. Macroplastique is a newer vulcanized silicone microimplant suspended in a povidine gel designed to resist absorption and provide more long-term urethral bulking for the treatment of SUI. However in a prospective randomized comparative study in women with ISD stress incontinence of Macroplastique vs the pubovaginal sling[44] we found that the initial 6 months subjective response was good in both the Macroplastique and sling groups (77% vs 90%), but at 5 years postoperatively the continence success (21% vs 69%) and satisfaction rates (29% vs 69%) were in favor of the sling procedure. With low morbidity the injectables continue to have a role in selected cases of women with stress urinary incontinence and ISD, but will need to be repeated in many cases.

The Zuidex system comprises four pre-filled syringes of non-animal stabilized hyaluronic acid/dextranomer (NASHA/Dx) gel and a guiding urethral instrument (the Implacer) (Figure 13.24). Transurethral injection can be performed for stress urinary incontinence without the need for cystourethroscopic visualization. In a study of 142 women with stress urinary incontinence (of mean age of 55 years old) treated with Zuidex, the response rate was 77% at 12 months, with significant reductions in 24-hour pad-weight test leakage and number of incontinence episodes/24 hours.[40]

Botulinum A toxin

Botulinum toxin (BTX), the product of the Gram-positive rod-shaped anaerobic bacteria *Clostridium botulinum*, was first isolated in 1897 and remains today one of the most

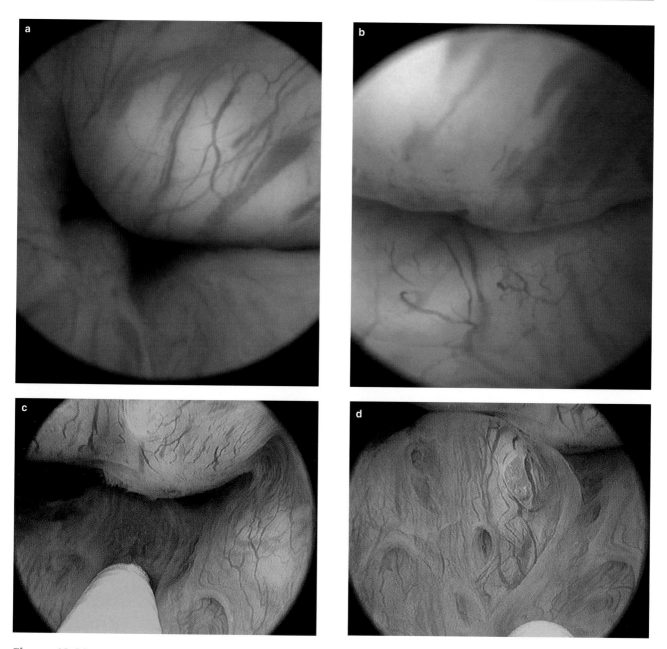

Figure 13.23
Collagen injected through a long needle into the anterior (a) and then posterior wall of the mid-urethra to provide a cough leakproof urethral closure (b). (c,d). Macroplastique urethral injection.

powerful neurotoxins known to man. A number of serotypes have been isolated from types A to G. Types A and B have been found to be of clinical value, with only type A used in urogynecological practice, as it has a longer duration of action and less side effects. Type A is available as Botox (Allergan Inc.) or Dysport (Ipsen). Botox is administered in a standard dosage of 100 units and Dysport in 500 units. Botulinum toxin is a neurotoxin which inhibits release of acetylcholine (ACH) from motor nerve neuromuscular junctions, causing relaxation and chemical denervation of skeletal and smooth muscle. It also inhibits release of transmitters of sensory nerves, modulating afferent C-fiber

activity in the bladder wall. These effects are temporary but can last between 6 and 12 months. BTX has been used in the treatment of strabismus, spastic neurological diseases, and diseases of the autonomic nervous system. In female urology, it has been used for neurogenic and non-neurogenic overactive bladder, detrusor sphincter dyssynergia and urinary retention, and the painful bladder syndrome.

BTX is normally administered as a cystoscopic injection into the intramuscular or submucosal layer of the posterior bladder wall (Figure 13.25a) in the form of 20–30 aliquots of 1 ml of diluted BTX. A long 20 Fr gauge needle is passed through the operating channel with a 30° cystoscope to

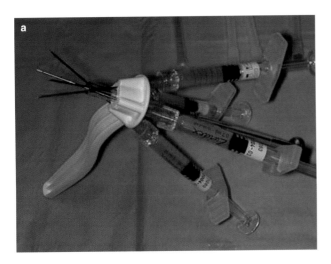
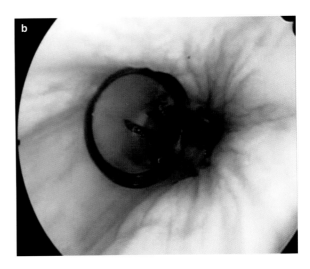

Figure 13.24
(a) The Zuidex system comprises four pre-filled syringes of non-animal stabilized hyaluronic acid/dextranomer (NASHA/Dx) gel and a guiding urethral instrument (the Implacer) and is used for transurethral injection for stress urinary incontinence. (b.) The Implacer is in place within the urethra.

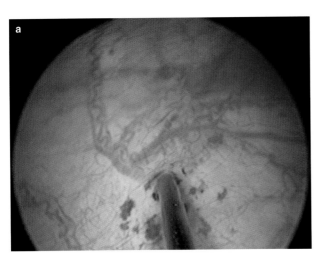
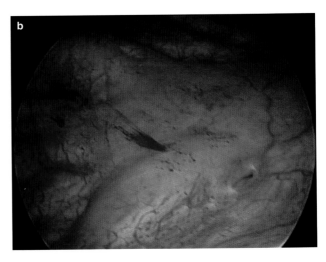

Figure 13.25
(a) Transvesical injection of Botox A into the posterior bladder wall in a woman with an overactive bladder. (b) Post-injection the bladder mucosa is raised, with a small amount of bleeding from the injection site. The trigone and ureter were not injected.

visualize the bladder base. The trigone and the ureteric orifices are avoided because of the fear of creating ureteric obstruction or reflux (Figure 13.25b). BTX has also been administered in an intravesical infusion. Transvesical injection can be performed as an outpatient procedure using lidocaine gel, although general anesthesia may be necessary in women with interstitial cystitis.

Published studies on the use of BTX have mainly been retrospective in nature and uncontrolled. Reitz et al,[45] in a large multicenter study of 231 patients with neurogenic detrusor overactivity (NDO) treated with Botox 300 units, found a significant improvement in bladder function with a

low incidence of complications. Popat et al[46] compared 44 patients with NDO with 31 patients with idiopathic detrusor overactivity (IDO). Owing to the increased risk of needing clean intermittent self-catheterization reported in previous studies, a lower dose of 200 units of Botox (20 injections of 1 ml) was used in the IDO group compared with 300 units (30 injections) in the NDO group. Assessment at 4 and 16 weeks was performed post-injection with urodynamic studies and bladder diaries. Both groups showed an excellent response to the treatment, with improved urodynamic parameters and reduced daytime frequency, urgency, and episodes of urine leak. No significant difference was noted between the groups. At 4 weeks, 25 of 39 patients with NDO (64.1%) and 13 of 24 patients with IDO (54.2%) were dry. At 16 weeks, these figures were 55.2% for patients with NDO and 57.1% for those with IDO. All but 2 patients reported at least an improvement in the number of incontinence episodes at both visits. There are only retrospective studies available on the use of BTX in women with interstitial cystitis (IC). Giannantoni et al[47] reported a pilot study of 12 women and 2 men with IC using 200 units of Botox, with improvement rates of 85% at 1 and 3 months.

Botox has shown considerable promise for the short-term treatment of neurogenic and non-neurogenic overactive bladder, improving continence in 50–90% of patients. It is safe and has a good duration of effect. Repeated treatments appear as effective as initial treatments. However, potential risks include urinary retention, so that a lower dose is advisable if there is urodynamic evidence of voiding dysfunction or a simultaneous injection of BTX into the urethral sphincter is being given. Few prospective randomized studies using validated instruments to assess effectiveness have been published to date.[48]

Management of suture injuries and intravesical foreign bodies following urogynecological surgery

As previously described and summarized in Table 13.1, most of the urogynecological procedures can result in LUT injuries. Intravesical sutures or slings may present with symptoms of recurrent UTI, irritable bladder symptoms (i.e. urinary frequency or incontinence), or pelvic pain or discomfort.[59–61] These foreign materials often develop incrustation and calculi (Figure 13.27).[61] Whether the suture material was placed incorrectly at the time of surgery and was not recognized intraoperatively or had eroded or pulled through into the urethra or bladder postoperatively is always a debatable issue. Non-absorbable sutures in these procedures suspend the vagina to the iliopectineal ligament or rectus sheath under tension and may erode into the bladder wall, especially if this has been damaged or weakened by repeated surgery. Jarvis[62] reported this complication in 3 of 200 (1.5%) Stamey operations and was of the opinion that the suture migrated through the bladder wall. Certainly, in cases where the suture with synthetic buffer is present in the bladder, migration of the suture placed under tension would appear likely in this complication. The question of whether the intravesical suture was pulled through the bladder wall or incorrectly placed at the time of surgery does have medicolegal implications but, in reality, it is difficult to say with certainty in any individual case. Performing a

routine intraoperative cystoscopy[52] will detect inappropriate placement of the tape or the suture, which can be then rectified. If there is full-thickness penetration of the bladder or urethra by suture or sling, removal and replacement is necessary. If the sling has been placed close to the bladder lumen, it should be replaced if possible to avoid secondary erosion (see Figure 13.10b). Endoscopic management of these complications with endourological forceps and scissors if possible will provide quicker recovery than open surgery. Removal of intravesical sutures can be performed without adversely affecting the patient's urinary continence.[4,63,65] Sutures (see Figure 13.27) and slings (Figure 13.28) can be grasped and gently pulled with endoscopic forceps and in many cases are easily removed without damage to the bladder. If there is significant resistance, the suture or synthetic material should be cut flush with the bladder mucosa, which will usually re-epithelialize. A follow-up cystoscopy may be appropriate to confirm this, particularly if urinary symptoms persist. If there is infection present in a multifilament sling, complete removal is frequently required either by transvaginal or retropubic exploration to successfully treat the infection (see Figure 13.14b).

Insertion of suprapubic catheters

Suprapubic catheters can be inserted using local analgesia once the bladder has been filled and distended above the symphysis pubis. However, if the bladder capacity is reduced or there has been significant previous pelvic or abdominal surgery, or the patient is having a general anesthetic for other surgery (e.g. stress incontinence or prolapse surgery), then insertion of the suprapubic catheter under cystoscopic vision is appropriate. Iatrogenic bowel damage can occur during suprapubic catheter insertion in difficult patients, even in experienced hands. If the bladder cannot be distended beyond 300 ml, due either to severe detrusor overactivity or fibrosis (e.g. radiation cystitis, interstitial cystitis), a suprapubic catheter should be inserted by open cystotomy by cutting down on a bladder sound passed transurethrally into the bladder.[65]

There are a variety of suprapubic catheters available for bladder drainage: the type used will vary with the indication. Postoperative bladder catheterization is not necessary following most of the newer minimally invasive sling procedures for stress incontinence. Urethral catheterization is usually all that is necessary for short-term bladder drainage following prolapse surgery. Postoperative voiding difficulty can be treated with intermittent self-catheterization or short-term continuous urethral catheterization. For long-term problems, intermittent self-catheterization may be necessary. However, in women who have more extensive pelvic reconstructive surgery or where there is significant preoperative voiding

Table 13.1   Frequency of urinary tract injuries during prolapse incontinence and stress surgery

Authors year	Operation	Number of operations	Number of urinary tract injuries	Percent of total urinary tract injuries	Number recognized intraop	Number recognized postop
Bai[49] 2006	POP surgery	?	5	?	3	2
Carey[a5] 2006	Burch colposuspension: • open • laparoscopic	200 104 96	6 intravesical sutures 1 5	3%	6	
Kitchener[6] 2006	Burch colposuspension: • open • laparoscopic	274 143 131	5 bladder injuries: 1 4	1.8% 0.7% 3%		
Barber[a 28] 2006	TVT (+/− POP surgery) Monarc sling (+/− POP surgery)	213 205	11 bladder injuries 0 ureteral injury 0 bladder injury 1 ureteral injury	5.1% 0.5%		
Abdel-Fattah[35] 2006	TOT (+/− POP surgery): • outside-in • inside-out	389 241 148	 2 urethral injuries 2 bladder injuries 0	1% 1.6% 0	 2 1	 1
Wang[a 50] 2006	SPARC sling Monarc sling	29 31	1 bladder injury 0 bladder injury	3.4% 0%		
Aronson[a 51] 2005	POP surgery USL fixation +/− VH +/− ant or post colporraphy	411	11 injuries: 3 ureteral injuries 7 bladder injuries 1 urethral injury	2.6%	11	
Kwon[a 52] 2002	POP +/− SUI surgery POP surgery SUI surgery	526 526 447	15 7 injuries: 6 ureteral obstructions 1 puckering bladder mucosa 8 bladder injuries: 2 intravesical suture 1 puckering bladder mucosa 2 bladder perforations 2 unrecognized cystotomy 1 insufficient cystotomy repair	2.8% 1.3% 1.8%	15	
Handa[a 53] 2001	POP surgery	157	0 unsuspected bladder injury 1 ureteral ligation 4 chronic ureteral obstruction			
Jabs[a 54] 2001	POP surgery	224	9 ureteral injuries 3 bladder injuries	5.3%	11	
Gill[a 8] 2001	Burch procedure +/− POP surgery	181	5 cystotomies 1 obstructed ureter (due to PVR)	3.3%		
Speights[a 55] 2000	Laparoscopic Burch +/− PVR	171	0 ureteral injury 4 bladder injuries	2.3%		

Table 13.1   (Continued)

Authors year	Operation	Number of operations	Number of urinary tract injuries	Percent of total urinary tract injuries	Number recognized intraop	Number recognized postop
Tulikangas[a][56] 2000	SUI surgery: • Burch procedure • pubovaginal sling	347 186 161	9 bladder injuries 4 4 (+1 previous surgery)	2.6% 2.1% 2.4%	9	
Dwyer[a][4] 1999	SUI surgery: • Stamey procedure • open Burch • laparoscopic Burch	1164 61 925 178	10 injuries: 1 intravesical suture 3 intravesical suture 3 intravsical suture 3 ureteric ligations	0.85% 1.6% 0.3% 3.3%	 1 1 3 2	 0 2 0 1
Sze[57] (review) 1997	SSF Endopelvic fascia fixation Iliococcygeal fixation	1080 367 155	4 bladder lacerations 2 bladder lacerations 1 bladder laceration	0.37% 0.54% 0.86%		
Harris[a][7] 1997	POP +/− SUI surgery	224	6 ureteral injuries 3 bladder injuries	4%		
	Colpopexy: • vaginal (USL or iliococcygeous susp) • abdominal (sacral mesh colpopexy)	80 21 59	2 ureteral ligations	9.5%		
	Other repairs SUI surgery: • Burch	69 75 60	0 4 ureteral injuries 2 intravesical sutures	0 10%		
	• fascia lata sling • needle urethropexy	13 2	1 intravesical sling	7.7% 0		
Jenkins[58] 1997	Bilateral intraperitoneal USL	50	2 bladder injuries	4%	2	

[a]Routine use of intraoperative cystoscopy.
POP = pelvic organ prolapse, Ant = anterior, Post = posterior, USL = uterosacral suspension, VH = vaginal hysterectomy, SUI = stress urinary incontinence, intraop = intraoperatively, postop = postoperatively, PVR = paravaginal repair, TOT = transobturator tape; SSF, sacrospinous fixation.

dysfunction present, a suprapubic catheter would be appropriate especially if the patient was unwilling or unable to perform intermittent self-catheterization. Suprapubic catheterization has a lower incidence of bacteriuria during the postoperative period[66] and may be more comfortable, as patients can void with the catheter in situ and have residual urine measured without further repeated urethral catheterization. However, there is the risk of infection of the suprapubic site and potential viscus or vessel injury during insertion.

The Bonanno suprapubic catheter (Becton Dickinson Ltd) is a narrow-diameter pigtail catheter (Figure 13.29) that is sutured to the abdominal wall. The Stamey (Cook Urological Inc.) and Cystocath (Dow Corning Corporation) (Figure

13.30) have mallecot tails, which are further secured by suturing or using an adhesive device to the suprapubic area: both are narrow-diameter catheters and may be prone to blockage in the presence of heavy hematuria. The Add-a-Cath (Femcare Ltd) uses a standard Foley catheter, which is placed through a peelaway trocar inserter. The Foley catheter is secured by the inflated catheter balloon. The catheters are more appropriate for long-term bladder drainage in women with chronic urinary retention (Figure 13.31). A permanent fistulous tract is created after a month, which allows easy catheter change by nursing or medical staff. Silicone elastomer coated or all-silicone catheter or hydrogel catheters would be appropriate for long-term use.

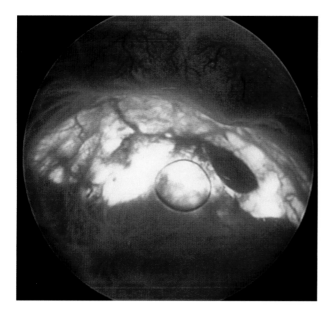

Figure 13.26
Cystoscopic view of the bladder dome with the symphysis pubis anterior to the bubble at the top of the picture. The bladder wall is transparent and thin from repeated previous retropubic surgery of a previous Burch colposuspension and fascial Aldridge sling. The abdominal surgeon's finger can be seen through the bladder wall to the right of the dome bubble.

Retrograde ureteric catheterization

For gynecologists, retrograde catheterization is used to exclude the possibility of ureteric obstruction postoperatively or to place ureteric stents to lessen the possibility of ureteric damage intraoperatively. This can be performed by a 30° lens with a 17–22 Fr rigid cystoscope or 15 Fr flexible cystoscope usually under intravenous antibiotic cover using gentamicin and amoxicillin, or gentamicin and cefuroxime or a third-generation cephalosporin. Ureteric catheters are available in various diameters, ranging from 3 Fr to 10 Fr with the 4–6 Fr open-ended catheters the most useful for diagnostic purposes. There are 1 cm graduations on the catheter, with thicker markings placed every 5 cm (the number of lines indicating the length of catheter), inserted from the ureteric orifice (Figure 13.32). Passage of the ureteric catheter 10–15 cm should take the catheter above the pelvic brim and exclude most gynecological causes of iatrogenic ureteric obstruction. The renal pelvis will be reached at 25–30 cm catheter insertion. Entry of the catheter into the ureteric orifices can be facilitated by using an Albarran bridge deflecting mechanism (see Figure 3.4). Although this

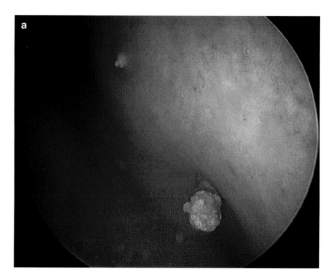

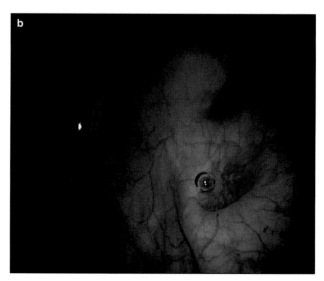

Figure 13.27
Remnants of a Burch colposuspension suture with encrustation before (a) and after removal (b).

is not always needed, it is useful particularly when the trigonal area and bladder base has been distorted by surgery or some other pathological process such as infection or a tumor (Figure 13.33). Once the ureteric catheter has been inserted, urine can be collected from the ureter for microscopy and culture. Contrast material can be injected through the ureteric catheter using a 1:1 mix of normal saline and contrast; an image intensifier is used to detect any obstruction and to determine the course of the ureter.

When there is difficulty in passing the ureteric catheter, the following maneuvers may help:

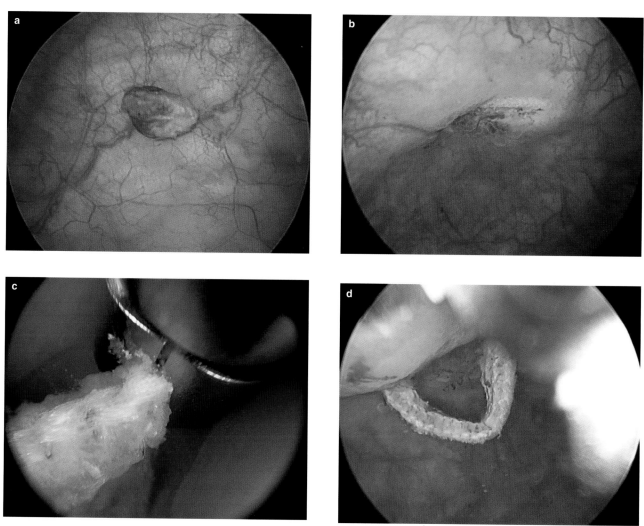

Figure 13.28
Calculus present on the dome of the bladder (a). Calculus has been removed to reveal underlying exposed IVS sling (b). Sling grasped with biopsy forceps (c) and pulled (d). Only a small defect (e) was present after sling removal. A urethral catheter was used to drain the bladder overnight.

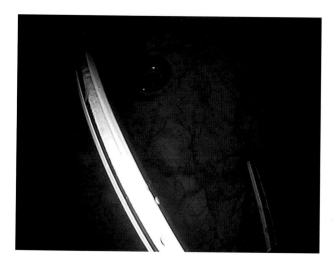

Figure 13.29
Cystoscopic view of Bonanno pigtail catheter.

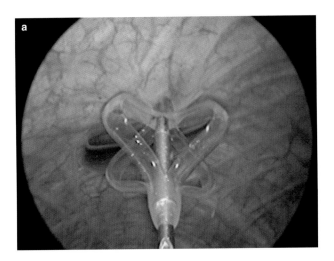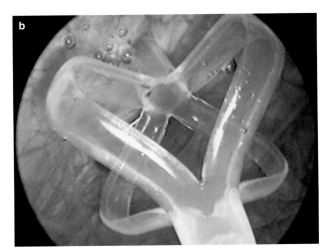

Figure 13.30(a,b)
Cystoscopic view of insertion of Stamey catheter with mallecot tail.

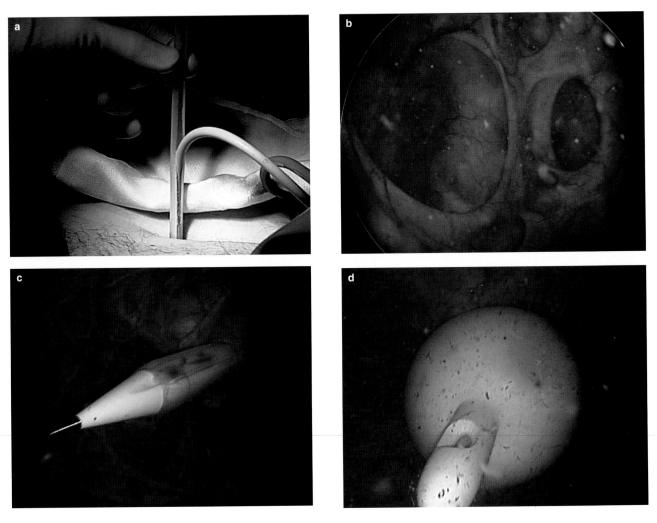

Figure 13.31
The Add-a-Cath (Femcare Ltd) with a standard silicone Foley catheter which is placed through a peelaway trocar inserter (a) in a 79-year-old woman with chronic urinary retention. There was gross trabeculation of the bladder wall (b). The dome of the bladder can be viewed during insertion of the trocar (c). The Foley catheter is secured by the inflated catheter balloon (d).

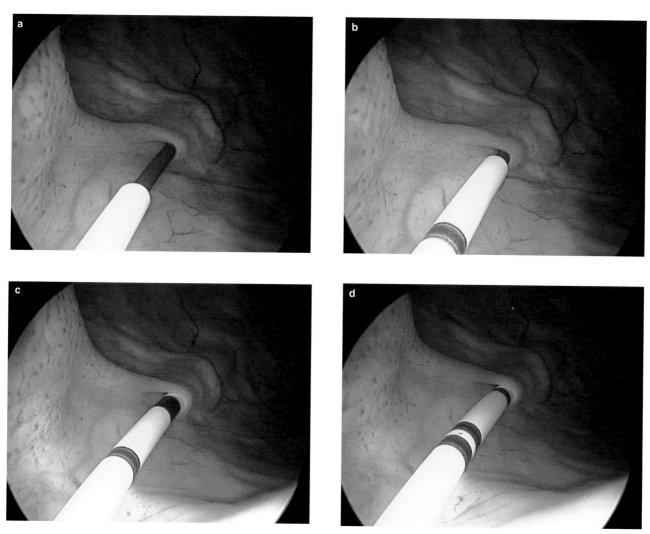

Figure 13.32
A 4 Fr ureteric catheter has been passed over a guide wire through the operating channel with a 30° cystoscope. The 1 cm markings can be seen on the catheter, with the thicker markings indicating 5 cm. The three lines indicate that this catheter has been passed 15 cm from the ureteric orifice.

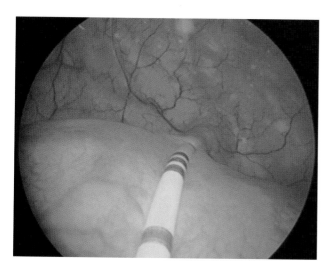

Figure 13.33
A ureteric catheter was passed to 15 cm preoperatively prior to removal of a mass under the trigone to aid ureteric identification during the surgery.

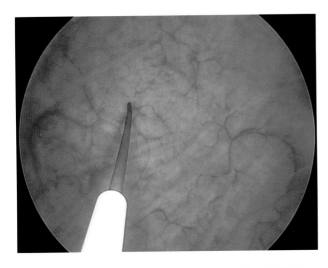

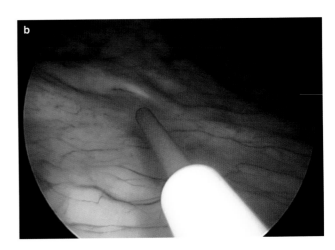

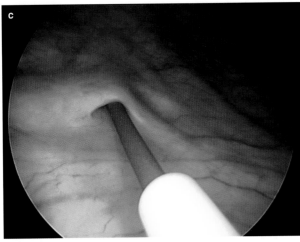

Figure 13.34
(a) Open-ended ureteric catheter with superslippery guide wire passed through its lumen. (b) The open-ended ureteric catheter is gently placed near the ureteric orifice and the guide wire is introduced (b) and passed up the ureter (c). The ureteric catheter or stent can be passed over the guide wire.

1. Using a guide wire (Figure 13.34a). Pass the open-ended catheter gently into the ureteric orifice (Figure 13.34b) and then introduce the guide wire through the catheter passed any obstruction (Figure 13.34c). Ureteric guide wires in common use are PTFE or hydrophilic coated (superslippery) to enable easier passage with low ureteric resistance.

2. Performing the cystoscopy with ≤100 ml in the bladder straightens the intravesical intramural ureter and reduces intraureteric pressure.

3. Injection of lidocaine gel or contrast mixture to act as a lubricant and to minimize friction or trauma during the passage of the ureteric catheter.

Once the guide wire is in place, the stent can be passed over the guide wire. A double J stent once passed retrograde, can be left in situ for 6 weeks.

Complications of ureteric catheterization are uncommon, but perforation[67] and ureteric colic can occur, emphasizing the need for care.

References

1. Gallaher WT. The Marshall–Marchetti operation: a review. Am J Obstet Gynecol 1952; 63: 842–6.
2. Burch JC. Urethrovesical fixation to Cooper's ligament for correction of stress incontinence, cystocele, and prolapse. Am J Obstet Gynecol 1961; 81: 281–90.
3. Vancaille TG, Schuessler W. Laparoscopic bladder neck suspension. J Laparoendosc Surg 1991; 1: 169–73.
4. Dwyer PL, Carey MP, Rosamilia A. Suture injury to the urinary tract in urethral suspension procedures for stress incontinence. Int Urogynecol J Pelvic Floor Dysfunct 1999; 10: 15–21.
5. Carey MP, Goh JT, Rosamilia A et al. Laparoscopic versus open Burch colposuspension: a randomised controlled trial. BJOG 2006; 113: 999–1006.
6. Kitchener HC, Dunn G, Lawton V et al. COLPO Study Group. Laparoscopic versus open colposuspension – results of a prospective randomised controlled trial. BJOG 2006; 113: 1007–13.
7. Harris RL, Cundiff GW, Theofrastous JP et al. The value of intraoperative cystoscopy in urogynecologic and reconstructive pelvic surgery. Am J Obstet Gynecol 1997; 177: 1367–9.

8. Gill EJ, Elser DM, Bonidie MJ, Roberts KM, Hurt WG. The routine use of cystoscopy with the Burch procedure. Am J Obstet Gynecol 2001; 185: 345–8.

9. Demirci F, Yildirim U, Demirci E et al. Ten-year results of Marshall Marchetti Krantz and anterior colporrhaphy procedures. Aust N Z J Obstet Gynaecol 2002; 42: 513–14.

10. Colombo M, Scalambrino S, Maggioni A, Milani R. Burch colposuspension versus modified Marshall–Marchetti–Krantz urethropexy for primary genuine stress urinary incontinence: a prospective, randomized clinical trial. Am J Obstet Gynecol 1994; 171: 1573–9.

11. Persky L, Guerriere K. Complications of Marshall–Marchetti–Krantz urethropexy. Urology 1976; 8: 469–71.

12. Lee RA, Symmonds RE, Goldstein RA. Surgical complications and results of modified Marshall–Marchetti–Krantz procedure for urinary incontinence. Obstet Gynecol 1979; 53: 447–50.

13. Kammerer-Doak DN, Cornella JL, Magrina JF, Stanhope CR, Smilack J. Osteitis pubis after Marshall–Marchetti–Krantz urethropexy: a pubic osteomyelitis. Am J Obstet Gynecol 1998; 179: 586–90.

14. Stamey TA. Endoscopic suspension of the vesical neck for urinary incontinence. Surg Gynecol Obstet 1973; 136: 547–54.

15. Karram MM, Bhatia NN. Transvaginal needle bladder neck suspension procedures for stress urinary incontinence: a comprehensive review. Obstet Gynecol 1989; 73: 906–14.

16. Abouassally R, Steinberg JR, Lemieux M et al. Complications of tension-free vaginal tape surgery: a multi-institutional review. BJU Int 2004; 94: 110–13.

17. Kuuva N, Nilsson CG. A nationwide analysis of complications associated with the tension-free vaginal tape (TVT) procedure. Acta Obstet Gynecol Scand 2002; 81: 72–7.

18. Peschers UM, Tunn R, Buczkowski M, Perucchini D. Tension-free vaginal tape for the treatment of stress urinary incontinence. Clin Obstet Gynecol 2000; 43: 670–5.

19. Lord HE, Taylor JD, Finn JC et al. A randomized controlled equivalence trial of short-term complications and efficacy of tension-free vaginal tape and suprapubic urethral support sling for treating stress incontinence. BJU Int 2006; 98: 367–76.

20. Clemens JQ, DeLancey JO, Faerber GJ, Westney OL, Mcguire EJ. Urinary tract erosions after synthetic pubovaginal slings: diagnosis and management strategy. Urology 2000; 56: 589–94.

21. Amundsen CL, Flynn BJ, Webster GD. Urethral erosion after synthetic and nonsynthetic pubovaginal slings: differences in management and continence outcome. J Urol 2003; 170: 134–7.

22. Koelbl H, Stoerer S, Seliger G, Wolters M. Transurethral penetration of a tension-free vaginal tape. BJOG 2001; 108: 763–5.

23. Bafghi A, Benizri EL, Trastour C et al. Multifilament polypropylene mesh for urinary incontinence: 10 cases of infections requiring removal of the sling. BJOG 2005; 112: 376–8.

24. Pifarotti P, Meschia M, Gattei U, Bernasconi F, Vigano R. Multicenter randomized trial of tension free vaginal tape (TVT) and intravaginal slingoplasty (IVS) for the treatment of stress urinary incontinence in women. Neurol Urodynam 2004; 23: 494–5.

25. Delorme E. [Transobturator urethral suspension: mini-invasive procedure in the treatment of stress urinary incontinence in women]. Prog Urol 2001; 11: 1306–13. [in French]

26. Delorme E, Droupy S, de Tayrac R, Delmas V. Transobturator tape (Uratape): a new minimally-invasive procedure to treat female urinary incontinence. Eur Urol 2004; 45: 203–7.

27. de Leval J. Novel surgical technique for the treatment of female stress urinary incontinence: transobturator vaginal tape inside-out. Eur Urol 2003; 44: 724–30.

28. Barber MD, Gustilo-Ashby AM, Chen CC et al. Perioperative complications and adverse events of the MONARC transobturator tape, compared with the tension-free vaginal tape. Am J Obstet Gynecol 2006; 195: 1820–5.

29. Miller JJR, Botros SM, Akl MN et al. Is transobturator tape as effective as tension-free vaginal tape with borderline maximum urethral closure pressure. Am J Obstet Gynecol 2006; 195: 1799–804.

30. Liapis A, Bakas P, Giner M, Creatsas G. Tension-free vaginal tape versus tension-free vaginal tape obturator in women with stress urinary incontinence. Gynecol Obstet Invest 2006; 62: 160–4.

31. De Tayrac R, Deffieux X, Droupy S et al. A prospective randomized trial comparing tension-free vaginal tape and transobturator suburethral tape for surgical treatment of stress urinary incontinence. Am J Obstet Gynecol 2004; 190: 602–8.

32. Minaglia S, Ozel B, Klutke C, Ballard C, Klutke J. Bladder injury during transobturator sling. Urology 2004; 64: 376–7.

33. Hermieu JF, Messas A, Delmas V et al. [Bladder injury after TVT transobturator]. Prog Urol 2003; 13: 115–17. [in French]

34. Smith PP, Appell RA. Transobturator tape, bladder perforation, and paravaginal defect: a case report. Int Urogynecol J Pelvic Floor Dysfunct 2007; 18: 99–101.

35. Abdel-Fattah M, Ramsay I, Pringle S. Lower urinary tract injuries after transobturator tape insertion by different routes: a large retrospective study. BJOG 2006; 113: 1377–81.

36. Schierlitz L, Dwyer P, Murray C et al. A randomized controlled study to compare tension free vaginal tape (TVT) and Monarc transobturator tape in the treatment of women with urodynamic stress incontinence (USI) and intrinsic sphincter deficiency (ISD). International Urogynecological Association Annual Scientific Meeting, Cancun, Mexico, 2007.

37. Wall LL, Stanton SL. Transvesical phenol injection of pelvic nerve plexuses in females with refractory urge incontinence. Br J Urol 1989; 63: 465–8.

38. Shortliffe LM, Freiha FS, Kressler R, Stamey TA, Constantinou CE. Treatment of urinary incontinence by the periurethral injection of glutaraldehyde cross-linked collagen. J Urol 1989; 111: 583–41.

39. ter Meulen PH, Berghmans LC, van Kerrebroeck PE. Systematic review: efficacy of silicone microimplants (Macroplastique) therapy for stress urinary incontinence in adult women. Eur Urol 2003; 44: 573–82.

40. Chapple CR, Haab F, Cervigni M et al. An open, multicentre study of NASHA/Dx Gel (Zuidex) for the treatment of stress urinary incontinence. Eur Urol 2005; 48: 488–94.

41. Madjar S, Sharma AK, Waltzer WC, Frischer Z, Secrest CL. Periurethral mass formations following bulking agent injection for the treatment of urinary incontinence. J Urol 2006; 175: 1408–10.

42. McLennan MT, Bent AE. Suburethral abscess: a complication of periurethral collagen injection therapy. Obstet Gynecol 1998; 92: 650–2.

43. Pannek J, Brands FH, Senge T. Particle migration after transurethral injection of carbon coated beads for stress urinary incontinence. J Urol 2001; 166: 1350–3.

44. Maher C, O'Reilly BA, Dwyer PL et al. Pubovaginal sling or transurethral Macroplastique for stress urinary incontinence and intrinsic sphincter deficiency: a prospective randomized trial. BJOG 2005; 112: 797–801.

45. Reitz A, Stohrer M Kramer G et al. European experience of 200 cases treated with botulinum-A toxin injections into the detrusor muscle for urinary incontinence due to neurogenic detrusor overactivity. Eur Urol 2004; 45: 510–15.

46. Popat R, Apostolidis A, Kalsi V et al. A comparison between the response of patients with idiopathic detrusor overactivity and neurogenic detrusor overactivity to the first intradetrusor injection of botulinum-A toxin. J Urol 2005; 174: 984–9.

47. Giannantoni A, Costantini E, Di Stasi SM et al. Botulinum A toxin intravesical injections for the treatment of painful bladder syndrome: a pilot study. Eur Urol 2006; 49: 704–9.

48. Schurch B. Botulinum toxin for the management of bladder dysfunction. Drugs 2006; 66: 1301–18.

49. Bai SW, Huh EH, Jung da J et al. Urinary tract injuries during pelvic surgery: incidence rates and predisposing factors. Int Urogynecol J Pelvic Floor Dysfunct 2006; 17: 360–4.

50. Wang AC, Lin YH, Tseng LH, Chih SY, Lee CJ. Prospective randomized comparison of transobturator suburethral sling (Monarc) vs suprapubic arc (Sparc) sling procedures for female urodynamic stress incontinence. Int Urogynecol J Pelvic Floor Dysfunct 2006; 17: 439–43.

51. Aronson MP, Aronson PK, Howard AE et al. Low risk of ureteral obstruction with "deep" (dorsal/posterior) uterosacral ligament suture placement for transvaginal apical suspension. Am J Obstet Gynecol 2005; 192: 1530–6.

52. Kwon CH, Goldberg RP, Koduri S, Sand PK. The use of intraoperative cystoscopy in major vaginal and urogynecologic surgeries. Am J Obstet Gynecol 2002; 187: 1466–71.

53. Handa VL, Maddox MD. Diagnosis of ureteral obstruction during complex urogynecologic surgery. Int Urogynecol J Pelvic Floor Dysfunct 2001; 12: 345–8.

54. Jabs CF, Drutz HP. The role of intraoperative cystoscopy in prolapse and incontinence surgery. Am J Obstet Gynecol 2001; 185: 1368–71.

55. Speights SE, Moore RD, Miklos JR. Frequency of lower urinary tract injury at laparoscopic Burch and paravaginal repair. J Am Assoc Gynecol Laparosc 2000; 7: 515–18.

56. Tulikangas PK, Weber AM, Larive AB, Walters MD. Intraoperative cystoscopy in conjunction with anti-incontinence surgery. Obstet Gynecol 2000; 95: 794–6.

57. Sze EH, Karram MM. Transvaginal repair of vault prolapse: a review. Obstet Gynecol 1997; 89: 466–75.

58. Jenkins VR 2nd. Uterosacral ligament fixation for vaginal vault suspension in uterine and vaginal vault prolapse. Am J Obstet Gynecol 1997; 177: 1337–43.

59. Athanasopoulos A, Liatsikos EN, Perimenis P, Barbalias GA. Delayed suture intravesical migration as a complication of a Stamey endoscopic bladder neck suspension. Int Urol Nephrol 2002; 34: 5–7.

60. Biyani CS, Upsdell SM. An unusual foreign body in the bladder 7 years after a Stamey endoscopic bladder neck suspension. Int Urogynecol J Pelvic Floor Dysfunct 1998; 9: 303–4.

61. Evans JW, Chapple CR, Ralph DJ, Milroy EJ. Bladder calculus formation as a complication of the Stamey procedure. Br J Urol 1990; 65: 580–2.

62. Jarvis GJ. Re: Erosion of buttress following bladder neck suspension. Br J Urol 1992; 70: 695.

63. Nabi G, Hemal AK, Khaitan A. Endoscopic management of an unusual foreign body in the urinary bladder leading to intractable symptoms. Int Urol Nephrol 2001; 33: 351–2.

64. Smith A, Rovner E. Long-term chronic complications from Stamey endoscopic bladder neck suspension: a case series. Int Urogynecol J Pelvic Floor Dysfunct 2006; 17: 290–4.

65. Feneley RC. The management of female incontinence by suprapubic catheterization with and without urethral closure. Br J Urol 1983; 55: 203–7.

66. Schiotz HA. Urinary tract infection after vaginal repair surgery. Int Urogynecol J 1992; 3: 185–90.

67. Al-Awadi K, Kehinde EO, Al-Hunayan A, Al-Khayat A. Iatrogenic ureteric injuries: incidence, aetiological factors and the effect of early management on subsequent outcome. Int Urol Nephrol 2005; 37: 235–41.

14

Intraoperative cystourethroscopy in the prevention and treatment of urinary tract injury in gynecological surgery

Peter L Dwyer

Introduction

Intraoperative injury to the urinary tract during gynecological surgery is a well-known complication and can involve the ureter, bladder, or urethra. If detected at the time of surgery, repair can be performed without significant consequence to postoperative recovery or urinary tract function. If undiagnosed, significant consequences can occur with the development of urinary fistulae and possible loss of kidney function. Secondary repair usually involves multiple outpatient visits and surgery, which results in loss of quality of life and possible long-term disability and medicolegal sequelae. At present, only 1 in 10 ureteric injuries and 1 in 2 bladder injuries are detected intraoperatively.[1] A recent Canadian study[2] showed the risk of litigation was increased 91-fold if a woman received a urinary tract injury compared with other complications during hysterectomy and tubo-ovarian surgery.

The use of cystoscopy at the conclusion of the operation will detect many of these injuries, allow intraoperative repair, and reduce postoperative morbidity. Patients with undiagnosed ureteral injuries may present with flank pain, fever, costovertebral angle tenderness, ureterovaginal fistula, ileus, urinary peritonitis, pyelonephritis, and (if untreated) loss of renal function and eventual renal failure. Patients may have oliguria, or (if bilateral ureteral injury) anuria. It is still being debated whether cystourethroscopy should be performed routinely at the time of some gynecological procedures such as hysterectomy. It could be argued that the routine use of cystoscopy adds to the duration and cost of surgery, which needs to be balanced with the potential benefits. However, a surgeon who considers that the risk of ureteric or bladder injury is increased because of the difficulty of the surgery – e.g. adhesions, hemorrhage, or pelvic pathology (e.g. cervical fibroids, endometriosis) – should have the skills to confirm the safety and integrity of the upper and lower urinary tracts before the patient leaves the operating room.

Injury to the urinary tract has been reported in most gynecological procedures. The risk of urinary tract injury in specific gynecological operations varies considerably between studies, which is a reflection perhaps of the variation in surgical techniques, experience, and skill of the surgeon performing the procedure and accuracy in reporting this complication.

This chapter reviews the incidence of urinary tract injury, possible etiological and risk factors, and the anatomy of the urinary tract with special reference to possible sites of injury. The role of cystourethroscopy in prevention of urinary tract injury and intraoperative detection and repair will be discussed.

Anatomical considerations and site of injury

The ureter is a contractile fibromuscular tube 22–30 cm in length, extending extraperitoneally from the pelvis of the kidney to the interior aspect of the bladder. It has an inner mucous membrane of transitional epithelium and submucosa surrounded by a layer of helical interlacing smooth muscle with an outer adventitia of loose areolar tissue containing its vascular and nervous supply. Having both an abdominal and pelvic course, the ureter receives its blood supply in the abdomen from the renal and inguinal arteries, abdominal aorta, and common iliac artery, and in the pelvis from the internal artery and its branches. Therefore, the arterial branches of the abdominal ureter come from the medial aspect, whereas the arterial supply in the pelvis is from a lateral direction. To minimize ischemic damage to the ureters, any peritoneal incision for identification and

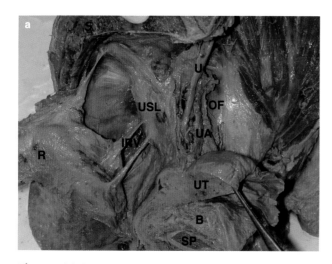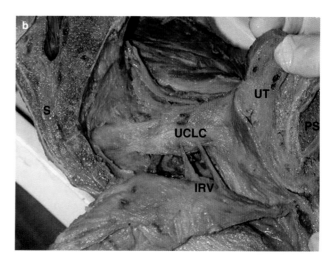

Figure 14.1
Left hemipelvis displaying uterosacral/lateral cervical ligament complex (UCLC) and its relationship to the left ureter (U), the uterine artery (UA), and the uterus (UT). The pelvis is tilted in the normal standing position to demonstrate the suspensory nature of this fibromuscular complex. The UCLC has a broad lateral origin over the lateral sacrum and sacroiliac articulation and converges medially to insert onto the posteriolateral cervix and upper third of the vagina. The ureter descends into the pelvis with the obturator fossa (OF) laterally and with the UCLC in increasing proximity medially. Other structures are sacrum (S), rectum (R), inferior rectal vessels (IRV), bladder (B), and pubic symphysis (SP). (b) Lateral view of UCLC with a blue pin marking the position of the ischial spine under the intermediate segment of the ligament. (Courtesy of C Achtari and P Dwyer.)

mobilization should be lateral to the ureter in the abdomen and medial in the pelvis,[3] while the adventitial sheath and overlying peritoneum should be left intact.

The abdominal ureters run anterior to the psoas muscle, crossing near the bifurcation of the common iliac vessel into the external and internal iliac (hypogastric) arteries. Once in the pelvis, the ureter lies medial to the branches of the internal iliac artery, lateral to the pouch of Douglas, anterior to the sacroiliac joints, and posterior to the ovaries. The ureter descends anteromedially into the pelvis, the obturator vessels and obturator fossa lying laterally and the uterosacral/lateral cervical ligamentous complex anteromedially (Figure 14.1). The mean distances of the ureter from the sacral, intermediate, and cervical portions of the cardinal ligament have been estimated by Buller et al[4] to be 4.1, 2.3, and 0.9 cm, respectively. The ureter continues anteromedially and passes under the uterine artery approximately 2 cm above and lateral to the vaginal fornix to reach the base of the bladder anterior to the vagina where it traverses the bladder wall for 1.5–2 cm before opening into the interior aspect of the bladder at the superior lateral border of the trigone.

Ureteric injury can result from incorrect placement of the forceps, suture ligation, transection with a scalpel, diathermy injury (open or laparoscopic), or kinking or ischemia from devascularization of the ureter. Gynecological injury is usually to the pelvic ureter and can occur anywhere in its 12–15 cm course from the ureteric bladder orifice to the pelvic brim.

However, the ureter is at most risk of injury at the following anatomical sites:

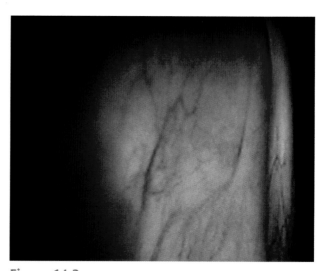

Figure 14.2
Woman with voiding difficulty and recurrent stress incontinence 2 years following a Burch colposuspension. Left suspension suture incorrectly placed, suspending the left ureter, which potentially can cause kinking and obstruction.

1. The intramural portion of the ureter as it traverses the bladder wall, where it can be ligated by deep lateral plication sutures during anterior colporrhaphy.
2. As the ureter enters the bladder during placement of vaginal suspension sutures for the Burch colposuspension (Figure 14.2) or Marshall–Marchetti–Krantz procedure.
3. During clamping of the uterine pedicle in hysterectomy at the base of the broad ligament as the ureter passes under the uterine artery before inserting into the bladder.

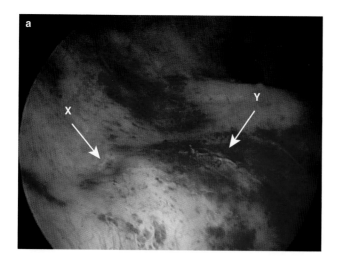

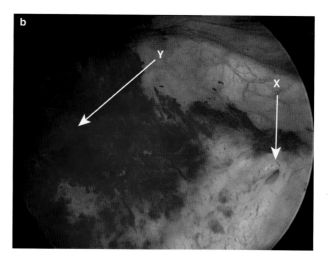

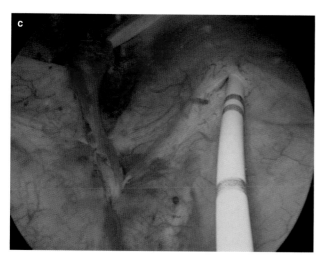

Figure 14.3(a,b,c)
Cystoscopic view of repaired cystotomy inadvertently made above the interureteric ridge (Y) during anterior colporrhaphy and uterosacral vault suspension. Cystoscopy confirmed the watertight closure of the two-layer repair and the patency of both ureters. Note bluish efflux from ureters (X) following indigo carmine injection. (c) Bladder injury, which occurred during laparoscopic hysterectomy was repaired transvaginally. Postoperative cystoscopy confirmed adequate repair and ureteric patency with a catheter passed 10 cms up the right ureter.

4. Close to the uterosacral ligaments during endometriosis ablation surgery or placement of uterosacral suspension sutures.
5. At the pelvic brim or lateral pelvic side wall when the ovarian vessels in the infundibulopelvic pedicle are clamped during oophorectomy; or during ligation of the internal iliac artery (hypogastric) for severe pelvic bleeding. The distance from the ureter to the infundibular pedicle is on average 1 cm when the ovary and tube are removed.

In a study of cases of ureteric injuries in gynecological surgery over 15 years, Liapis et al[5] identified 18 ureteric injuries from 5122 major gynecological operations (0.35%). In 9 of the 18 cases, the injury was detected intraoperatively, either by following the path of the ureter (5 cases) or seeing leakage of urine (4 cases). Intraoperative cystoscopy was not routinely performed. The site of the ureteric injury was in 4 cases near the infundibulopelvic pedicle during ligation, in 4 cases near the lateral cervical ligament, in 8 cases at the level of uterine artery ligation, in 1 case at the level of

uterosacral ligament ligation, and in 1 case the site of injury was not stated.

The anatomy of the bladder and urethra is discussed in Chapter 2. The most likely site of bladder injury and fistula development is above the trigone on the base of the bladder in the uterovesical space during dissection of the bladder off the cervix at the time of abdominal or vaginal hysterectomy, or during anterior colporrhaphy (Figure 14.3). The anterior wall of the bladder and bladder neck are the common sites of injury during sling procedures (Figure 14.4) or urethral suspension surgery in the retropubic space. Injury to the bladder can result in a vesicovaginal fistula (see Figure 14.4), which may result in immediate vaginal leakage of urine or delayed leakage (7–14 days) if ischemia, necrosis, and infection play a secondary role. Presentation of intraoperative bladder injury may be delayed with the patient having recurrent urinary tract infection (UTI) or irritable bladder symptoms from erosion of synthetic mesh or sutures in the bladder, after prolapse (Figure 14.5) or stress incontinence surgery (Figure 14.6).

The risk of injury to the ureter or bladder is increased when the normal anatomy of the pelvis or urinary tract is

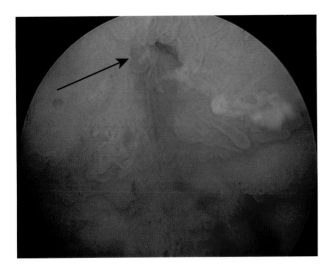

Figure 14.4
Cystoscopy was performed in a woman with an infected Silastic sling and a vesicovaginal fistula present at 12 o'clock above bladder neck (arrow) extruding purulent material and blood.

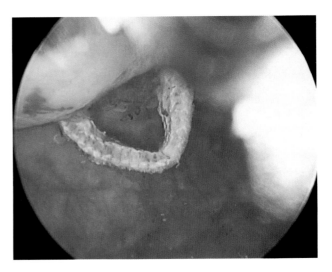

Figure 14.6
Intravaginal slingplasty (IVS) multifilament polypropylene sling penetrating the dome of the bladder in a woman with recurrent stress incontinence and irritable bladder symptoms.

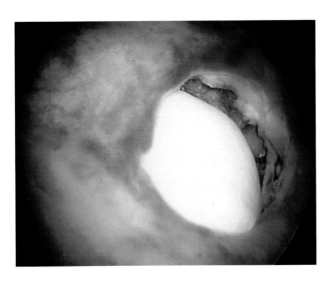

Figure 14.5
Cystoscopic view of the bladder following transvaginal excision of polypropylene mesh found protruding into the bladder in a women with recurrent urinary tract infection (UTI) and pelvic pain 3 years following abdominal mesh colposacropexy.

Pelvic surgery and urinary tract injury

Hysterectomy

Hysterectomy, is one of the most commonly performed gynecological procedures, and is also a common cause of injury to the ureter and bladder. The choice of surgical approach to the same operation has an influence on the risk of injury. In a systematic MEDLINE search for all ureteric injuries at gynecological surgery between 1966 and 2004, Gilmour et al[1,6] found the ureteric injury rate per 1000 operations for vaginal hysterectomy was 0.2, subtotal abdominal hysterectomy was 0.6, total abdominal hysterectomy was 1.3, and laparoscopic hysterectomy was 7.8. Although the trend in incidence of injury is convincing, the cause for these differences at this stage is conjecture. Vaginal hysterectomy has the lowest risk of ureteric injury. The reason for this in the author's opinion is the more effective removal of the bladder and ureters from the operative field. During vaginal hysterectomy, the bladder is dissected from the cervix with opening of the pelvic peritoneum in the vesicouterine space. The bladder and ureters are lifted anteriorly by a Breisky–Navratil retractor (Figure 14.8), while the cervix and uterus are pulled downwards. This removal of the ureters and bladder from the operative field is more difficult to achieve with abdominal hysterectomy. The bladder is dissected off the cervix and upper vagina but not completely. In subtotal hysterectomy, the cervix is conserved and clamping of the cervical angles is avoided, lowering the risk to the ureters. The risk of ureteric injury is highest in this systematic review with laparoscopic hysterectomy. The commonest cause of ureteric damage during laparoscopic surgery has been by electrocoagulation, but

abnormal or when surgical access is poor. The relationship of the ureter to cervix and uterus can be altered as a result of uterocervical enlargement from fibroids, hematometra (Figure 14.7), or by an ovarian mass. Surgical access can be inhibited by patient obesity or by use of an inappropriate or small incision. Other pelvic conditions such as endometriosis, previous radiation, or pelvic adhesions from previous infection or surgery can make surgery more difficult and place the urinary tract at risk.

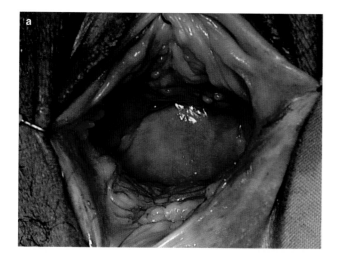

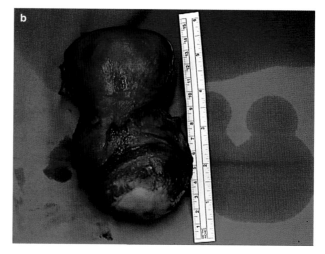

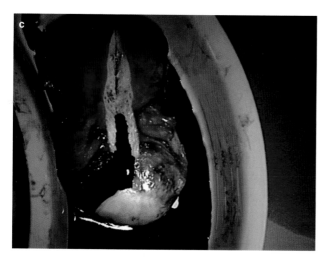

Figure 14.7

A 35-year-old women with a 16-week size hematometra caused by cervical stenosis following a Manchester repair with cervical excision. Repeated cervical exploration failed to adequately drain the uterus. On vaginal examination the cervix was grossly distended with no cervical os visable (a). The left ureter was injured during hysterectomy and was reimplanted into the bladder with a psoas hitch. Ureteric injury was only detected when postoperative cystoscopy failed to confirm ureteric efflux of indigo carmine. The ureter was placed at risk by cervical distention (b,c), which in hindsight may have been avoided if the hematometra had been drained abdominally prior to hysterectomy.

injuries from clamping, misplaced sutures, and trocar entry have been reported.[7] Assimos et al[8] also reported that the incidence of major iatrogenic ureteric injuries in gynecology rose from 13 to 41 per 10 000 gynecological cases with the introduction of operative gynecological laparoscopy. The injury rate is also high for malignant disease, depending on the radical nature of the surgery and experience of the surgeon, with some reports of 10% for the Wertheim–Meigs hysterectomy.[6] Subspecialization in this area of gynecology is well accepted and has significantly lowered the incidence of urinary tract injury during radical hysterectomy.

However, in half of all ureteric injuries, there are no predisposing factors that can be identified and the surgery performed is described as routine.[7] Ureteric injury in these cases is a reflection of the intrinsic risk of operating in this area of the pelvis where the urinary and genital tracts are so closely aligned both anatomically and functionally.

The risk of bladder injuries also varies between different modes of hysterectomy. In a systematic MEDLINE search for all bladder injuries at hysterectomy reported in the literature between 1966 and 2004,[1,6] the injury rate per 1000

operations for vaginal hysterectomy was 3.6, subtotal abdominal hysterectomy 0.3, total abdominal hysterectomy 2.6, and laparoscopic hysterectomy was 6.4. On these figures, subtotal abdominal hysterectomy is the safest method for bladder injury. However, vaginal hysterectomy is commonly performed with anterior colporrhaphy for anterior vaginal wall prolapse which would have increased the risk of injury to the bladder. Laparoscopic hysterectomy was again the highest, with an incidence of bladder injury almost double open abdominal and vaginal hysterectomy. Although laparoscopy is said to improve visualization in pelvic surgery, this has not resulted in improved safety for the urinary tract. These injuries are presumably a result of the greater technical difficulty of laparoscopic surgery and the longer learning curve, and emphasize the need for intraoperative cystoscopy in these higher-risk cases.

Bladder injuries are more likely to be recognized at the time of surgery and repaired than ureteric injury if intraoperative cystoscopy is not performed. A laceration to the bladder usually results in immediate leakage of urine, which does not occur in most instances if a ureter is clamped or ligated.

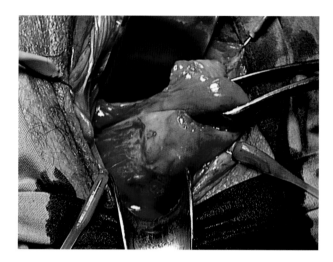

Figure 14.8
Vaginal hysterectomy performed with removal of the bladder and ureters from the operative field by a Breisky–Navratil retractor.

Prolapse surgery

Anterior compartment

Anterior colporrhaphy with or without bladder neck plication (Kelly) has traditionally been used to treat anterior vaginal wall prolapse and stress incontinence. Intraoperative cystoscopy has not been considered by most gynecologists to be necessary following this operation as the risk of urinary tract injury is believed to be low. However, injury can and does occur to urethra, bladder, or ureters. During dissection of the bladder from the lateral vaginal wall or the vaginal vault, the bladder may be inadvertently opened. Clear urine may be seen, which should be quickly differentiated from peritoneal fluid by examination of the bladder interior and recognition of the trigone and ureteric orifices. Closure of the bladder wall in two layers with postoperative bladder drainage gives a universally successful repair. However, if the bladder injury is missed because no urine leakage is seen, or if repair is inadequate, a vesicovaginal fistula (VVF) can result. In Hilton's series[9] of 135 urogenital fistula (VVF or urethrovaginal fistula [UVF]) in the North of England, 2 followed anterior colporrhaphy and 4 followed vaginal hysterectomy. Cystoscopy after a surgical repair should detect any unsuspected injury. If the bladder is inadvertently opened, a cystoscopy following repair is appropriate to confirm both a watertight closure and ureteric patency, as the intravesical course of the ureters is usually close to the transvaginal injury site (see Figure 14.2).

Ureteric injury can also occur during anterior compartment prolapse surgery. During anterior colporrhaphy, the

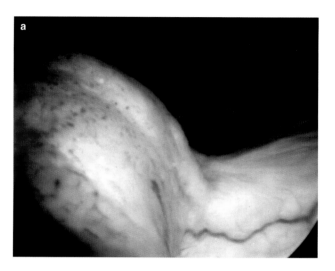

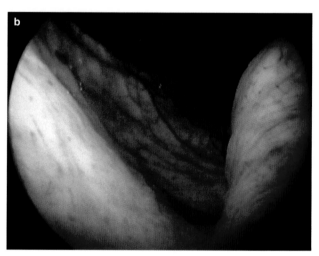

Figure 14.9 (a,b)
Cystoscopic view of the bladder base following an anterior colporrhaphy with midline plication of pubovaginal fascia. Note distortion of the trigone and indrawing of the ureteric orifices.

intramural sections of the ureters are close to the midline plication sutures, estimated by Stanhope et al[10] to be a mean distance of 0.9 cm from the sutures. The ureters are at risk, particularly with wide lateral dissection where deep fascial sutures are placed into the wall of the bladder. This creates an infolding of the trigone and base of the bladder (Figure 14.9) with a ureteric orifice in close proximity. Jabs et al[11] reported a series of 224 intraoperative cystoscopies performed with various gynecological procedures and found that 7 of the 9 cases with ureteric blockage had an anterior colporrhaphy performed. In 6 cases the obstruction was relieved by removing the bladder neck or fascial plication sutures and 1 had an intraoperative stent passed. A study by Kwon et al[12] on the use of intraoperative cystoscopy in major vaginal and urogynecological surgery

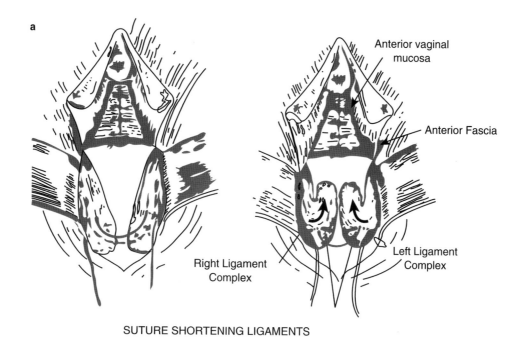

SUTURE SHORTENING LIGAMENTS

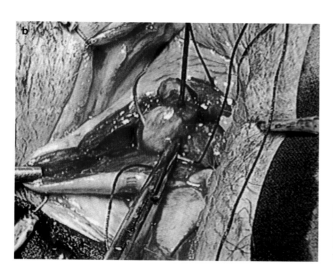

Figure 14.10
McCall procedure with his original drawing (a) and operative view
(b) of the McCall suture suspending the posthysterectomy vaginal
vault to the uterosacral ligaments.

found that anterior colporrhaphy had the highest rate of
ureteric injury of all gynecological operations, occurring in
7 of the 346 (2%) anterior colporrhaphies performed,
resulting in suture removal and replacement.

The ureters can be palpated vaginally in a similar way
to abdominally once their location is identified. The
intravesical ureter can be palpated in the bladder wall and
more proximal pelvic ureter by placing traction on the
pelvic peritoneum. Palpation using the thumb and
forefinger gives a typical 'snap' of the cord-like ureteric
structure. The avoidance of placing plication sutures
too laterally and deep is also important in prevention,
as the intravesical ureters are in close proximity (see
Figure 14.9b).

Middle compartment for apical prolapse

Vaginal vault prolapse is a common problem following
hysterectomy, with the incidence varying between 0.2%
and 43% and most reports in the order of less than 5%.[13]
The most effective technique for resupporting the upper
vagina, either at the time of vaginal hysterectomy or for
posthysterectomy vault prolapse repair, continues to be
debated. In 1957 McCall[14] described a posterior culdoplasty technique where sutures are placed through the
vagina, uterosacral ligaments, and peritoneum to close the
cul-de-sac and support the vaginal vault (Figure 14.10).
Numerous modifications using the cardinal/uterosacral

complex to prevent or treat posthysterectomy vault prolapse have been described. The vaginal apex can be attached to the pelvis, either directly by suturing or indirectly by using autologous or synthetic material. The two most commonly used pelvic wall sites for direct transvaginal suture fixation of the vaginal apex are the sacrospinous ligament and iliococcygeal fascia. Sacrospinous and iliococcygeal fixation are procedures with a low risk of urinary tract injury when not combined with surgery for anterior vaginal wall prolapse. However, a high incidence of postoperative cystocele of 30% has been reported and has decreased the popularity of these procedures.[15]

The proximity of the ureters to the uterosacral ligaments has placed them at risk of injury, particularly with the uterosacral ligament suspension procedures. The risk will vary with the placement of the suture into the uterosacral ligament complex and whether the bladder and ureter can be safely removed from the operative field. The risk is low with the McCall procedure performed with vaginal hysterectomy (see Figure 14.10), as suture placement is into the cervical portion of the ligament once the bladder with ureters has been dissected free of the cervix. In women with posthysterectomy vault prolapse, the ligamentous complex can only be found with certainty higher and more laterally in the pelvis and can be approached either intra- or extraperitoneally. Most of the studies reported are intraperitoneal suspension procedures with reported incidences of ureteric injury from 1% to 10.9% (Table 14.1). The extraperitoneal approach we believe is safer with a low risk of ureteric injury.[16] Injury may be caused by suture ligation or ureteric kinking from the suspension sutures. The high incidence of ureteric injury has made intraoperative cystoscopy an integral part of uterosacral suspension procedures. In most of the recent series, when ureteric obstruction is detected on cystoscopy, it is simply treated with removal of the offending suspension suture as apposed to ureteric reimplantation if diagnosed following surgery.

Prevention of urinary tract injury

Urinary complications are reduced by good surgical technique and a sound knowledge of the anatomy and sites of risk to the ureter. An awareness of the position of the ureter and bladder at all times during surgery, particularly when clamping pedicles, the use of electrocautery, or during surgical dissection is fundamental in reducing the risk of injury. Ideally, the urinary tract should be removed from the field of surgery by retraction. The ureter can normally be easily found crossing the pelvic brim at or near the bifurcation of the common iliac vessel into the external and internal iliac (hypogastric) arteries before descending into the pelvis in the posterior leaf of the broad ligament. Identification of the ureter is appropriate prior to ovarian

cystectomy or clamping of the ovarian vessels in the infundibulopelvic pedicle during oophorectomy or ovarian cystectomy. The course of the ureter is more difficult to see in the broad ligament where it passes under the uterine artery and into the base of the bladder, unless extensive dissection is performed more laterally, as in a Wertheim hysterectomy where the whole course of the uterine artery and ureter are identified. Ureteric safety is ensured by the reflection of the bladder and ureter off the cervix and upper vagina, thereby removing them from the operative field before clamping the uterine vessels.

The routine use of preoperative imaging of the urinary tract using ultrasound, intravenous pyelography, and computed tomography has not been shown to be effective or cost-efficient in the prevention of urinary tract injury.[11] The ureteric course will be altered by fibroids larger than 12 weeks' gestation and ovarian cysts greater than 5 cm, especially if the cyst protrudes posteriorly into the broad ligament. However, in these cases, the ureter is known to be at greater risk, so it should be displayed during dissection and before the infundibulo-ovarian pedicle is clamped. Impaired or absent renal function may be diagnosed with these tests in a small number of cases. In Jabs and Drutz's series[11] of 224 patients with preoperative imaging, 3 patients (1%) had congenital or surgical absence of a kidney and 2 patients (1%) had mild bilateral hydronephosis; 8 women also had benign ovarian cysts. The routine use of prophylactic ureteric catheterization in gynecological surgery to help identify and protect the ureter has not been shown to affect the rate of ureteric injury[19] and may cause injury (see discussion in Chapter 11). However, when the ureter is at high risk of injury or ligation, the prophylactic placement of a ureteric catheter would seem warranted. Examples of this would be in a woman with a VVF close to the ureteric orifice during transvaginal closure (Figure 14.11), and during the transvaginal excision of a vaginal fibroid situated under the urethra and bladder (Figure 14.12).

The risk of urinary tract injury is higher in certain types of stress incontinence and prolapse surgery, and intraoperative cystourethroscopy has been incorporated into the procedure as an essential part. The Stamey bladder neck suspension and the tension-free vaginal sling for stress incontinence procedures (Figure 14.13) and the intraperitoneal bilateral uterosacral ligament vault suspension for prolapse would be examples of this. In other procedures, such as the Burch colposuspension and transobturator sling procedure, opinion is divided whether intraoperative cystoscopy is necessary, although reports of urinary tract injury are common.[18,19] These operations are covered in more detail in Chapter 13.

Early detection of injury to the ureter, bladder, or urethra intraoperatively will allow any injury to be repaired without significant sequelae. Intraoperative detection of damage can be performed by inspection of the urinary tract

Table 14.1 Frequency of ureteral injuries during pelvic organ prolapse and SUI surgery[a]

Authors year	Surgery type	Number of operations	Number of ureteral injuries	Percent of ureteral injuries	Number recognized intraop	Number recognized postop
Gustilo-Ashby[b 21] 2006	POP vaginal surgery:	700	36	5.10%	34	2
	Bilat intraperitoneal USL	355	21	5.9%		
	Proximal McCall culdoplasty	204	9	4.4%		
	Distal McCall culdoplasty	185	1	0.5%		
	Colpocleisis	48	2	4.2%		
	Anterior colporraphy	574	2	0.4%		
	Indeterminate		1	1%		
Aronson[b 22] 2005	Mayo culdoplasty USL fixation +/− vaginal hysterectomy +/− ant and post colporraphy	411	3 1 due to USL 1 due to VH 1 to AC		3	
von Pechmann[23] 2003	Colpocleisis + high levator plication	92	4	4.3%		
	Prior hysterectomy	55	1			
	Concurrent VH	37	3			
Dandolu[24] 2003	Pelvic reconstructive surgery	858	3	0.34%	1	2 (partial obstruction – normal intraop cystoscopy)
Kwon[b 12] 2002	Anterior colporraphy	346	6	1.7%		
	Vaginal culdoplasties	237	0	0		
	SSF	152	0	0		
	Iliococcygeus suspension	34	0	0		
Jabs[b 11] 2001	POP surgery (abdominal or vaginal approach)	224	9	4%	9	
Karram[b 25] 2001	Bilateral intraperitoneal USL suspension	202	5	2.4%	5	
Barber[b 26] 2000	Bilateral intraperitoneal USL suspension (1 unilateral)	46	5	10.8%	5	
Shull[27] 2000	Bilateral intraperitoneal USL suspension (3 extraperitoneal)	302	3	1%		
Dwyer[b 18] 1999	Stamey suspension	61	0	0		
	Burch colposuspension:	1103	3	0.27%		
	open	925	0	0		
	laparoscopic	178	3	1.6%	2	1
Webb[28] 1998	POP surgery:	693	4	0.6%		
	Mayo culdoplasty	660				
	SSF	2				
	Abdo mesh SCP	31				
Harris[29] 1997	POP +/− SUI surgery	224	6	2.7%	6	
Pettit[b 30] 1994	McCall culdoplasty	83	3	3.6%		
Dwyer[16]	Bilateral extraperitoneal USL suspension	123	2	1.6%	2	0

[a] Courtesy of B. Fatton.

[b] Routine intraoperative cystoscopy.

POP = pelvic organ prolapse, Ant = anterior, Post = posterior, Abdo = abdominal, USL = uterosacral suspension, VH = vaginal hysterectomy, SUI = stress urinary incontinence, AC = anterior colporraphy, SCP = sacrocolpopexy, intraop = intraoperatively, postop = postoperatively.

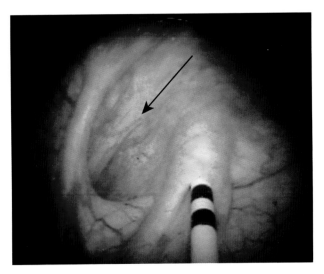

Figure 14.11
Vesicovaginal fistula (arrow) above interureteric ridge and to left of right ureteric orifice. Ureteric catheter passed to 10 cm (2 bar marker on catheter) to protect ureter during surgical repair.

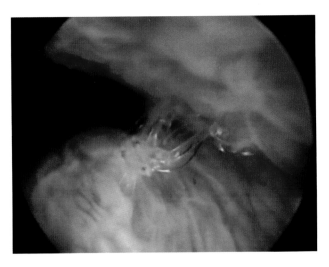

Figure 14.13
Urethroscopic view of urethral injury in a 30-year-old woman who had a tension-free vaginal tape (TVT) sling inserted for stress incontinence 8 months earlier. She had a previous history of urethral diverticulectomy.

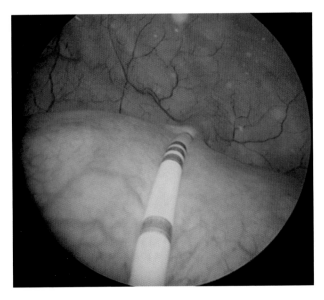

Figure 14.12
Ureteric catheter passed prior to transvaginal removal of a vaginal fibroid that was present under the bladder trigone.

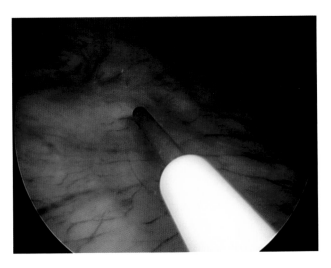

Figure 14.14
Open-ended ureteric catheter with slippery guide wire ready to be passed into left ureteric orifice.

during and after surgery, or more reliably by endoscopic observation of ureteric patency and function and inspection of the lower urinary tract.

Routine cystoscopy can miss some urinary injuries and misdiagnose long-standing obstruction as being caused intraoperatively. Injury associated with necrosis or ischemia, especially in the presence of infection, can be associated with

the development of late vesicovaginal or ureteric fistulae. Also, at times, ureteric efflux may be sluggish or absent despite being unobstructed, especially if the patient has preoperative impaired renal function or is oliguric intraoperatively from hypovolemia. Ureteric catheterization may be needed to confirm ureteric patency. This can be made more difficult by distortion and edema of the bladder base, which occurs during surgery, particularly in the anterior compartment with cystocele repair (see Figure 14.9).

Injection of 5 ml of indigo carmine dye 8–10 minutes prior to ureteric visualization will enhance vision of the ureteric orifices and urine jets. A guide wire can be passed through the open-ended ureteric catheter to confirm patency (Figure 14.14) or bypass an obstruction or kinking in the intravesical ureter. The guide wire can be introduced into the ureteric orifice and the open-ended ureteric catheter passed over it. If there is concern about the integrity and viability of the ureter, a ureteric stent can be inserted over the guide wire for more long-term drainage. The use of guide wires and ureteric catheterization is discussed in Chapter 13.

In a study by Kwon et al[12] the incidence of false-positive ureteric obstruction was 0.6%, where patency was confirmed by ureteric catheterization. Visco et al[20] constructed a decision analysis model to evaluate the cost-effectiveness of intraoperative cystoscopy at the time of abdominal, vaginal, and laparoscopic hysterectomy. They found that the incidence of ureteric injury rates at or above 1.5% for abdominal hysterectomy and 2% for vaginal hysterectomy made intraoperative cystoscopy a cost saving. However, this analysis was performed on the basis of the cost of treatment of repair of ureteric damage and did not include the potential cost of litigation. Other potential benefits – such as the diagnosis of bladder injury and other bladder pathology (e.g. undiagnosed bladder cancer), or the benefit of routine cystoscopy enhancing the endoscopic skills of gynecologists – were not included or considered.

References

1. Gilmour DT, Dwyer PL, Carey M. Lower urinary tract injury during gynecologic surgery and its detection by intraoperative cystoscopy. Obstet Gynecol 1999; 94(5): 883–9.
2. Gilmour DT, Baskett TF. Disability and litigation from urinary tract injury at benign gynecological surgery in Canada. Obstet Gyecol 2005; 105: 109–14.
3. Chan JK, Morrow J, Manetta A. Prevention of ureteral injuries in gynecological surgery. Am J Obstet Gynecol 2003; 188 (5): 1273–8.
4. Buller JL, Thompson JR, Cundiff GA et al. Uterosacral ligament: description of anatomical relationships to optimize surgical safety. Obstet Gynecol 2001; 97 (6): 873–9.
5. Liapis A, Bakas P, Giannopoulos V, Creatsas G. Ureteral injuries during gynecological surgery. Int Urogynecol J Pelvic Floor Dysfunct 2001; 12: 391–4.
6. Gilmour DT, Das S, Flowerdew G. Rates of urinary tract injury from gynecologic surgery and the role of intraoperative cystoscopy. Obstet Gynecol 2006; 107: 1366–72.
7. Drake MJ, Noble JG. Ureteric trauma in gynecological surgery. Int Urogynecol J Pelvic Floor Dysfunct 1998; 9: 108–17.
8. Assimos DG, Patterson LC, Taylor CL. Changing incidence and etiology of iatrogenic ureteral injuries. J Urol 1994; 152: 2240–6.
9. Hilton P. Fistulae. In: Shaw R, Soutter WP, Stanton SL, eds. Gynaecology, 3rd edn. London: Churchill Livingstone, 2003: 835–56.
10. Stanhope CR, Wilson TO, Utz WJ, Smith LH, O'Brien PC. Suture entrapment and secondary ureteric obstruction. Am J Obstet Gynecol 1991; 164: 1519–19.
11. Jabs CF, Drutz HP. The role of intraoperative cystoscopy in prolapse and incontinence surgery. Am J Obstet Gynecol 2001; 185(6): 1368–71.
12. Kwon CH, Goldberg RP, Koduri S, Sand PK. The use of cystoscopy in major vaginal and urogynecological surgeries. Am J Obstet Gynecol 2002; 187(6): 1466–71.
13. Dwyer PL, Schraffordt S. Iliococcygeal fixation – middle compartment prolapse. In: Stanton SL, Zimmern PE, eds. Female Pelvic Reconstructive Surgery. London: Springer-Verlag, 2002.
14. McCall ML. Posterior culdoplasty; surgical correction of enterocele during vaginal hysterectomy; a preliminary report. Obstet Gynecol 1957; 10: 595–602.
15. Maher C, Murray C, Carey M, Dwyer PL, Agoni AM. Iliococcygeus or sacrospinous fixation for vaginal vault prolapse. Obstet Gynecol 2001; 98: 40–4.
16. Dwyer PL, Fatton B. Bilateral extraperitoneal uterosacral suspension: a new approach to correct post-hysterectomy vaginal vault prolapse. Int Urogynecol J Pelvic Floor Dysfunct. 2007 August (Epub).
17. Kuno K, Menzin A, Kauder HH, Sison C, Gal D. Prophylactic ureteral catheterization in gynecologic surgery. J Urol 1999; 162: 1563–8.
18. Dwyer PL, Carey MP, Rosamilia A. Suture injury to the urinary tract in urethral suspension procedures for stress incontinence. Int Urogynecol J Pelvic Floor Dysfunct 1999; 10: 15–21.
19. Abdel-Fattah M, Ramsay I, Pringle S. Lower urinary tract injuries after transobturator tape insertion by different routes: a large retrospective study. Obstet Gynecol Surv 2007; 62: 172–3.
20. Visco AG, Taber KH, Weidner AC, Barber MD, Myers ER. Cost-effectiveness of universal cystoscopy to identify ureteral injury at hysterectomy. Obstet Gynecol 2001; 97: 685–92.
21. Gustilo-Ashby AM, Jelovsek JE, Barber MD et al. The incidence of ureteral obstruction and the value of intraoperative cystoscopy during vaginal surgery for pelvic organ prolapse. Am J Obstet Gynecol 2006; 194: 1478–85.
22. Aronson MP, Aronson PK, Howard AE et al. Low risk of ureteral obstruction with 'deep' (dorsal/posterior) uterosacral ligament suture placement for transvaginal apical suspension. Am J Obstet Gynecol 2005; 192: 1530–6.
23. von Pechmann WS, Mutone M, Fyffe J, Hale DS. Total colpocleisis with high levator plication for the treatment of advanced pelvic organ prolapse. Am J Obstet Gynecol 2003; 189: 121–6.
24. Dandolu V, Mathai E, Chatwani A et al. Accuracy of cystoscopy in the diagnosis of ureteral injury in benign gynecologic surgery. Int Urogynecol J Pelvic Floor Dysfunct 2003; 14: 427–31.
25. Karram M, Goldwasser S, Kleeman S et al. High uterosacral vaginal vault suspension with fascial reconstruction for vaginal repair of enterocele and vaginal vault prolapse. Am J Obstet Gynecol 2001; 185: 1339–42.

26. Barber MD, Visco AG, Weidner AC, Amundsen CL, Bump RC. Bilateral uterosacral ligament vaginal vault suspension with site-specific endopelvic fascia defect repair for treatment of pelvic organ prolapse. Am J Obstet Gynecol 2000; 183(6): 1402–10.

27. Shull BL, Bachofen C, Coates KW, Kuehl TJ. A transvaginal approach to repair of apical and other associated sites of pelvic organ prolapse with uterosacral ligaments. Am J Obstet Gynecol 2000; 183: 1365–73.

27. Webb MJ, Aronson MP, Ferguson LK, Lee RA. Post-hysterectomy vaginal vault prolapse: primary repair in 693 patients. Obstet Gynecol 1998; 92: 281–5.

29. Harris RL, Cundiff GW, Theofrastous JP et al. The value of intraoperative cystoscopy in urogynecologic and reconstructive pelvic surgery. Am J Obstet Gynecol 1997; 177: 1367–9.

30. Pettit PD, Petrou SP. The value of cystoscopy in major vaginal surgery. Obstet Gynecol 1994; 84: 318–20.

15

Training requirements for endoscopy of the urinary tract in female pelvic medicine

Peter L Dwyer

Introduction

In the past, female pelvic floor disorders have been a somewhat neglected area of women's healthcare and the prevalence of the problem has been underestimated. A recent North American prevalence study revealed that women have an 11% lifetime risk of having surgery for vaginal prolapse or stress incontinence, with 1 in 3 requiring more than one operation.[1] In an Australian study MacLellan et al[2] found that half the women surveyed aged 15–95 years had symptoms of pelvic floor dysfunction defined as stress or urge incontinence, flatus or fecal incontinence, symptoms of vaginal prolapse, or a previous pelvic floor repair. With an aging population, the prevalence of pelvic floor disorders will increase, so there is a need for greater emphasis on these conditions in our undergraduate and postgraduate training programs and to develop more effective diagnostic and treatment strategies. Knowledge of endoscopy of the lower urinary tract is central to diagnosis and management of pelvic floor disorders.

Education in cystourethroscopy in obstetric and gynecological training programs

Traditionally, gynecologists have not been trained in the use of endoscopy of the urinary tract, and no emphasis has been put on this area in the curriculum, training program, or examination process by most colleges or societies of obstetrics and gynecology around the world. In the United States the requirements for residency programs certified by the American Board of Obstetrics and Gynecology make no mention of training in cystoscopy.[3,4] The Royal Australian and New Zealand College of Obstetricians and Gynaecologists have a detailed curriculum of requirements for their fellows to achieve by the end of training, which includes diagnostic, therapeutic, and surgical skills (www.ranzcog.edu.au). In obstetrics, fellows are expected to be able to manage urinary incontinence, urinary retention, and injury to the urinary tract as a result of pregnancy and delivery. In gynecology, fellows should be able to investigate and manage urinary incontinence and uterovaginal prolapse, diagnose and plan appropriate management of gynecological fistula, and assess and manage women with urogynecological disorders. Intraoperative surgical skills required are:

- identification of the ureter abdominally intraoperatively
- recognition of injuries to the ureter, including those which become apparent postoperatively
- recognition of bladder and bowel trauma during surgery and being able to manage these problems under supervision.

Fellows are required to have detailed knowledge of 58 specific surgical procedures with credentialing at three levels: namely, understand (not perform), perform with assistance, and perform unassisted. There are 12 operations under the heading of hysteroscopic surgery and 12 operations under laparoscopic surgery. The only mention cystoscopy gets in the 60-page curriculum document is one line on page 45 that cystoscopy should be able to be performed unassisted. What seems not to be recognized, or at least not stated, is that to diagnose and manage urinary incontinence, uterovaginal prolapse, urinary fistula, and intraoperative urinary tract injury, a high level of skill in cystourethroscopy is required. This means understanding the equipment and how it is used, what is normal and abnormal in the urinary tract, how to do simple procedures such as bladder biopsy and removing foreign bodies, and diagnosing ureteric patency. As well as having this stated in the curriculum of every college or society of obstetrics and gynecology, a process is needed to implement this into the training program.

The specialties of urology and gynecology have a long history of a common interest in the lower urinary tract in the female. Historically, gynecologists have played an important role in the development of cystourethroscopy (see Chapter 1) and many eminent gynecologists and urologists have believed that a good knowledge of endoscopy of the urinary tract is essential for all gynecological pelvic surgeons. The urinary and genital tracts are too inter-related functionally, anatomically, and embryologically to be separated by artificial barriers of the medical specialties of female urology and gynecology. Howard Kelly, Professor of Obstetrics and Gynecology at Johns Hopkins Hospital in Baltimore, was a pioneer in female urology, developing operations for stress incontinence and vaginal prolapse. During the 1880s in the United States, he also introduced cystoscopy and ureteric catheterization.[5] His successor at Johns Hopkins, Guy Hunner, continued his work in female urology and was the first to clearly describe the condition of interstitial cystitis. However, it seems that these skills and interest were lost to most gynecologists until Jack Robertson pioneered the air cystourethroscope and its use in the evaluation of urinary incontinence and urethral pathology in the 1960s.[6] Another professor of gynecology at Johns Hopkins, Richard Te Linde, said in 1978: 'it is difficult for me to conceive doing first class gynecology without knowledge of female urology'.

Urologists with an interest in female urology and pelvic floor disorders also acknowledge the need for a broader education. Vaginal prolapse surgery, previously the province of the gynecologist, is increasingly being performed by urologists. In my own practice, a third of my patients undergoing prolapse surgery have a stress incontinence procedure. Therefore, if you are managing women with pelvic floor problems, you need expertise in all aspects of diagnosis and treatment. In an editorial[7] in the *International Urogynecology Journal*, Gerry Blaivas, Professor of Urology at Cornell University, New York, and past Editor-in-Chief of *Neurology and Urodynamics* wrote that, 'all training programs in Urogynecology and Reconstructive Pelvic Surgery (URPS) should enjoy approximately equal input from Urology and Gynecology.' It is important that gynecologists and urologists and their colleges recognize these deficiencies. Better leadership is needed to provide broader multidisciplinary training involving both specialties, particularly for younger pelvic surgeons – rather than maintaining boundaries and the status quo to the detriment of patient care.

The learning process in cystoscopy for many gynecologists has been by an informal apprenticeship observing mentors performing cystourethroscopy and other urogynecological procedures, and dealing with difficult urinary problems as they arise. However, for most gynecologists, exposure to cystoscopic training has been limited and so they feel uncomfortable in using this equipment when the need arises. Calling in urogynecological or urological colleagues may be time consuming, unnecessary for simple benign conditions (e.g. squamous metaplasia), and at times not possible. Gynecologists generally have had an excellent training in endoscopy and endoscopic equipment in the areas of abdominal and pelvic laparoscopic surgery and genital endoscopy (e.g. hysteroscopy) where endoscopic surgical procedures, including the resection of submucous fibroids (Figure 15.1), is commonplace for many gynecologists.

Gynecologists performing pelvic surgery should be able to perform diagnostic cystoscopy, recognize normal and abnormal findings, and perform intraoperative cystourethroscopy to exclude intravesical and intraurethral injury or penetration of foreign material and to confirm ureteric patency. It is our hope that this book will help enable gynecologists to have these skills.

Guidelines for training in urogynecology and endoscopy

A good understanding of urogynecology and pelvic floor disorders is important in the undergraduate training of medical students to produce well-informed general practitioners and primary care community doctors, and in the postgraduate training of obstetrician gynecologists and subspecialists in urogynecology to ensure the highest level of specialist care for women with pelvic floor disorders. With this need in mind, the International Urogynecological Association (IUGA) decided to establish educational guidelines that would be universally acceptable for governing boards and licensing bodies around the world. A consensus statement by the Education Committee of IUGA produced guidelines for the training programs in urogynecology and reconstructive pelvic surgery (URPS) for undergraduate medical students, postgraduate trainees in obstetrics and gynecology, and subspecialist urogynecologists. The committee felt that the guidelines were recommendations for minimal levels of knowledge and skills in URPS which should be adapted by national societies and licensing bodies to suit their own national and regional needs.

Three sets of guidelines were provided for each of the three different levels:

- undergraduate medical student
- obstetrician/gynecologist
- subspecialist.

These guidelines specified knowledge requirements in urinary tract and pelvic floor anatomy and physiology and in pelvic floor disorders; they outlined the diagnostic and clinical skills required to achieve the appropriate standard

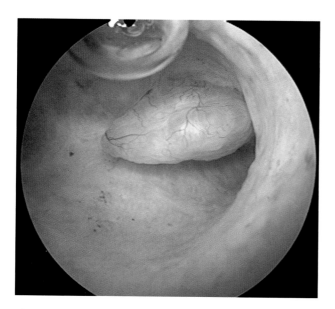

Figure 15.1
Hysteroscopic view of the endometrial cavity following distention with glycine. There is a pale healthy endometrial lining, a central bubble at the dome, and a small submucous fibroid awaiting resection; not too different a picture from cystoscopy.

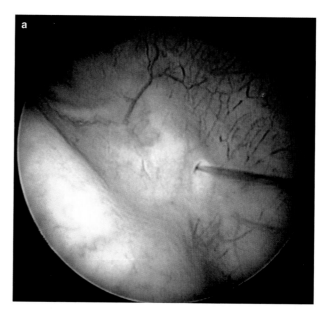

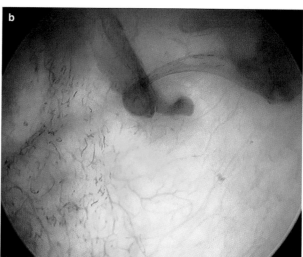

Figure 15.2
Ureteric jet of indigo carmine confirming ureteric patency.

for pre- or postgraduate medical training program, leading to a general license to practice medicine at this level. Following the guidelines, the consensus statement provides mandatory and encouraged levels of knowledge and skill requirements appropriate and desirable in a person becoming a practising general practitioner, obstetrician/gynecologist, or subspecialist in urogynecology. These guidelines have been published[8] and can also be accessed on the Internet (www.IUGA.com.).

Gynecologists are increasingly asking for training in cystourethroscopy, and hospital administrations and health authorities are also asking for evidence of training and experience for accreditation purposes.

Guidelines for training in cystourethroscopy have recently been proposed by Hibbert et al.[3] In their program, cystoscopy was performed with most major gynecological procedures, which enabled the residents to obtain enough experience to justify granting certification and hospital credentialing in cystoscopy. Residents in training were given lectures on the principles of urinary tract evaluation, prevention of injury, and detection and treatment of complications, and a video produced by the hospital on cystoscopy. The residents were then required to observe and assist with five or more cystourethroscopies. Once the observational requirements were completed, residents had to perform at least 10 procedures and demonstrate to their supervisor the ability to appropriately use the equipment and adequately visualize the urethra, bladder, and ureteric orifices to confirm patency with and without the injection of indigo carmine dye (Figure 15.2). Once residents have reached the appropriate level of expertise determined by the consultant staff, the residency program director provides them with documentation of certification in competence in cystoscopy to perform intraoperative diagnostic urinary tract cystoscopic evaluation. The authors of this study concluded that performing routine cystoscopy for evaluation of potential urinary tract injury during major gynecological surgery did provide sufficient experience and training to justify credentialing residents in diagnostic cystoscopy. These guidelines and training protocol could be extended to include some or all the urogynecological procedures performed by subspecialist urogynecologists and be used in the training of generalist gynecologists (Table 15.1).

Table 15.1 Guidelines of the International Urogynecological Association for postgraduate training programs and educational objectives for subspecialty training in urogynecology and reconstructive pelvic surgery (URPS)

Medical therapy and surgical skills

Management options:
- catheterization (urethral, suprapubic, and clean intermittent self-catheterization)
- devices (mechanical and electronic)
- aids, appliances, pants, and pads.

Non-surgical treatment:
- urinary and GI tract disorders, including incontinence
- physiotherapeutic techniques and aids, including biofeedback
- electrical and magnetic therapy
- behavioral therapy, including bladder and bowel retraining and acupuncture
- role of pharmacological agents to treat pelvic floor disorders
- role of hormonal therapy.

Surgical procedures:
- urethral dilatation
- urethrotomy
- suprapubic cystotomy
- bladder neck buttress, TVT
- vaginal repair of genital tract prolapse, including anterior colporrhaphy, posterior colpoperineorrhaphy, vaginal hysterectomy and repair, enterocele repair, Manchester repair, sacrospinous fixation, iliococcygeous fixation, paravaginal repairs
- vaginal and abdominal repair of recurrent prolapse, including sacrocolpopexy, rectopexy, uterosacral ligament complication, sacrohysteropexy, Moscowitz procedure, colposuspension and similar suprapubic suspension operations (both open and through minimal invasive techniques)
- sling procedures
- long needle suspension procedures
- para- and transurethral injection procedures
- vaginal plastic surgery
- implantation of artificial urinary sphincter
- repair of vesicovaginal, ureterovaginal, urethrovaginal, and rectovaginal fistulas
- Martius graft technique
- augmentation cystoplasty
- urinary diversion and undiversion
- urethral diverticulectomy and excision of paraurethral cysts
- urethral reconstruction
- urethral closure techniques
- rectal mucosal prolapse surgery (abdominal – Ripstein procedure, and rectal approach)
- post-anal repair
- anal sphincter repair – primary and secondary
- sacral nerve stimulation and implantation
- dynamic gracilis plasty
- recognition and treatment of intraoperative bladder and bowel injuries.

References

1. Olsen A, Smith VJ, Bergstrom JO, Colling JC, Clark AL. Epidemiology of surgically managed organ prolapse and urinary incontinence. Obstet Gynecol 1997; 89: 501–6.
2. MacLellan AH, Taylor AW, Wilson DH, Wilson D. The prevalence of pelvic floor disorders and relationship to gender, age, parity and mode of delivery. Br J Obstet Gynaecol 2000; 107: 1460–70.
3. Hibbert ML, Salminen ER, Danty LA, Davis GD, Perez RP. Credentialing residence for intraoperative cystoscopy. Obstet Gynecol 2000; 96: 1014–16.
4. Karram M, Kleeman S. Cysturethroscopy and the gynecologist. Int Urogynecol J Pelvic Floor Dysfunct 2005; 16: 329.
5. Kelly HA. The direct examination of the female bladder with elevated pelvis: the catheterization of the ureters under direct inspection, with or without elevation of the pelvis. Am J Obstet Dis Woman Child 1894; 25: 1.
6. Robertson JR. Air cystoscopy. Obstet Gynecol 1968; 32: 328.
7. Blaivas JG. Filling in the blanks. Int J Urogynecol 2003; 14: 295.
8. Drutz HP, Riss PA, Halaska M et al. IUGA Guidelines for Training in Urogynecology and Reconstructive Pelvic Surgery (URPS). Int J Urogynecol J Pelvic Floor Dysfunct 2002; 13: 386–95.

Index

Note: Page numbers in italics refer to Figures and Tables